T0298807

Cambridge History of Medicine

EDITORS: CHARLES WEBSTER AND CHARLES ROSENBERG

Legal medicine in history

This collection of essays presents fresh interpretations of the growth of medico-legal ideas, institutions and practices in Britain, Europe and America over the past four hundred years. Based on a wealth of new research, it brings the historical study of legal medicine firmly into the realm of social history.

Case studies of infanticide, abortion, coroners' inquests and criminal insanity show that legal medicine has often been the focus of social change and political controversy. The contributors also emphasize the formative influence of legal systems on medico-legal knowledge and practice. *Legal medicine in history* enlarges our understanding of the public role of medicine in modern western societies, while opening up new perspectives on social, cultural and political history.

Cambridge History of Medicine

EDITED BY

CHARLES WEBSTER

Reader in the History of Medicine, University of Oxford, and Fellow of All Souls College

CHARLES ROSENBERG

Professor of History and Sociology of Science, University of Pennsylvania

For a list of titles in the series, see end of book

Legal medicine in history

EDITED BY

MICHAEL CLARK

Wellcome Trust, London

AND

CATHERINE CRAWFORD

University of Essex

CAMBRIDGE
UNIVERSITY PRESS

Published by the Press Syndicate of the University of Cambridge
The Pitt Building, Trumpington Street, Cambridge, CB2 1RP
40 West 20th Street, New York, NY 10011–4211, USA
10 Stamford Road, Oakleigh, Melbourne 3166, Australia

© Cambridge University Press 1994

First published 1994

A catalogue record for this book is available from the British Library

Library of Congress cataloguing in publication data

Legal medicine in history / edited by Michael Clark and
Catherine Crawford.
p. cm. – (Cambridge history of medicine)
Includes index.
ISBN 0 521 39514 3 (hc)
1. Medical jurisprudence – History.
I. Clark, Michael, 1954– .
II. Crawford, Catherine. III. Series.
[DNLM: 1. Forensic Medicine – history. W 611.1 L496 1994]
RA1021.L44 1994
614'.1'09 – dc20
DNLM/DLC
for Library of Congress 93–11582 CIP

ISBN 0 521 39514 3 hardback

Transferred to digital printing 2004

CE

Contents

III Special offenders

IV The politics of post-mortems

V Medical authority in question

Notes on contributors

NORMAN AMBAGE is a former graduate student of the Department of History, University of Lancaster, where in 1987 he completed his Ph.D thesis on 'The Development of the Home Office Forensic Science Service, 1931–1967'. Since 1988, he has worked in the National Health Service as Information Officer for the Trafford and Macclesfield Health Authorities.

HELEN BROCK, who has a Ph.D in zoology, retired in 1981 from an honorary research fellowship in the Department of the History of Science, Glasgow University. Her research was on eighteenth-century British medicine, centred around William Hunter, with an additional interest in medicine in colonial North America, and she has publications in both these fields.

BARBARA BROOKES is a Lecturer in History at the University of Otago, New Zealand, and the author of *Abortion in England, 1900–1967* (1988). She has published a number of articles on women's history and on medical history and is co-editor of two books on New Zealand women's history. She is currently working on a book examining how the supposedly 'natural desires' of marriage, home and family have shaped New Zealand women's past.

MICHAEL CLARK is a former research fellow of the Department of History, University of Lancaster and the Centre de Recherche en Histoire des Sciences et des Techniques, La Villette, Paris. He has published articles on the history of psychiatry, and is currently working on a history of English forensic medicine during the past 150 years. Since 1990, he has managed the Wellcome Trust's collection of medical and medical-historical films and videos.

CATHERINE CRAWFORD is a lecturer in the Department of History, University of Essex. After completing an Oxford D.Phil. thesis on medical testimony in English courts in the eighteenth and nineteenth centuries, she was a research fellow at the Wellcome Institute for the History of Medicine. She is currently working on relations between law and medicine in England and France in the early modern period.

JOEL PETER EIGEN is Professor of Sociology at Franklin and Marshall College in Lancaster, Pennsylvania. He has written on forensic testimony bearing on insanity in early modern England, and on contemporary developments in American jurisprudence concerning the certification of new forensic specialists in medical psychology. A past visiting fellow at the Institute of Criminology at Cambridge University and Leonard Slater Fellow at Durham University, he is currently completing a book on medicine, madness, and criminal responsibility in late eighteenth- and early nineteenth-century England.

DAVID HARLEY teaches the history of medicine in Oxford. He is especially interested in the religious and professional aspects of early modern medicine. He has published articles on tobacco, midwifery, spa medicine, demonic possession, professional disputes, and the influence of Calvinist theology on medicine.

RUTH HARRIS is a fellow and tutor of Modern History at New College Oxford. She is the author of *Murders and Madness: Medicine, Law and Society in the Fin de Siècle*, and is currently writing a history of Lourdes, as well as a history of nineteenth-century France for Penguin.

MARK JACKSON qualified as a doctor at St Thomas' Hospital, London, in 1985. After a brief clinical career, he completed a doctoral dissertation at the University of Leeds on newborn-child murder in the eighteenth century. Now a research officer at the Wellcome Unit for the History of Medicine at Manchester, he is working on the recent history of medicine and mental handicap, and on the history of immunology.

JULIE JOHNSON is Associate Director of the Center for the History of Business, Technology, and Society at the Hagley Museum and Library in Wilmington, Delaware. She received her Ph.D in the History and Sociology of Science from the University of Pennsylvania, where she now lectures. She is currently expanding her dissertation, 'Speaking for the dead: forensic scientists and American justice in the twentieth century', into a book which will examine the use of scientific evidence as a means of rationalizing criminal and civil litigation in the United States.

PAUL ROTH first trained as a classicist, completing a Ph.D in Greek at Bryn Mawr College. For his law degree, awarded in 1988, he completed a study of the legal implications of testing for HIV. He has published articles on Greek philology and on labour law. He is a Barrister and Solicitor of the High Court of New Zealand and lectures in law at the University of Otago, New Zealand.

JOE SIM is Professor of Criminology, John Moores University, Liverpool, in the Institute of Crime, Justice and Welfare Studies. He is the author of *Medical Power in Prisons* (Open University Press, 1990) and co-author of *British Prisons* (with Mike Fitzgerald, Basil Blackwell, 1982) and *Prisons Under Protest* (with Phil Scraton and Paula Skidmore, Open University Press, 1991).

TONY WARD is a barrister and Lecturer in Law at De Montfort University, Leicester. He was formerly joint organizer of INQUEST, which campaigns about coroners' courts and deaths in custody, and offers advice and support to the bereaved. His publications include *Privatization and the Penal System* (with Mick Ryan, 1989) and several articles on coroners' law, prisons and policing. He is currently engaged in a study of psychiatry and criminal justice in the twentieth century and is co-editor, with Alison Liebling, of *Deaths in Custody: International Perspectives*, to be published by David Whiting in 1994.

STEPHEN WATSON gained his Ph.D from Lancaster University for a thesis on the development of definitions of moral imbecility, which was supervised by Roger Smith. He has taught the history of medicine at Sheffield City Polytechnic and Sunderland Polytechnic.

MARY NAGLE WESSLING studies aspects of medicine, law and gender in German history between 1730 and 1830. She did her Ph.D research at the University of Michigan, and has taught at Michigan, Stanford, and the University of Essex, where she was a visiting research fellow in 1992. She is currently affiliated with the Historical Center for the Health Sciences at the University of Michigan.

BRENDA WHITE is a research fellow in the Department of History, University of Stirling, and formerly in the Department of Economic and Social History, University of Glasgow, where she was assistant editor and contributor to the *Dictionary of Scottish Business Biography*. She has written several articles on the history of legal medicine and public health in Scotland, is co-author with M. Anne Crowther of *On Soul and Conscience: The Medical Expert and Crime*, and is now working on Scottish health policy in the interwar period.

Preface

This book was conceived at a conference on the history of legal medicine held at the University of Lancaster in 1987, organized by Michael Clark and Roger Smith and funded by the Nuffield Foundation and the Wellcome Trust. The aim of the meeting was to bring together scholars working on various aspects of the history of medico-legal relations in order to develop comparative perspectives and stimulate further research. Four of the papers in this book were first presented at the Lancaster conference; the rest are the fruit of research conducted since then.

The Wellcome Trust has provided both of us with research fellowships in recent years, and without that support this book would probably not exist. We are also indebted to Charles Webster, Carol Jones and John Keown, who made valuable suggestions at an early stage. Our warm thanks go also to Anne Goldgar, who advised and occasionally arbitrated on editorial questions, and to Marie Williams, who helped prepare the text. Most of all, though, we would like to thank the contributors. Their commitment to the project and their constant good humour were a great help to us.

Introduction

MICHAEL CLARK and CATHERINE CRAWFORD

This book presents new research on the history of legal medicine from the early seventeenth century to the 1960s. It ranges widely in subject matter, from abortion and infanticide to medico-legal education and the politics of the coronership, while its geographical scope extends from colonial Maryland and Enlightenment Germany to *Belle Epoque* Paris and twentieth-century England. However, this book is not just a sampler of current historical work on legal medicine. It is intended to form a coherent historiographical intervention in a field which has long been studied largely in isolation from social, political, and even legal history.

Much existing historical work on legal medicine lacks a sufficiently strong sense of the ways in which particular historical settings have affected the development of medico-legal knowledge and practice. For want of adequate contextualization, scientific and technical advances have usually been understood in self-referential terms.[1] At the same time, historians' view of not only the history of criminal justice but also, for example, the history of women and the family, of local government, and of health and safety at work has been limited by lack of awareness of their medico-legal aspects.[2] Our aim in this book is to show what the history of legal medicine stands to gain from new approaches to the social history of law and medicine, and to explore some of the ways in which medico-legal history can enrich our understanding of history in general. *Legal Medicine in History* is thus not so much a history *of* legal medicine as a set of studies of the place of legal medicine *in* the social, legal, administrative and political histories of societies in which it has been practised.

The terms of reference in this field present a problem which we do not pretend to have 'solved'. Rather, the terminological difficulties which have beset all attempts to define the field of medico-legal knowledge and practice are themselves revealing, for they reflect its great historical variety and contingency. As part of their ongoing struggle to achieve greater professional recognition, medico-legal practitioners have repeatedly sought to define more precisely their sphere of competence, and to standardize the usage of the various terms used to denote their areas of knowledge and expertise. Much ink has been spilt over what William J. Curran has called 'The confusion of titles in the medico-legal field' (1975),[3] but as the medico-legal bibliographer Jaroslav Nemec observed in 1973, 'All efforts ... to define the scope or even agree upon the name of our subject have been in vain'.[4] The problem is not one of semantics, but of the different ways in which the field of medico-legal relations has been conceived and organized in different jurisdictions and at different times. In many countries, legal medicine was long regarded not as a specialty but as part of the professional duties of every medical practitioner, while as several of the papers in this volume illustrate, what is now usually termed 'legal' or 'forensic' medicine has at various times and places included not only what we know as clinical forensic medicine and forensic pathology, but also elements of medical law and ethics, 'medical police', public health and poor-law medicine. With the growth of medical and scientific specialization during the past 150 years, much of what formerly belonged to legal medicine has gradually been hived off to form separate disciplines or specialties, but the definition of 'legal medicine' still retains a considerable degree of ambiguity.

In this book, 'legal' or 'forensic' medicine is taken to be the application of medical knowledge in the broadest sense to help solve legal problems or satisfy legal requirements. This definition is intended to include: (1) all manner of clinical and post-mortem investigations carried out by surgeons, apothecaries, midwives and physicians on the instructions of legal officers or tribunals; (2) all kinds of medical evidence presented to investigating magistrates, coroners' courts, and civil, criminal or ecclesiastical tribunals, whether in the form of written reports or as oral testimony; and (3) the provision of medical certificates and testimonials for legal or quasi-judicial purposes, including those of penal administration. Medical matters which were merely the *subject* of legal proceedings – such as disputes over fees, medical ethics or alleged malpractice – have been excluded, with the partial exception of abortion, which features in these pages as the subject of both medical testimony and legal argument. Like all definitions in this hybrid field, this one is somewhat arbitrary, but it provides a basis on which to distinguish a set of institutionally and professionally organized medico-legal relations from all the more-or-less accidental encounters between law and medicine in the past.

With a few exceptions, notably Stanford Emerson Chaillé's 'Origins and progress of medical jurisprudence, 1776–1876' (1876/1949) and Erwin Ackerknecht's 'Early history of legal medicine' (1950–1), the Anglo-American historiography of legal medicine remained slight up to 1960.[5] During the 1960s and 1970s, growth of interest among practitioners was reflected in a number of brief general outlines of the history of legal medicine intended primarily for medical audiences.[6] The fruits of more serious historical research also began to appear in such works as J. D. J. Havard's *The Detection of Secret Homicide* (1960), Nigel Walker's *Crime and Insanity in England* (1968, 1973) and the historical bibliographies of R. P. Brittain (1962, 1970) and Jaroslav Nemec (1969, 1973).[7] But with the notable exception of the history of forensic psychiatry, the history of legal medicine still remained largely in the hands of senior or retired medico-legal practitioners and crime journalists, and, as Brittain and Myers observed in 1968, much of what passed for 'research' in the subject in fact consisted of the reproduction of anecdotal materials and unverified hypotheses gleaned third- or fourth-hand from a few, usually unacknowledged, 'classic' sources.[8] The rapid growth of scholarship in medical history from the early 1970s onwards left the history of legal medicine largely untouched, while the upsurge of interest in the social history of crime and criminal justice during the same period was not at first matched by any corresponding growth of interest in the history of medico-legal practice.

In the late 1970s this picture began to change, partly due to Thomas Forbes's numerous empirical studies of causes of death and early instances of medical testimony recorded in London and Middlesex coroner's inquests and the Old Bailey Sessions Papers.[9] Forbes did not advance any new interpretations of the historical development of English legal medicine, but the richness of his source materials undoubtedly helped to stimulate interest in the subject. In 'Crowner's Quest' (1978) and *Surgeons at the Bailey* (1985), Forbes showed that there was a considerable amount of medico-legal practice in London during the eighteenth and early nineteenth centuries.[10] But as Forbes himself pointed out, despite his forays into the pre-1750 era, little was known about the nature or extent of English medico-legal practice in the early modern period. This was in marked contrast to the wealth of information on medico-legal doctrine and practice in Renaissance and Enlightenment Germany presented by Esther Fischer-Homberger in her 1983 monograph, *Medizin vor Gericht*.[11]

During the past decade, however, social historians of medicine have begun to exploit legal records for the glimpses they provide of the activities of medical practitioners in the sixteenth, seventeenth and eighteenth centuries, and some of these investigations have yielded important evidence of early medico-legal practice in England. All three of the papers in the first part of this book implicitly call into question the longstanding assumption of England's relative 'backwardness' in legal medicine by comparison with continental Europe in the early modern period. Helen Brock and Catherine Crawford's study of seventeenth-century Maryland – a small, isolated community with no medical institutions and only basic legal ones – shows that even in a frontier society it was not unusual for medical practitioners to provide expert testimony in cases of suspected abortion, infanticide, homicide and suicide, and to carry out medico-legal dissections as early as the 1640s. This evidence from a remote English colony suggests that medico-legal practice was probably far more common in England itself during this period than has generally been assumed, an expectation which is supported by David Harley's study of medico-legal practice in Lancashire and Cheshire between 1660 and 1760. Drawing on a wide range of sources, including the records of both civil and ecclesiastical courts, Harley shows surgeons, midwives, apothecaries and physicians carrying out a variety of medico-legal tasks, ranging from the provision of medical certificates and testimonials to the post-mortem examination of the victims of suspected poisoning. Both these papers highlight the leading role played by midwives as experts on sexual and obstetrical questions, not only in cases of suspected infanticide, abortion and rape, but also in legal proceedings brought to determine the paternity of bastard children and impose maintenance orders on illegitimate fathers.[12]

The first three papers in this volume also suggest a need to reappraise the role of the coronership in early English forensic medicine. Medico-legal practitioners and historians have long enjoyed something of a love–hate relationship with the coronership and the inquest. As the traditional centrepiece of the Anglo–American medico-legal investigative system, the coronership has inspired a grudging affection on the part of even its fiercest critics on account of its sheer antiquity and the many bizarre features of its history.[13] Yet at the same time it has generally been seen as one of the main obstacles to the achievement of an efficient and 'rational' system of medico-legal investigation, and thus as one of the chief causes of the alleged backwardness of Anglo–American forensic medicine.[14] This overriding concern with the functional efficiency of the coronership as a system of medico-legal investigation has arguably resulted in a narrow and distorted view of its past, and has led practitioners and historians to underestimate the constructive role which it may have played in the development of medico-legal practice in the early modern period. In the nineteenth century, coroners were frequently denounced by medical writers for their reluctance to employ medical witnesses to carry out post-mortems or present medical evidence at inquests. But as Brock and Crawford's, Harley's and Jackson's papers all suggest, in the seventeenth and eighteenth centuries some – perhaps a good deal – of the demand for more medical evidence at inquests came from coroners themselves rather than medical practitioners. Moreover, Brock and Crawford show that in some Maryland inquests where the coroner does not appear to have summoned any medical assistance, the inquest juries included men who can be identified as surgeons, whom the coroner very likely chose because of their medical knowledge and experience. This suggests that we may need to reassess the role of the coroner and his jury in the development of medico-legal practice in the early modern period. Although the English criminal trial jury has been the focus of considerable historical research,[15] the coroner's jury has received much less attention. However, Michael Macdonald's work on suicide in seventeenth- and eighteenth-century England ascribes a key role to coroner's juries in the apparent 'secularization of suicide' during this period indicated by the massive decline of *felo de se* verdicts in favour of findings of accidental death, death by act of God, or blameless self-destruction while of unsound mind.[16] In this case a major secular shift in attitudes was translated into concrete forms of social practice via the deliberations and decisions of coroner's juries, who thus appear as important mediators between public opinion and legal practice in the early modern period.

A comparable shift in attitudes and practices is documented in Mark Jackson's study of infanticide investigations in the north of England during the seventeenth and eighteenth centuries. Jackson shows how statute law, judicial opinion, pre-trial practice and public opinion interacted to produce two distinct phases in the medical evidence of infanticide between 1624 and 1803. He demonstrates widespread familiarity with the special presumption of childmurder enacted by the statute of 1624, and an equally widespread and growing dissatisfaction with its severity, which eventually led to the statutory presumption being discreetly set aside not only by juries but by magistrates and judges. By the 1760s, legal authorities at all levels were setting aside the statute and prosecuting infanticide according to the common-law standards of proof that were applied to most other crimes. This shift from statute back to common law was reflected in, among other things, more frequent recourse to medical testimony and a growing interest in tests of live-birth (especially floating the infant's lungs), as opposed to the previous emphasis on indications of still-birth, such as signs of foetal immaturity. The validity of the hydrostatic lung test became the subject of debate both inside and outside the courtroom, and the technical sources of medical uncertainty were given considerable publicity. As will become apparent from Mary Wessling's paper later in this book, similar concerns played a part in the intensification of research on the lung test in Württemberg towards the end of the eighteenth century. Humanitarian sentiment appears to have been profoundly implicated in the legal and scientific history of infanticide evidence and, arguably, in the growth of forensic medicine generally in both England and continental Europe at this time.

While all three of these papers substantially modify our picture of Anglo–American 'backwardness' in matters medico-legal in the early modern period, it nevertheless remains the case that medico-legal scholarship was remarkably slow to develop in England by comparison with Italy, France and Germany.[17] Indeed, it is largely the contrast between the steady production of continental treatises on legal medicine from the seventeenth century onwards and the relative paucity of English contributions before the nineteenth century which has led historians to assume that there was little medico-legal practice to be discovered in early modern England. But while several commentators have suggested that the English legal system must have retarded the growth of medico-legal science in England, they have tended merely to cite the differences between 'inquisitorial' and 'accusatorial' legal systems without exploring their respective effects on the development of legal medicine.[18] Catherine Crawford's comparative study of the place of medical expertise in continental Roman-canon and Anglo–American common-law systems during the early modern period argues that the differing methods and standards of proof that characterized the two systems had important implications for legal medicine. Not only the legal status of medical experts, but the ways in which medical expertise was obtained and incorporated into legal proceedings, strongly encouraged the development of medico-legal science in Roman-canon jurisdictions. In particular, the absence of juries, the obligation to record all proceedings in writing, and the need to justify decisions by reference to authority led to the creation of an extensive literature on legal proof of which forensic medicine formed an integral part. Moreover, the German procedure of officially consulting university professors in difficult legal cases stimulated the production of scholarly commentaries on medico-legal problems by virtually commissioning them. In the English case, Crawford argues, it was not so much the coroner system as common-law trial by jury and common-sense standards of legal proof which militated against a formally privileged position for medical expertise and against the development of scholarship on questions of medico-legal proof.

Mary Wessling's study of the medical evidence of infanticide in eighteenth-century Württemberg exemplifies many aspects of this analysis of continental procedures, while recalling some of the themes of Mark Jackson's paper. In Württemberg, too, the infanticide question focused attention on forensic medicine generally in the later eighteenth century and greatly stimulated medical interest in the problems associated with physical evidence of live-birth. Wessling shows how the Enlightenment drive to minimize the use of torture in criminal proceedings generally and in infanticide trials in particular, in the interests of a more rational and humane administration of justice, increased the pressure on medical evidence to provide the courts with certainty. Under this pressure, existing standards of medical knowledge and inference in the conduct of post-mortem examinations of infants and in the preparation of initial medical reports were increasingly found wanting. In a series of cases tried in the 1770s, physicians at the University in Tübingen made detailed technical criticisms of hydrostatic lung tests for the duchy's high court, which they backed up by experimental and pathological investigations intended to identify potential sources of error and suggest more reliable alternatives to the test. Wessling suggests that it was their involvement in these cases and the increasingly critical role of the physical evidence that led the Tübingen medical faculty to extend its teaching of legal medicine and to produce a series of influential monographs on the medical evidence of infanticide.

As in England, so in Württemberg, a major force behind the growth of medico-legal knowledge at this time seems to have been a widespread opposition to the death penalty for infanticide. This opposition found its way into criminal proceedings in quite different ways in each jurisdiction, but had remarkably similar effects in stimulating the growth of forensic medicine in each case. Jackson's and Wessling's papers suggest that one role of forensic medicine at this time was to provide systems of criminal justice with greater flexibility by effectively enlarging the scope for judicial discretion and providing opportunities for more humane attitudes to punishment to affect legal practice. In seventeenth- and eighteenth-century England, one way of evading the rigours of the infanticide statute was by what Hoffer and Hull have called 'benefit of linen'.[19] Evidence that clothes had been prepared for an infant came to be accepted as proof that its mother had not intended to kill or conceal it; this exempted the case from the 1624 statute and allowed the woman to be tried according to ordinary common-law rules. In France, flexibility in the direction of leniency could be achieved by adjourning an infanticide trial 'for further enquiry' and releasing the accused while the 'enquiry' was fictitiously and endlessly conducted.[20] By such means, in both adversarial and inquisitorial systems, the rigidity of the law could be informally softened in cases where it seemed unduly harsh. We suggest that medical evidence, too, could be useful in this way. In England, medical testimony could contradict the 1624 statutory presumption in particular cases, while in Württemberg, expert scrutiny of the medical evidence could produce the hint of doubt that justified refusing to authorize torture in order to complete the proof of a capital crime.

The law against infanticide was not the only criminal statute thought to be too harsh in eighteenth-century England. The 'pious perjury' whereby juries deliberately undervalued stolen goods to bring thefts below the statutory threshold of felony was an accepted method of adapting the law to fit contemporary notions of reasonableness.[21] Another was the gradual extension to all and sundry of benefit of clergy, the medieval privilege exempting clergymen from capital punishment by secular courts.[22] Viewed in this context, forensic medicine offered additional opportunities for tempering justice with humanity, by means that were more congenial to Enlightenment and Benthamite thinking than white lies and institutionalized evasions. The potential of medical evidence to introduce *doubt* as well as clarity into legal proceedings may well have enhanced its judicial role in an era when certain capital statutes and the use of torture were becoming increasingly unacceptable to public opinion.[23] This is not to say that late eighteenth-century medical witnesses were necessarily predisposed towards leniency, nor to impute disingenuousness to other trial participants, but to suggest that medical evidence had a historical significance which may or may not have been apparent at the time.

Enlightened reformers of the late eighteenth and early nineteenth centuries such as Johann Peter Frank saw forensic medicine and its complement medical police as having important roles to play in public health work and in the administration of the civil law.[24] These ideas were especially influential in Scotland, where the growth of legal medicine throughout the nineteenth century faithfully reflected the philanthropic ideas of the Whig–Liberal reformers who first introduced it from the Continent around 1800.[25] Brenda White's paper shows how, in less than forty years after Andrew Duncan, Sr, began teaching the subject in 1792, medical jurisprudence in Scotland advanced from being considered an obscure and politically controversial subject of doubtful relevance to achieving the status of an integral part of Scottish medical education. The Scottish system of teaching forensic medicine and medical police together arguably made Scottish doctors more aware than their English-trained counterparts of the broader socio-legal and moral implications of their practice. The fact that the two subjects were taught jointly helped give legal medicine a higher profile in Scotland than in England, and it prepared Scottish medical graduates to play an active part in public health administration as well as in medico-legal practice generally. In conjunction with the Scottish pattern of police and public health reform, this led to the emergence in Scotland of the distinctive figure of the 'medical policeman', who combined the offices of burgh police surgeon and medical officer of health.

In England, too, the early nineteenth century saw a rapid expansion of medico-legal education. But there was never any English equivalent to the Scottish system of teaching forensic medicine together with medical police, and whereas in Scotland medical jurisprudence gradually built up a solid institutional presence in the university legal and medical faculties, in England it never gained more than a precarious foothold in the teaching hospitals and university medical schools. There were no English teaching posts in forensic medicine as prestigious as the regius professorships at

Glasgow and Edinburgh, and legal medicine never achieved the same importance in English as it did in Scottish medical education.[26] Nor did English medico-legal practice succeed in developing the intimate working relationship with everyday legal and medical practice that it came to have in Scotland.[27] During the twentieth century, English medico-legal practitioners have made a number of attempts to enhance the academic status of their subject and create a strong institutional focus for the development of medico-legal expertise. But none of these efforts have been very successful, and even today, English forensic medicine does not enjoy the professional standing or moral authority of its Scottish counterpart.

Much of the history of legal medicine has been written in terms of the gradual emergence and increasing recognition of medico-legal expertise, usually identified with forensic-pathological and toxicological expertise and interpreted very much in the light of present-day assumptions about what constitutes expert knowledge and who possesses it.[28] Historically, though, medico-legal expertise has been anything but a fixed quantity. The meaning of such expertise has varied enormously from one historical setting and period to another, and as several of the papers in this collection show, the history of legal medicine features a more numerous and varied cast of experts – including midwives, surgeons, apothecaries, general practitioners, prison medical officers and police surgeons – than does current medico-legal practice. The sources of expertise and the qualifications required for the performance of various medico-legal functions have also varied widely, and have seldom been the subject of universal agreement at any given time.

Throughout the history of legal medicine, expert status has regularly been contested by different occupational groups and specialties. In her 1977 essay 'Hebammen und Hymen' (Midwives and the hymen), Esther Fischer-Homberger has shown how during the sixteenth, seventeenth and eighteenth centuries, scientific opinion on the hymen varied with the relative status and competing medico-legal interests of medical men and midwives. In the sixteenth century, medical men denied the existence of the hymen in an attempt to discredit midwives as medico-legal authorities on the question of virginity. But during the seventeenth century medical men again became curious about the hymen, and in the eighteenth century they decided that it did exist and was indeed an indication of virginity, thus belatedly acknowledging the validity of midwives' traditional knowledge. But by this time the authority of medical men on such matters was firmly entrenched.[29] This example serves to introduce a theme which will be met with more than once in the remainder of this book, namely the close reciprocal relationship between medico-legal expertise and its objects of knowledge and practice. Expertise is not entirely relative, but its multiple historical meanings can only be grasped if expertise itself is made the object of historical enquiry, rather than being treated as an absolute standard by which to judge the shortcomings and achievements of the past.

Of all the various medico-legal specialties, forensic psychiatry is the one where medical authority has met with most resistance. Two papers in our section on 'Special offenders' are case studies of the ways in which psychiatric expertise established its authority in the courtroom. Joel Eigen's paper on medical evidence in criminal trials involving the insanity defence during the half-century before the McNaughtan Rules (1843) shows how medical men persuaded Old Bailey judges and jurors to accept counter-intuitive and psychologically complex views of criminal insanity. By examining the transcripts of many obscure trials involving the insanity defence, Eigen shows how esoteric psychiatric concepts such as partial insanity first gained acceptance in the criminal courtroom. During the eighteenth century, the 'facts' of insanity were the common property of laymen and doctors alike, for they consisted of overt behavioural phenomena, such as incoherent conversation, indicative of total loss of reason. However, from about 1800, medical men with special experience of insanity began to challenge the lay view that sanity, and hence criminal responsibility, could be inferred unproblematically from behaviour. Armed with new psychological concepts such as 'lesion of the will', they claimed that certain forms of mental abnormality were imperceptible to laymen and that sustained professional contact with the mad made it possible for medical experts to detect insanity in persons whose conduct appeared entirely rational. In his analysis of five cases in which attempts were made to enlarge the conceptual scope of the insanity defence, Eigen shows how mad-doctors sought to persuade judges and jurors of the validity of these novel insights.

Eigen's study also provides a corrective to a theme which has dominated nearly all previous work on the history of forensic psychiatry – that of *conflict* between the law and medicine over the definition of insanity.[30] He suggests that, at least in this period, there was active *collaboration* between law and medicine in this area, based on a conjunction of interests. The late eighteenth and early nineteenth centuries saw the decisive development both of defence advocacy in English criminal trials and of psychiatry as a medical specialty.[31] In Eigen's cases we see defence lawyers, mad-doctors and judges effectively colluding to facilitate the introduction of new medical-psychological concepts into English legal practice. This contrasts with the more familiar story of long-sustained conflict between the law and medicine over the framing and application of the insanity defence. The McNaughtan Rules, formulated after the controversial trial of Daniel McNaughtan in 1843, set out precise legal criteria for deciding on the criminal responsibility of mentally abnormal offenders.[32] The Rules have been variously portrayed as a restatement of the traditional legal view of the relation between moral awareness and culpability,[33] as an *ad hoc* solution to the problems posed by one especially difficult case,[34] or, more recently, as an exercise in political damage limitation at a time of revolutionary upheaval.[35] Eigen's study suggests another reading. The McNaughtan Rules may represent an attempt to introduce greater flexibility into the adjudication of criminal insanity while at the same time limiting the potential for medical–legal collaboration to unduly expand the scope of the insanity defence.

Finally, it is worth noting with respect to Eigen's paper that, once again, creative innovation in legal medicine appears to have been associated with attempts to lessen the severity of laws requiring the death penalty for fairly minor offences. As Eigen's study shows, the concept of partial insanity was introduced into English legal practice to defend not serial killers but a man who stole silver spoons and a woman who forged a cheque – crimes for which the prescribed penalty was death. The broadening of the definition of legal insanity clearly allowed for greater humanitarian discretion in the enforcement of the law and the punishment of offenders, and in this respect it invites comparison with the near-contemporary growth of scientific interest in the hydrostatic lung test.

In a recent survey of the history of law–psychiatry relations in Britain and Europe, Roger Smith has drawn attention to the ways in which particular institutional settings and practices have shaped the development of psychiatry.[36] In Smith's view, modern psychiatry developed from numerous, essentially local, forms of knowledge and practice, and has only comparatively recently achieved the status of an independent medical specialty. Nowhere is this more apparent than in the case of forensic psychiatry, which 'developed as an occupation in the interstices of administrative and legal procedure',[37] and still bears many traces of its origins in penal and custodial practices. In this book, the papers by Joel Eigen and Stephen Watson show how the emergence of forensic-psychiatric expertise depended upon highly specific forms of knowledge that were developed in and for the courtroom and the prison. Eigen notes that prison surgeons appeared increasingly often as expert witnesses in the early nineteenth century. They acquired authority in criminal trials, he argues, because their unrivalled opportunities to observe prisoners awaiting trial made them particularly good at detecting feigned insanity.[38] By the late nineteenth century, as Stephen Watson relates, the English prison doctor's task of diagnosing feigned insanity had fed into a developing knowledge of the relationship between mental defect and crime, and had led to the creation of a new object of knowledge: the weakminded habitual criminal, or 'moral imbecile'. On the basis of his long experience of habitual criminals and the special facilities for observation which the prison afforded, the English prison medical officer of the late nineteenth and early twentieth centuries claimed an expertise in this variety of mental deficiency. The moral imbecile had no very obvious defect of intelligence, and did not exhibit many of the usual symptoms of certifiable insanity. His or her defect manifested itself in an inability to refrain from committing crimes, however slight the chances of gain and however strong the likelihood of punishment. Routine methods of prison discipline and punishment had no effect on such people; they were believed to lack the moral understanding to experience a punitive and deterrent effect, and were therefore literally 'unfit for discipline'. Though apparently very rare and notoriously difficult to identify outside the prison context, the moral imbecile was the subject of much professional and public debate from the 1880s down to the 1920s, and was recognized in the Mental Deficiency Act of 1913 as one of the main types of certifiable mental deficiency.

The prison medical officer's reputation as an expert in mental deficiency rested almost entirely on his alleged expertise in detecting this one rather special type of deviance. Yet, as Watson's paper shows, the moral imbecile category provided the basis for an expert status which was regularly recognized by the courts and the Home Office. This status was secure while the prison remained one of the principal 'surfaces of emergence' for the problem of mental defect and while assessments of intelligence remained largely subjective. It also depended upon the stereotype of the weakminded habitual criminal continuing to resonate with wider public concern about the care and control of the 'feebleminded'. Once these conditions ceased to hold, however, the moral imbecile category, and with it the prison medical officer's claim to expertise, rapidly ceased to have any relevance, and soon came to appear just as anomalous and outdated as the prison-bounded techniques of observation on which they were based.

Watson's paper suggests that the medico-legal expert does not simply provide a service or mediate between conflicting social interests, but actually helps to create new categories of deviance and new objects of medico-legal knowledge and practice. Like the hymen in early modern Europe, the moral imbecile's career as an object of knowledge depended on particular institutional needs and occupational practices. Just as recognition of the expertise of midwives in divorce and annulment proceedings depended on belief in the existence of the hymen and its relevance as a proof of virginity, so recognition of the prison medical officer's expertise in mental deficiency depended on belief in the existence and wider social relevance of the moral imbecile.

Like his distant cousin the psychopath, the moral imbecile generated a volume of medical and criminological debate and commentary quite out of relation to his numerical importance.[39] Ruth Harris's paper explores the debates that surrounded another very select and problematic group of offenders, the French anarchist terrorists of the 1890s. Most historical accounts of forensic psychiatry privilege the narratives constructed by medical experts which link abnormal mental states to criminal behaviour, but Harris's paper highlights the narratives that the anarchists themselves produced.[40] The Third Republic's inquisitorial criminal procedure, with its exhaustive preliminary inquiries, produced a kind of ongoing dialogue or negotiation between investigating magistrates, defendants, and lay and expert witnesses. Each trial participant offered a version of events and motivations, from which a single, definitive account was eventually constructed, which formed the basis for deciding on the accused's degree of criminal responsibility. In the anarchist trials, however, this process was subverted by the anarchists' refusal to see themselves as criminals or to allow any suggestion of diminished responsibility to detract from the political significance of their acts. Against the many voices which attempted to portray them as deranged fanatics, criminal degenerates or egotistical would-be martyrs, the anarchist terrorists articulated a heroic image of themselves as courageous defenders of society's weakest and most vulnerable members – an image which resonated powerfully with contemporary notions of masculine honour. Repeated legal and psychiatric interrogations only succeeded in producing detailed and often moving accounts of their impoverished lives and defiant political credos, which the bourgeois press then publicized, just as the anarchists had intended. The anarchists thus emerge as veritable co-authors of the courtroom dramas in which they starred. Their trials and even their executions became deliberately orchestrated acts of political propaganda.

Alienists did not attempt to distance themselves from the political issues raised by these trials. Though some expert commentators devised pathological explanations for anarchist terrorism, most of them invoked the language of pathology only rhetorically, in order to portray the anarchists as monsters of depravity. Shocked by what they saw as extremist attacks from both left and right, they rallied to the defence of the Republic, and sought to affirm and mediate what they considered to be its healthy social and political values through their own professional expertise. For once, medicine, law and public opinion were nearly unanimous in refusing to countenance any diminution of criminal responsibility.

The French anarchist terrorist trials are a particularly spectacular example of the politics of medico-legal practice. The next two papers explore this aspect of legal medicine with reference to the more mundane activity of establishing cause of death. In England, repeated reforms of the coroner system of medico-legal investigation have tended progressively to obscure the political implications of coroners' practice. Joe Sim and Tony Ward's paper on deaths in custody in Victorian England sets out to recover this dimension of the coronership by showing the highly controversial role that it had in the politics of local government, law enforcement and police custody. The nineteenth-century coronership was a kind of irregular or alternative magistracy, whose precise functions, jurisdictions and powers vis-à-vis the criminal justice system, the police, and local government remained loosely defined and subject to many local variations and disputes. The inquest and the coroner's jury (obligatory at all inquests until 1926) were essentially popular institutions, and inquest juries often held local authorities responsible for deaths in prisons, barracks, workhouses, asylums and police stations. The coronership and the inquest appeared increasingly anachronistic alongside the new Victorian institutions of local government, poor law and prison administration, while their potential to embarrass local elites and expose custodial institutions to unfavourable publicity made local officials more willing to think of possible alternatives to the coroner system. Sim and Ward show that in the 1850s and 1860s it was not doctors but magistrates who first proposed replacing the coroner's inquest by a kind of medical examiner system, and that the underlying motives for the proposed medicalization were as much financial and political as scientific. Coroners successfully countered this threat, however, by appealing to public fears that a more medicalized inquiry would also be less open and independent. Although subsequent legislation did gradually enlarge the role of medical evidence in coroner's inquests, this was achieved without much altering the traditional structure of coroners' practice. The gradual reform of the coronership in a steadily more medical direction thus represented a compromise which had political origins and meanings that have almost been lost sight of. But they still affect coroners' practice today – especially in cases of death in custody.[41]

In North America the coronership also enjoyed a high political profile, but for a rather different reason: its involvement in political corruption and the municipal spoils system. Julie Johnson's paper on the coroner system and forensic pathology in twentieth-century America describes the world of the political 'machines' which dominated urban American politics right down to the 1960s and 1970s, and shows how even the most determined attempts at reform, backed up by powerful medical-professional lobbying, and carried on against a background of widespread elite consensus in favour of medico-legal reform, could nevertheless be frustrated by a failure to grasp the political realities surrounding the coroner's office and those who worked in it. As Johnson clearly shows, even the eventual recognition of legal medicine (in fact, forensic pathology) as a fully-fledged academic discipline and professional specialty in America from the 1950s has not succeeded in overcoming these political problems, nor has it significantly improved its status within medicine. In basing their specialty in high-prestige university medical school departments rather than in the more practical, down-to-earth settings of the coroner's or medical examiner's office, American forensic pathologists unwittingly ensured that their specialty would remain marginal to the politics of medico-legal investigation, while nevertheless failing to secure the respect of academic medicine.

The final section of this book presents two case studies of the shifting boundaries of medical authority in England between the wars. The history of legal medicine is in many respects a story of medicalization, in the sense of the expansion of medical expertise and authority into new areas of social practice, especially those connected with the detection and management of crime and deviance. However, as several papers in this collection suggest, medicalization may respond as much to the needs of the law or social administration as to the professional aspirations of medicine.[42] Barbara Brookes and Paul Roth's analysis of the case of *Rex* v. *Bourne* (1938) and its significance for the development of modern English abortion law shows not only professional-medical interests working to liberalize the law, but the law itself playing a creative role in the medicalization of this controversial practice. In deliberately inviting prosecution for criminal abortion in a case bound to attract great public sympathy for the defence, the surgeon Aleck Bourne and his supporters in the Abortion Law Reform Association were seeking clarification of the circumstances in which medical practitioners acting in good faith could legitimately perform abortions. But by making it almost impossible for anyone other than doctors to meet the *bona fides* requirement for performing an abortion, Mr Justice Macnaghten's judgment in the Bourne case made them virtually the sole legal arbiters in abortion decisions. It thus effectively gave doctors a monopoly on legal abortion – even while failing, as it turned out, to give them the degree of legal protection from criminal prosecution which they had originally sought. In this case it was the law, rather than medical ambitions and strategies, that was ultimately responsible for the 'medicalization' of what remains, more than fifty years later, a highly sensitive issue.[43]

In the case of the campaign to establish a national medico-legal institute for England and Wales, described in Norman Ambage and Michael Clark's paper, even the very expansionist strategies of medico-legal reformers were unable to prevent an actual *de*-medicalization of scientific crime investigation in the interwar period. During the early decades of the twentieth century, English reformers made repeated attempts to improve standards of medico-legal training, to enhance the prestige of forensic medicine as an academic discipline, and to create a strong institutional focus for the development of medico-legal expertise. These efforts culminated in a campaign to establish a central medico-legal institute as part of the University of London during the 1920s and 1930s. But by the mid-1930s, when this public and professional agitation was reaching its peak, underlying trends were moving in the opposite direction. The growth of specialization and professional autonomy in both forensic science and forensic medicine meant that it was no longer practicable or even desirable to try to combine all the different sub-specialties involved under one roof and one single, medical authority. Moreover, the Home Office and the police wanted forensic science and clinical forensic medicine – not forensic pathology and toxicology – to help them boost detection rates in crimes against property and cases of sexual assault. At the same time, the ambitious scale on which the medico-legal institute had been conceived and the growing financial demands of rearmament made the scheme vulnerable to competition from the much less grandiose and apparently more cost-effective regional forensic science laboratories. In these circumstances, the medico-legal institute proposal, which had become the focus of so many of English forensic medicine's professional aspirations, seemed redundant to the Home Office and Treasury officials whose support was essential if it were to have any chance of success. Consequently, instead of the nascent forensic science service being placed under the auspices of forensic medicine, forensic medicine came to be seen as merely an appendage of forensic science.

Although in the post-1945 period forensic pathology did finally succeed in forging closer ties with the Home Office and the police, it did so on a much more decentralized and part-time basis than the medico-legal reformers of the 1920s and 1930s had envisaged, and has never succeeded in regaining authority over the forensic science service. Though repeated attempts have been made during the last fifty years to improve forensic medicine's professional organization and to provide better facilities for postgraduate study and research, English forensic pathologists have been no more successful than their American counterparts in raising their academic and professional standing, and the institutional and career structures of English forensic medicine have given rise to much concern over the past three decades.[44] Thus, in spite of the many historical differences between the English and American experiences, the conclusion suggested by Ambage and Clark's paper is similar to that of Johnson's: the authority of medico-legal expertise depends as much on favourable social, institutional and political conditions as on its technical efficacy or professional maturity. Several papers in the book support this view.

More generally, this book argues that the history of legal medicine is not just the history of a medical specialty or specialties, but part of a broader history of scientific and professional authority in society. It is in some respects a story of medicalization, but also of the ways in which non-medical factors such as the law, public opinion, and local and national politics have helped to shape medico-legal knowledge, institutions and practice. Moreover, legal medicine has itself often played an active part in shaping legal, political and social change. Legal medicine has today become institutionally and professionally structured in very specific ways, but its history is far more complex and less predictable than the present organization of medico-legal work would seem to suggest. We hope that the following pages will succeed in conveying some of this richness.

NOTES

1 See, for example, Keith Simpson, 'The development of forensic medicine', *Guy's Hospital Gazette*, 78 (1964), 384–90; J. Malcolm Cameron, 'The changing face of forensic medicine and its contribution to clinical medicine', *London Hospital Gazette*, 73 (1970), Supplement, ii–ix; William G. Eckert and Neil Garland, 'The history of the forensic applications in radiology', *American Journal of Forensic Medicine and Pathology*, 5 (1984), 53–6. The chapter headings in Thomas Forbes's *Surgeons at the Bailey: English Forensic Medicine to 1878* (New Haven and London: Yale University Press, 1985) read as if the book were a textbook of forensic medicine, rather than a history.

2 Some examples of medico-legal history which have shed light on these topics are Esther Fischer-Homberger, *Die traumatische Neurose: vom somatischen zum sozialen Leiden* (Berne: Hans Huber, 1975); Karl Figlio, 'How does illness mediate social relations? Workmen's compensation and medico-legal practices, 1890–1940', in Peter Wright and Andrew Treacher, eds., *The Problem of Medical Knowledge: Examining the Social Construction of Medicine* (Edinburgh: Edinburgh University Press, 1982), pp. 174–224; Figlio, 'What is an accident?', *Bulletin of the Society for the Social History of Medicine*, 33 (December 1983), 27–9; Peter Bartrip, *Workmen's Compensation in Twentieth-Century Britain: Law, History, and Social Policy* (Aldershot: Avebury, 1987); Elizabeth Cawthon, 'Thomas Wakley and the medical coronership – occupational death and the judicial process', *Medical History*, 30 (1986), 191–202.

3 W. J. Curran, 'The confusion of titles in the medicolegal field: an historical analysis and a proposal for reform', *Medicine, Science and the Law*, 15 (1975), 270–5. Cf. Oliver C. Schroeder, Jr, 'Forensic medicine: yesterday, today and tomorrow', *Postgraduate Medicine*, 28 (1960), A60–A70; Jaroslav Nemec, *International Bibliography of Medicolegal Serials 1736–1967* (Bethesda, MD: National Library of Medicine, 1969), p. 1.

4 J. Nemec, *International Bibliography of the History of Legal Medicine* (Bethesda, MD: US Department of Health, Education and Welfare, 1973), p. v.

5 S. E. Chaillé, 'Origins and progress of medical jurisprudence, 1776–1876', *Transactions of the Medical Congress of Philadelphia* (1876), reprinted, with a biographical sketch of Chaillé, in *Journal of Criminal Law and Criminology*, 40 (1949), 397–444; E. Ackerknecht, 'Early history of legal medicine', *Ciba Symposia*, 11 (1950–1), 1288–1304, 1313–16, reprinted in Chester R. Burns, ed., *Legacies in Law and Medicine* (New York: Science History Publications, 1977), pp. 249–71. See also Sydney Smith, 'The history and development of forensic medicine', *British Medical Journal*, 1 (1951), 599–607; Smith, 'The development of forensic medicine and law–science relations', *Journal of Public Law*, 3 (1954), 304–19; Albert Rosenberg, 'The Sarah Stout murder case: an early example of the doctor as expert witness', *Journal of the History of Medicine and Allied Sciences*, 12 (1957), 61–70, reprinted in Burns, ed., *Legacies in Law and Medicine*, pp. 230–9.

6 Le Moyne Snyder, 'Medicine and the law – retrospect and prospect', *Journal of the American Medical Association*, 171 (1959), 644–8; J. A. Gorsky, 'The history of forensic medicine', *Charing Cross Hospital Gazette*, 58 (1960), 31–6; R. P. Brittain and R. O. Myers, 'The history of legal medicine', in Francis E. Camps et al., eds., *Gradwohl's Legal Medicine*, 2nd edn (Bristol: John Wright, 1968), pp. 1–14; Cameron, 'Changing face of forensic medicine'; H. L. Taylor, 'The evolution of legal medicine', *Medico-Legal Bulletin*, 252 (1974), 1–7; Bernard J. Ficarra, 'History of legal medicine', *Legal Medicine Annual 1976* (New York: Appleton-Century-Crofts, 1977), 3–27.

7 J. D. J. Havard, *The Detection of Secret Homicide: A Study of the Medico-Legal Investigation of Sudden Death* (London: Macmillan, 1960); N. Walker, *Crime and Insanity in England. Vol. I: The Historical Perspective* (Edinburgh: Edinburgh University Press, 1968); N. Walker and S. McCabe, *Crime and Insanity in England. Vol. II: New Solutions and New Problems* (Edinburgh: Edinburgh University Press, 1973); R. P. Brittain, *Bibliography of Medico-Legal Works in English* (London: Sweet & Maxwell, 1962); R. P. Brittain, A. Saury and M.-R. Guidet, *Bibliographie des travaux français de médecine légale* (Paris: Masson, 1970); Nemec, *International Bibliography of Medicolegal Serials*; Nemec, *International Bibliography of the History of Legal Medicine*.

8 Brittain and Myers, 'History of legal medicine', p. 1. One such source is Chaillé, 'Origins and progress of medical jurisprudence'; others are Ludwig Julius Caspar Mende, *Ausführliches Handbuch der gerichtlichen Medizin für Gesetzgeber, Rechtsgelehrte, Arzte und Wundärzte. Erster Theil: Kurze Geschichte der gerichtlichen Medizin* (Leipzig, 1819) and Victor Janovsky, 'Die geschichtliche Entwicklung der gerichtlichen Medizin', in Josef Maschka, ed., *Handbuch der gerichtlichen Medizin* (Tübingen, 1881), vol. I, pp. 1–32.

9 See, for example, T. Forbes, 'By what disease or casualty: the changing face of death in London', *Journal of the History of Medicine and Allied Sciences*, 31 (1976), 395–420; Forbes, 'Coroners' inquests in the County of Middlesex, England, 1819–1842', *Journal of the History of Medicine and Allied Sciences*, 32 (1977), 375–94; Forbes, 'Inquests into London and Middlesex homicides, 1673–1782', *Yale Journal of Biology and Medicine*, 50 (1977), 207–20. See also Gary I. Greenwald and Maria White Greenwald, 'Medico-legal progress in inquests of

felonious deaths: Westminster, 1761–1866', *Journal of Legal Medicine*, 2 (1981), 193–264; Greenwald and Greenwald, 'Coroner's inquests, a source of vital statistics: Westminster, 1761–1866', *Journal of Legal Medicine*, 4 (1983), 51–86.

10 Thomas Forbes, 'Crowner's Quest', *Transactions of the American Philosophical Society*, 68 (1978), 1–52.

11 Esther Fischer-Homberger, *Medizin vor Gericht: Gerichtsmedizin von der Renaissance bis zur Aufklärung* (Berne: Hans Huber, 1983).

12 For an introduction to the medico-legal role of midwives, see Erwin H. Ackerknecht, 'Midwives as experts in court', *Bulletin of the New York Academy of Medicine*, 52 (1976), 1224–8.

13 Such as deodands and inquests upon treasure trove and royal fish. See F. J. Waldo, 'The ancient office of coroner', *Transactions of the Medico-Legal Society*, 8 (1910–11), 101–29; William Wynn Westcott, 'A note upon deodands', *Transactions of the Medico-Legal Society*, 7 (1909–10), 91–7; R. F. Hunnisett, *The Mediaeval Coroner* (Cambridge: Cambridge University Press, 1961); Paul Knapman and Michael J. Powers, *The Law and Practice on Coronership (Thurston's Coronership: 3rd Edition)* (Chichester: Barry Rose, 1985), pp. 1–15.

14 On this theme, see especially Havard, *Detection of Secret Homicide*, passim, and Jürgen Thorwald, *Dead Men Tell Tales* (London: Thames & Hudson, 1966), p. 90.

15 John H. Langbein, 'The criminal trial before the lawyers', *University of Chicago Law Review*, 45 (1978), 263–316; P. J. R. King, 'Decision-makers and decision-making in the English criminal law, 1750–1800', *Historical Journal*, 27 (1984), 25–58; Thomas Andrew Green, *Verdict According to Conscience: Perspectives on the English Criminal Trial Jury, 1200–1800* (Chicago and London: University of Chicago Press, 1985); J. S. Cockburn and T. A. Green, eds., *Twelve Good Men and True: The Criminal Trial Jury in England, 1200–1800* (Princeton: Princeton University Press, 1988).

16 Michael Macdonald, 'The secularization of suicide in England 1660–1800', *Past & Present* 111 (May 1986), 50–97; Macdonald and Terence R. Murphy, *Sleepless Souls: Suicide in Early Modern England* (Oxford: Clarendon Press, 1990).

17 Nemec, 'II. Origins of medicolegal literature and the development of medicolegal serials', in his *International Bibliography of Medicolegal Serials*, pp. 2–9; Fischer-Homberger, *Medizin vor Gericht*.

18 See J. B. Speer, Jr, essay review of 'Crowner's Quest' by Thomas R. Forbes, *Annals of Science*, 37 (1980), 353–6, at p. 355.

19 Peter C. Hoffer and N. E. H. Hull, *Murdering Mothers: Infanticide in England and New England, 1558–1803* (New York: New York University Press, 1981).

20 Gérard Aubry, *La jurisprudence criminelle du Châtelet de Paris sous le règne de Louis XVI* (Paris: Pichon et Durand-Auzias, 1971), pp. 35, 37, 59–60.

21 John Beattie, *Crime and the Courts in England, 1660–1800* (Oxford: Clarendon Press, 1986; Princeton: Princeton University Press, 1986), pp. 423–9.

22 J. H. Baker, *An Introduction to English Legal History*, 3rd edn (London: Butterworths, 1990), pp. 586–9.

23 The capacity of medical testimony to generate doubt, thereby serving the interests of defendants, is discussed in Catherine Crawford, 'The emergence of English medical jurisprudence: medical evidence in common-law courts, 1730–1830', Ph.D thesis, University of Oxford, 1987, ch. 3.

24 See Leona Baumgartner and Elizabeth M. Ramsey, 'Johann Peter Frank and his "System einer vollständigen medicinischen Polizey"', *Annals of Medical History*, n.s., 5 (1933), 525–32, 6 (1934), 69–90; George Rosen, 'Cameralism and the concept of medical police', *Bulletin of the History of Medicine*, 27 (1953), 21–42; Rosen, 'The fate of the concept of medical police 1780–1890', *Centaurus*, 5 (1957), 97–113; Ludmilla Jordanova, 'Policing public health in France 1780–1815', in Teizo Ogawa, ed., *Public Health. Proceedings of the 5th International Symposium on the Comparative History of Medicine – East and West* (Tokyo: Taniguchi Foundation, 1981), pp. 12–32.

25 On Scottish forensic medicine generally, see M. Anne Crowther and Brenda White, *On Soul and Conscience: The Medical Expert and Crime. 150 Years of Forensic Medicine in Glasgow* (Aberdeen: Aberdeen University Press, 1988).

26 Sydney Smith, 'History and development of forensic medicine', pp. 604–5; F. N. L. Poynter, 'Medical education in England since 1600', in C. D. O'Malley, ed., *The History of Medical Education* (Berkeley and London: University of California Press, 1970), pp. 235–49, at pp. 244–6.

27 A. V. Sheehan, *Criminal Procedure in Scotland and France* (Edinburgh: HMSO, 1975), pp. 113, 121–2, 129–30, 221–5.

28 See, for example, Snyder, 'Medicine and the law'; J. Malcolm Cameron, 'The medico-legal expert – past, present and future', *Medicine, Science and the Law*, 20 (1980), 3–13; and Forbes, *Surgeons at the Bailey*. On expertise and the law generally, see Anthony Kenny, 'The expert in court', *Law Quarterly Review*, 99 (1983), 197–216 and Roger Smith and Brian Wynne, eds., *Expert Evidence: Interpreting Science in the Law* (London and New York: Routledge, 1989).

29 Esther Fischer-Homberger, 'Hebammen und Hymen', *Sudhoffs Archiv*, 61 (1977), 75–94, reprinted in Fischer-Homberger, *Krankheit Frau und andere Arbeiten zur Medizingeschichte der Frau* (Berne: Hans Huber, 1979), pp. 85–105, 146–50. Londa Schiebinger kindly provided us with an English summary of this paper.

30 See especially Roger Smith, *Trial by Medicine: Insanity and Responsibility in Victorian Trials* (Edinburgh: Edinburgh University Press, 1981); Walker, *Crime and Insanity*, vol. I; Jacques Quen, 'Anglo-American criminal insanity: an historical perspective', *Journal of the History of the Behavioural Sciences*, 10 (1974), 313–23; Jan Goldstein, *Console and Classify: The French Psychiatric Profession in the Nineteenth Century* (Cambridge: Cambridge University Press, 1987), ch. 5.

31 Langbein, 'Criminal trial', pp. 307–16; J. M. Beattie, 'Scales of justice: defense counsel and the English criminal trial in the eighteenth and nineteenth centuries', *Law and History Review*, 9 (1991), 221–67; Andrew T. Scull, *Museums of Madness: The Social Organization of Insanity in Nineteenth-Century Britain* (London: Allen Lane, 1979), chs. 4 and 5; Roger Smith, *Trial by Medicine*, chs. 1–3.

32 A full transcription of McNaughtan's trial is reprinted in D. J. West and Alexander Walk, eds., *Daniel McNaughton: His Trial and the Aftermath* (London: Gaskell, 1977), pp. 12–73. For the text of the McNaughtan Rules, see ibid., pp. 74–81. On the many versions of the man's surname, see Bernard L. Diamond, 'On the spelling of Daniel M'Naghten's name', *Ohio State Law Journal*, 25 (1964), 84–8.

33 Walker, *Crime and Insanity*, vol. I, chs. 5 and 6; Roger Smith, *Trial by Medicine*, pp. 14–17, 19, 76, 88–9, 107, 170.

34 Roger Smith, *Trial by Medicine*, pp. 14, 76.

35 See especially Richard Moran, *Knowing Right from Wrong: The Insanity Defense of Daniel McNaughtan* (London: Collier-Macmillan, 1981), passim.

36 Roger Smith, 'The law and insanity in Great Britain, with comments on continental Europe', in F. Koenraadt, ed., *Ziek of Schuldig? Twee eeuwen Forensische Psychiatrie en Psychologie* (Utrecht: Rodopi, 1991), pp. 247–81.

37 Ibid., p. 261.

38 See also Joel Peter Eigen and Gregory Andoll, 'From mad-doctor to forensic witness: the evolution of early English court psychiatry', *International Journal of Law and Psychiatry*, 9 (1986), 159–69.

39 Henry Werlinder, *Psychopathy: A History of the Concepts. Analysis of the Origin and Development of a Family of Concepts in Psychopathology* (Philadelphia: Coronet Books for Uppsala University Press, 1978).

40 See also Roger Smith, 'Defining murder and madness: an introduction to medico-legal belief in the case of Mary Ann Brough, 1854', *Knowledge and Society: Studies in the Sociology of Culture Past and Present*, 4 (1983), ed. Robert Alun Jones and Henrika Kuklik, 173–225.

41 On this point, see Lindsay Prior, *The Social Organization of Death: Medical Discourse and Social Practices in Belfast* (Basingstoke and London: Macmillan, 1989; New York: St Martin's Press, 1989).

42 See also Benjamin Spector, 'The growth of medicine and the letter of the law', *Bulletin of the History of Medicine*, 26 (1952), 499–525, reprinted in Burns, ed., *Legacies in Law and Medicine*, pp. 272–98.

43 A different reading of the Bourne trial can be found in John Keown, *Abortion, Doctors and the Law: Some Aspects of the Legal Regulation of Abortion in England from 1803 to 1982* (Cambridge: Cambridge University Press, 1988), ch. 3.

44 A. K. Mant, 'A survey of forensic pathology in England since 1945', *Journal of the Forensic Science Society*, 13 (1973), 17–24; Cameron, 'Medico-legal expert'; Mant, 'Changes in the practice of forensic pathology, 1950–85', *Medicine, Science and the Law*, 26 (1986), 149–57.

I

Early modern practice

1

Forensic medicine in early colonial Maryland, 1633–83

HELEN BROCK and CATHERINE CRAWFORD

By a royal charter of 1632, Lord Baltimore, a Roman Catholic, became proprietor of the colony of Maryland in North America. He was also granted the right to 'ordain, make and enact laws of whatsoever kind' for its government, but only 'with the advice assent and aprobation of the freemen of the said province'. Maryland was first settled in 1633 by some 150 immigrants, twenty of whom were 'gentlemen of good fortune', all but one of them Roman Catholics. The rest were, for the most part, Protestant indentured servants committed to about five years' servitude before obtaining their freedom. Lord Baltimore appointed his brother, Leonard Calvert, governor of the colony, to administer its affairs with the help of an advisory council and civil, judicial and military officers appointed from amongst the gentlemen.[1]

Despite these provisions, the new colony had few men capable of administering even the most rudimentary system of criminal justice. Only one of the first settlers, Jerome Hawley, a gentleman and former member of the Inner Temple, had any legal training, and his stay in the colony was very short. Indeed, by 1640 most of the gentleman colonists had either died or returned to England, and were not replaced.[2] In the absence of anyone of comparable education or social standing, Governor Calvert therefore had to recruit new law officers from among the freemen and freed servants, who were for the most part men of little or no education or experience of criminal justice administration. Moreover, the level of criminal proceedings in the colony was such that the governor had difficulty in finding men to appoint as justices and sheriffs who had not themselves faced criminal charges.[3] It was even more difficult to find suitable men to serve on inquest or trial juries, and cases were often decided by men unable to sign their own names, who may have had little understanding of their duties. In seventeenth-century Maryland, life expectancy was very low and the turnover in office-holders correspondingly high, so that few lived long enough to profit from their experience. Although by 1670 there were two more trained lawyers in the colony, for the most part the law continued to be administered by amateurs.

Unlike the proprietors of Virginia and Massachusetts, Lord Baltimore neither made provision for the health care of his settlers nor actively encouraged medical men to migrate to the new colony. However, by 1637 three had arrived as freemen, and by 1640 four more, while another three had been brought in as servants, and thereafter there was a steady flow of medical men, most of them surgeons, into the colony.[4] In later years, some men born in the colony may also have entered the profession, but it was overwhelmingly immigrants who provided medical services. Three of the earliest medical men were Catholics, but little is known about the religion of the later arrivals. Nor is anything known about their education or social status. They probably came hoping to better themselves, but this was not yet possible by the practice of medicine alone. In spite of the high incidence of disease in the colony, the population was too small and too poor to support the number of medical men who made their way to Maryland. Some forsook medicine, and the rest had to become planters, merchants or paid government officials as well as medical practitioners in order to survive.

The early colonists were mainly engaged in the production of tobacco, which became the currency of the colony. They settled on widely separated plantations along riverbanks. Under such conditions, with people living in small, isolated communities, the authorities were not always able to exercise much control over behaviour. Maryland gained a reputation for violence and lawlessness,[5] which seems to have been justified. It was up to private individuals, if they suspected or had knowledge of any misdemeanours or felonies, to bring them to the notice of the courts. Doubtless, in these circumstances, many crimes went unreported.

In the colony's early years, all criminal cases came before the provincial court. As the population increased and the settled area expanded, the colony became divided into counties, the first of which, St Mary's, was formed in 1638. Each county came to have its own county court able to try less important civil and criminal cases. But more important cases, especially those whose punishment involved loss of life or limb, continued to be referred to the provincial court. Cases were normally tried according to Maryland law but when, as in the case of abortion and infanticide, no specific colonial law or precedent existed, reference was made to English law.

The proceedings of the provincial and county courts, published in the *Archives of Maryland*, are incomplete for the seventeenth century. Records for the provincial court run only from 1637 to 1683, while records of proceedings have survived for only four of the eleven county courts that had been established by the end of the century.[6] But the surviving records nevertheless contain a good deal of information about the use of medical evidence in the early Maryland courts. Cases of murder, suicide, infanticide, rape, and abortion were often sent for trial, and despite the relative unsophistication of Maryland's administrative and judicial systems, medical testimony seems to have been a fairly common feature of inquests and criminal trials from the colony's earliest years.

Thomas Forbes found no record of an investigative post-mortem being carried out in England before 1635, when William Harvey dissected Thomas Parr. This was not done in relation to a court case, but to find out how Parr had allegedly managed to live for 152 years.[7] But the practice of obtaining information from post-mortem examinations about cause of death in possible homicide cases must already have been well established, for it was taken to North America by early settlers. The first recorded post-mortem in colonial America was carried out in Massachusetts in 1639, where it was shown that the death of an 'ill disposed boy' had resulted from a fractured skull caused by the correction given to him by his master; the first in Maryland was probably one performed in 1643.[8] Whether any Maryland surgeon had had previous experience of carrying out post-mortem examinations, formulating an opinion as to the cause of death, and giving evidence in court is not known. There was one substantial guide in English, a translation of the sixteenth-century French surgeon Ambroise Paré's work on forensic medicine, *How to Make Reports, and to Embalme the Dead* (1634), which could have given them useful advice, but it is doubtful whether any Maryland surgeon possessed a copy.[9] However, the existence of this translation suggests a need for such a work and supports the view that medico-legal post-mortems were by no means uncommon in early seventeenth-century England.

In Maryland, as in England, whenever an unexplained death occurred, particularly if the body showed any injuries or if a murder was suspected, a coroner was responsible for appointing a jury of inquest to view the body and determine the cause of death. The first Maryland coroner was appointed in 1637 and in 1640 a full description of his duties was drawn up.[10] Occasionally, when an appointment had lapsed, it fell to the sheriff of the county in which the death had taken place to appoint the jury and hold an inquest. A jury of inquest might or might not include a surgeon. Where external injuries were extensive, laymen were considered capable of giving a reasonable opinion as to the cause of death. But if there was some doubt, and no surgeon on the jury of inquest, a surgeon was often directed to carry out a post-mortem.

Between 1635 and 1683 some forty-five trials for homicide took place at the provincial court. The first was for the murder of an Indian, the King of

Yowocomoco, by three men, one of whom, John Elkin, confessed to the killing so that there was no need for a jury of inquest.[11] His trial in 1642 demonstrates the reluctance of juries to convict a settler for the murder of an Indian. The first jury brought in a verdict of 'not guilty',

> explaining themselves that they delivered that verdict because they understood the last not to have beene committed ag[ain]st his Lo[rdshi]ps peace or the kings, because the party was a pagan, & because they had no president [*sic*] in the neighbour colony of virginea, to make such fact murther &c.

The governor, before whom the case was tried, told them

> that those Indians were in the peace of the king & his Lo[rdshi]p & that they ought not to take notice of what other colonies did, but of the Law of England, &c. and thereupon dismissed them to consider better of it.
>
> And then they returned, that they found him guilty of murther in his owne defence. and being told that this implied a contradiction they returned to consider better of it: and then they returned for their verdict, that they found that he killed the Indian in his owne defence.
>
> And the Gov[erno]r willed that the verdict be not entred as a verdict, but that another Jury be charged to enquire & try [the case] by the same evidence.

The second jury found Elkin 'guilty of manslaughter'.[12]

In 1643 an Indian boy was shot by John Dandy and died a few days later. A post-mortem dissection was carried out, probably by the surgeon George Binx, who was the foreman of the coroner's jury, possibly aided by another surgeon, Robert Ellyson, who, like Binx, later appears as a member of the grand jury on this case.[13] Tracing the passage of the bullet through the boy's body, the coroner's jury reported that it had

> ent[e]red the epigastrium neare the navell on the right side, obliquely descending, & peircing the gutts, glancing on the last vertebra of the back, and was lodged in the side of Ano.

Dandy was convicted of murder and sentenced to death but his punishment was reduced to seven years' service to the Lord Proprietor – as colony hangman.[14]

Indigenous Indians found themselves subject to Maryland law and were tried in the courts for crimes they were believed to have committed against settlers. Several settlers were murdered by Indians and, if caught and convicted, the Indians were hung. Only in one of these cases was medical evidence called for. An Indian had hit Benjamin Price on the head, but there was some doubt as to whether this was the cause of Price's death two weeks later when, having been swimming, he came out of the river 'shaken with ague, vomited and died'. The surgeons John Stansby and John Pearce were ordered to dissect Price's head in the presence of the Indian chief

Monatquund so that no unjust blame could be placed on the Indian, but the result of the post-mortem is not recorded.[15]

Richard Morton was shot by Patrick Due for stealing oysters, receiving injuries from which he subsequently died. Stephen Clifton attended him and when he died examined his body. He reported that Morton had been

> wounded in his left arme w[i]th small Burshott, soe th[a]t from the Elbow, to the upper part of the os humeris there were Eight Orifices. The greatest Orifice was uppon th^{e} musculus part, neare unto the musculus Byceps where a quantity of the shott had ent[e]red, making a large Orifice to the head of the os humeris, w[i]th severall Cavities missing the Bone, & penetrating into the Center of the Body. Likewise Two other shotts were placed, the one just above the Bastard Ribbs, penetrating the Lungs, the other betweene the third & ffowrth Ribbs, into the Body likewise, by means whereof his pulse was weake: His body (as hee complaynd) was extreame cold: Hee talked very idely, & was vexed with shortness of breth, & spitting of blood. Thereby is gathered th[a]t certaine and speedy Death is att hand, W[hi]ch followed on the 17th of the s[ai]d instant.[16]

Due was convicted of manslaughter. Pleading benefit of clergy,[17] he was only branded, but two friends had to stand surety for his good behaviour.[18]

Twenty of the forty-five trials for homicide were of masters accused of killing their servants; surprisingly, only two were of servants for killing their masters. Masters invested in servants and depended on them to cultivate the tobacco on which their livelihood depended. It might therefore be supposed that servants would have been well treated, but twenty-six of them went to court to complain of ill treatment, hoping that the courts might grant them their freedom, transfer them to new masters, or impose restraints on their masters. Probably more would have liked to do so but feared reprisals. Some servants undoubtedly were lazy and uncooperative, and under an Act of 1637, 'ill servants' could legally be punished by whipping with up to thirty-nine lashes.[19] The most common complaints were of excessive and repeated beatings, but shortage of food, inadequate clothing (which was the responsibility of the master), and excessive work loads were also claimed.

The high level of disease in the colony, with malaria affecting nearly the whole population,[20] meant that servants were often sickly and incapable of doing much work. Frustration with their inefficiency and a suspicion that they were malingering seem to have provoked much of the abuse of servants, sometimes leading to their death. It was a problem, then, for the courts to decide whether it was physical punishment or ill health that was the cause of death.

Lack of visual evidence of physical abuse and a witness's account of the servant's strange behaviour exonerated Ralph Beane of causing his servant

Raphe Lee's death, even though he had brought suspicion on himself by rapidly burying the body. A surgeon must have examined the body, as payment for the examination was made to a surgeon's widow, but no report has survived. The servant was judged to have died from 'some impostume [i.e., abscess] or apoplexy'.[21] Nor were Thomas Ward and his wife held responsible for the death of their maid despite the severe beating they gave her for running away, after which they rubbed salt into her wounds. But they were fined 300 pounds of tobacco because their punishment was judged unreasonable 'considering her weake estate of body'.[22]

When James Wilson, servant to Thomas Bradnox, died in 1652 the coroner's jury concluded that

> the material cause of the said death was an intermitting fever with a dropsy or scurvy as commonly understood and further that the stripes given him by his master not long before his death were not material.[23]

No surgeon was called to give his opinion but William Fuller was a member of the jury. Though never described as a medical man, on two occasions he gave evidence as to the suitability of treatment being given to the sick, which suggests that he had some medical knowledge.[24] In this case he may have been responsible for the opinion.

While trial juries were prepared to listen to expert opinion, they could also be influenced by the traditional belief that a murdered corpse would bleed if the murderer came near or touched it – a phenomenon known as cruentation. This belief, which had formerly been widespread in Europe, was losing its credibility by the seventeenth century, but it still featured in some British trials of this period.[25] In one Maryland case, faith in the old customary test appears to have outweighed medical opinion. John Dandy (colony hangman 1643–50) was again on trial in 1657, this time for causing the death of one of his servants. The body of Henry Gouge had been seen floating naked in the river. Dandy had hauled him out and hastily buried him, but was observed and reported to the authorities. James Veitch, the County Sheriff, was sent by the provincial court to oversee the examination of the body by two surgeons, Richard Maddox and Emperor Smith, and to take evidence from neighbours. The surgeons did

> detest [*sic*] . . . that we can See nor find nothing about the Said head, but only two places of the Skin and flesh broke on the right Side of the head and the Scull perfect and Sound, and not anything doth or can appear to us to be any Cause of the Death of the Said Gouge, And alsoe we doe detest that we did Endeavour what possible in us lay to Search the body of the Said Corps, and Could not possibly do it; It being So Noysome to us all.[26]

But Dandy's neighbours were evidently not prepared to let him get away with murder again. Evidence was given of the beatings he had given to

Gouge, and Dandy's wife, along with several neighbours, came forward to swear that when Dandy pulled Gouge from the river the corpse bled from an old wound to the head that Dandy had given him with a hatchet. The trial jury apparently accepted this evidence as a sign of Dandy's guilt, for he was again convicted of murder and sentenced to be hanged. This time the sentence was carried out.[27]

In a similar case, an informal cruentation test that went in the favour of the accused was involved in his defence, apparently successfully. In 1661 Thomas Bradnox was again charged, along with his wife, with causing the death of one of their servants, Thomas Watson. Another of their servants, Sarah Taylor, gave evidence against them, saying that they gave Watson 'very bad usage which was not fitt for a Christian in his weake Condicion'.[28] Other evidence was given that Watson 'was very sick and much Swelld with the Scurvy'.[29] But one witness swore that Watson's corpse had not bled when Bradnox prodded it, which implied his innocence:

> Capt[ain] Thomas Bradnox did touch the Corps of Thomas Watson and did thrust his Thumb upon his body to shew how his flesh did dent[,] and stirrd and shogd the Corps ... [and] I did not in the leaste see any blood come from the Corps.[30]

Thomas Bradnox died before the case was heard in 1653, when the grand jury dismissed the charges against his wife.[31]

In another case, in 1660, the test of cruentation was performed at the request of the jury of inquest. Thomas Mertine was in court on suspicion of having killed his servant Catherine Lake; he had kicked her, after which she had had a fit and died. The coroner's jury found the corpse to be 'very cleare', but, not convinced of Mertine's innocence, they ordered

> the said Thomas Mertine and the Servants of the howse to ley their hands upon the dead Corps, and there was noe issue of bloud from the Corps, neither could they perceive any alteration in the Corps nor any action from any personall man that was the Cause of her Death but the providence of the Allmighty.[32]

A possible fourth example of cruentation concerned the death of a boy, Samuel Youngman, in 1665. Youngman was beaten up by his master, Francis Carpenter, and was dead next morning. At the inquest, evidence was given that when Carpenter touched the body it began to bleed from the ear. A surgeon, Thomas Goddard, who was foreman of the inquest jury, dissected the skull and found

> a depression in the Craneum in one place and another wound where all the musculous flesh was Corrupted and w[i]thall finding Corrupted blood between the dura mater[,] the pia mater & the braines, besides severall other bruses both in the head and the body.

The verdict of the inquest jury was that 'for want of Carefull looking after[,] the afores[ai]d Wounds in the head were the Cause of his death'.[33] This sort of qualified judgement – that certain wounds had proved fatal only through lack of care – was often used in early modern English trials to argue that the perpetrator of an assault should not be held responsible for a subsequent death,[34] but Youngman being Carpenter's indentured servant, Carpenter consequently *was* responsible for his care. There was no doubt that Carpenter had brutally beaten the man and deprived him of bedding and adequate shelter afterwards. The bleeding of the corpse may nevertheless have been seen as additional evidence that the death was Carpenter's doing. He was convicted of manslaughter, but pleading benefit of clergy, he suffered only branding on the hand.[35]

The conclusions of Maryland surgeons who performed medico-legal autopsies sometimes reflect the belief that death could be caused only if the vital organs were involved. This notion was clearly articulated and explained at the trial of John Grammer for the death of his servant, Thomas Simmons. The inquest jury found 'the impression of many stripes upon the body w[i]th a whipe which to the best of Our Judgm[en]ts might be a furtherance to his death'. The surgeons John Brooke and Stephen Clifton were ordered to open suspicious places on Simmons's body and reported that

> the Cutis and Cuticula layer layed bare[,] noe Contusion could be found upon the musculous part or ffleshy Pannicle [i.e., covering].[36]

The defendant himself then asked the surgeons to carry out a more extensive examination of the body because, he said, Simmons had been 'a diseased p[e]rson a twelve month'. The body when opened was found to be

> Cleere of inward bruises, either upon the Diaphrugma or w[i]thin the Ribbs, The lungs were of a livid Blewish Culler full of putrid ulcers, the liver not much putrid although it semed to be disafected by reason of it's pale & wann Couller: the Purse of the Heart was putrid and rotton by w[hi]ch we gather that this person by Course of Nature could not have lived long, Putrifaccion being gott soe neer unto that noble part the hart[,] even att the doore.[37]

It is not mentioned how long Simmons had been dead. The grand jury returned a verdict of *Ignoramus* (i.e., dismissed the case), a verdict that the court questioned and asked the grand jurors to justify. The reasons they gave were,

> First that noe Evidence [i.e., witness] which appeared before us and gave Evidence did possitively sweare that any blowes given by John Grammer or his man could touch his life ... Fourthly that the Chirurgeons swore that noe stripes given him had in the least toucht any principall part whereby in his Judgm[en]t according to the rules of physick his life could not be toucht.[38]

However, on another occasion, the inquest jurors were reluctant to apply the idea that only wounds in certain places could be fatal. When they viewed the body of Alice Sandford, servant to Pope Alvey, beaten for not moving when he told her to, they found:

> noe mortall wound, But the Body being beaten to a Jelly, The Intrayles being cleare from any inward disease, to the best of o[u]r Judgm[en]ts & the Doctors th[a]t was w[i]th us, But if it were possible that any Christian could bee beaten to death w[i]th stripes, wee think the afores[ai]d Servant was. And this is our Joynt Verdict.[39]

It was enough to convict Alvey of having 'feloniously killed' Alice Sandford, but, pleading benefit of clergy, he was merely branded.[40]

A tendency to classify wounds as being in themselves either 'mortal' or 'not mortal' was also evident at the inquest into the death of Jeffrey Hagman, servant to Joseph Fincher, who died in 1664, having been kicked and beaten after collapsing under the weight of tobacco plants that Fincher had loaded onto him. He was further belaboured by Fincher's wife when he went too slowly to fetch her some water. After a post-mortem by the surgeon Robert Lloyd, the inquest jury of which he was a member found that there was

> no mortall wound about him that did occasion his death but doe unanimously concurr and Judge that the s[ai]d Haggman being a diseased person died of the scurvey and an Imposthume.[41]

At his trial at the provincial court, however, Fincher was found guilty of murder and hanged.[42]

In 1664, John Grammer was again accused of having killed a servant. Though there was no surgeon on the inquest jury, they reported that

> having viewed the Corps [we] doe finde noe impression of any stripes upon his Body: But doe unanimously concurr in our Judgements that want of good dyett and lodging has been the Chiefe furtherance and Cause of his death.[43]

Grammer was imprisoned, but not sent for trial. After eight months in jail he petitioned for discharge and was freed.[44]

All the above cases relate to white indentured servants. During this period there was only one trial of a master for maltreatment of a black slave. Uncooperative and unwilling to work, the slave was beaten by his master, Simon Overzee, who then poured hot lard over him and chained him by his wrists to a ladder. The poor man, who did not understand a word of English, had been a constant source of trouble and had run away several times. No expert opinion was sought but the court tried to find out, without success, if, when chained to the ladder, the man's feet had touched the ground. However, witnesses said the slave was extremely unruly, and Overzee's behaviour went unpunished.[45]

The attitude to servants and their death at the hands of their masters was perhaps conditioned by the Old Testament:

> If a man smite his servant or his maid with a rod and he die under his hand he shall surely be punished. Notwithstanding if he [the servant] continue a day or two he [the master] shall not be punished for he [the servant] is his money. (Exodus 21:20–1)

In England, beating of servants and apprentices was an accepted punishment for disobedience and other misdemeanours and sometimes went beyond reasonable correction to physical abuse or death. But unlike their Maryland counterparts, English apprentices and servants often had parents or relations to support them against abuse by their masters, and this may have been a restraining influence. In the closer knit communities of England, public opinion also may have exercised some check on vicious behaviour.

The Maryland authorities recognized that there was an unacceptable level of violence towards servants which became worse with the arrival of increasing numbers of slaves in the colony from 1680 onwards. By the end of the century the Assembly was attempting to legislate against cruel masters, and in 1692 introduced an Act 'for the Relief of Negroes and Slaves from the barbarous and inhumane useage of unreasonable Masters too frequently practiced in this Province':

> Whereas some Masters Mistresses and Overseers void of humane pitty & Christian Comisseration have barbarously dismembered and Cauterized their Slaves not only to the Scandall of Christianity, but by such Cruelties keep them from Embracing the same[,] Be it therefore Enacted by the Authority aforesaid [the Assembly] That if any Master, Mistress or overseer ... shall after this Act dismember or Cauterize any such Slave, it shall be lawfull for the Justices of the County Court upon proof thereof to manumitt and set free such slave to all intents and purposes whatsoever. And in case any Master Mistress or overseer ... shall deny suffic[ien]t meat drink Lodging and Cloathing or shall unreasonably burthen them beyond their strength with labour or deny them necessary rest and sleep, be it to any English Servant or Slave, It shall be lawfull in such cases upon due proof thereof to the Justices of the County Court for the first & second Offence, to Fine the said Master Mistress or overseer as to them shall seem meet, and for the third offence to sett them free from their said servitude.[46]

But this Act by no means put an end to such cruelty, which continued on into the next century.

There were, of course, violent and rebellious servants in Maryland, but only two cases were reported that led to the death of a master. In one, two black slaves joined with three white servants and attacked their master, John Hawkins, with an axe, breaking his skull. One of the white servants, John Warry, confessed to the attack and no medical evidence was called for. One of the blacks, named only as Tony, was found not guilty, but the rest were condemned to be hanged with Tony acting as their hangman.[47]

In the other case Margaret Vyte was stabbed in the right arm by a black man, named only as Jacob, and the wound 'bled a day & a night'. Francis Stockett was called to attend her: when she died he gave it as his opinion that the wound was the cause of her death, and Jacob was condemned to hang.[48]

Between 1649 and 1670 the deaths of twelve servants were investigated as possible suicides, six by drowning. Witnesses said that John Clifford had not been abused by his master and therefore had no reason to drown himself, and that his body, when taken out of the river, was clean of marks. No verdict is recorded.[49] At the inquest into the death of Roger Evans after his body was found by the river, the jury was at first unable to decide whether he had drowned himself or had had 'a relapse of the sleepie diseas' and been overcome by the tide. But Evans was said to have been kindly treated by his master, and the jury concluded that he 'Came by his Death through his owne Idelnes and Rogish absentment'.[50] John Short was judged to have killed himself by rushing into the river, where he drowned, to escape a beating from his master.[51] In only one such case was medical opinion consulted, probably because a wound was plainly visible on the surface of the body. Ann Beetle was thrown out of bed by her mistress and sustained 'a great cut on her eye brow and her face all bloody and a great clot of blood on the wound', but a surgeon who examined her after she was found drowned said that her injuries were not the cause of her death, and the jury of inquest concluded that 'she drowned her selfe'.[52]

Three servants hanged themselves. Jane Copley, who ran away and was found dead under a tree, was judged to have starved to death.[53] Thomas Teestead cut his own throat,[54] while the inquest jury found that Ann Vaughan had

> Two wounds in her Throate with a payre of sizers & one in her Belly supposed to bee w[i]th a knife, & a small wound in her side, w[hi]ch s[ai]d wounds Wee doe suppose to bee the Immediate cause of her death. And wee doe ... suppose th[a]t shee gave her selfe the s[ai]d wounds & doe Endite her ... of willfull murther.[55]

No surgeon was called in either of these cases, but Richard Wells, a surgeon, was on both juries of inquest. It may be that in both cases the coroner made a point of having a surgeon on the jury because they involved wounds.

By English law, the property of suicides was forfeit to the Crown.

Servants, of course, had no goods to confiscate. In the few cases where free men committed suicide, the courts appear to have been concerned only with securing their property for the Proprietor. There were three cases of doubtful suicide. John Jerome was found drowned and as he was known to have suffered from 'melancholy discontent' the inquest jury reported that they 'rather beleive[d] th[a]t hee willfully drowned himselfe, Though Wee cannot say soe much upon our Oathes.'[56] David Anderson was found to have died 'by being surfitted with drinke', but the inquest jury concluded 'that drinke was accedentally the Cause of his death, and that he . . . Ought to have Christiall Buriall'.[57] William Styles, found dead in bed, had been drunk and had 'over gorged himselfe w[i]th Eating', and was judged to have 'Choaked in his sleepe'.[58] There is no sign of medical opinion being consulted at these inquests.

Servants came to the colony young and unmarried, and could not marry until their servitude was completed. The demand was for male servants to work on the plantations, and in the early years men outnumbered women six to one. Even at the end of the seventeenth century there were still two men to every woman, and many men never managed to acquire a wife. Sexual tensions ran high. Married women were not free from sexual overtures, while unmarried daughters and maid servants were subject to much greater pressures.[59] Surprisingly perhaps, there are only eight cases of alleged rape in the seventeenth-century records. In none of these cases does a physical examination of the alleged victim appear to have been carried out, and no one tried for rape was convicted.[60]

In 1650 an Act was passed making adultery and fornication punishable as the governor saw fit, and a considerable number of such cases were brought to court, mainly on the basis of hearsay and circumstantial evidence. If the offence was considered proven, the punishment for servants given by the court was whipping on the bare back. If the man was a free man he was fined.[61] The birth of a bastard was proof of illicit sex and was investigated as a crime but also because it was feared that the child would become a charge on the community. Under an Act of 1658, the penalty for both parties for producing a bastard was made to depend on whether the father was a freeman or a servant. If the father was named and confessed, and was a servant, he was made responsible for half the cost of maintaining the child. The only way that he could do this was by extended servitude. In such a case a mother, too, might have her servitude extended to make up for time lost looking after the child and for its maintenance. If the father was a free man he was made responsible for the whole maintenance of the child.[62] In only one bastardy case did opinion figure on a matter that might be considered 'medical': a servant claimed that a man she had slept with on the 1st of January was the father of a full-term child born on the 16th of

July. The court, 'upon Examination of sercumstances, and of the Judgement of divers persons, finding the Child being perfectly borne, Could nott bee the Child of the Reputted Father, being borne within the time before Limitted', cleared the man.[63] It is probable that the woman who delivered the infant was among the 'divers persons' whose judgement about its maturity was consulted. In spite of the penalties for producing bastards, they represented at least 10 per cent of children born in the colony during these years. Premarital pregnancy was theoretically a crime but although 30 per cent of women went to their marriages already pregnant, none were prosecuted.[64]

The penalties for producing bastards were such that some turned to abortion or infanticide. In earlier times in England the judicial opinion of abortion was that it was homicide if performed after 'ensoulment' or 'quickening'. But in 1644 it was stated in Edward Coke's *The Third Part of the Institutes of the Laws of England* that abortion was 'a great misprision and no murder'. From at least that date, then, it was a non-capital offence for which there was no stated punishment, and in England, through the seventeenth century, very few cases were brought to court.[65] How common abortion was in Maryland is impossible to tell, for it was a clandestine act which presumably often passed unnoticed. In the 1650s four cases came before the courts. Captain Mitchell was charged with having committed adultery with Susan Warren, a widow, and, when she became pregnant, attempting to induce an abortion by administering opium. Although abortion did not occur, Mrs Warren was eventually delivered of a dead child. Mitchell was brought to the provincial court charged also with being an atheist and fornicating with his pretended wife, Joan. The grand jury found a verdict of *billa vera* on all charges. Mitchell then elected to have his case decided by the judge, 'not desiring that the Court Should be troubl[e]d with impanelling another jury', and was fined 5,000 pounds of tobacco.[66]

Jacob Lumbrozo, a Jewish Portuguese medical practitioner, who also appears in the court records as an attorney and a frequent litigant, was charged with aborting the child he had begot (allegedly by force) on his servant Elizabeth Wiles. Several witnesses testified that he had 'told her that shee must take a strong purge to tacke away her swelling', and that he repeatedly 'gave her fisick to distroy it', until 'came sumthing downe as bige as her hand from her bodie'. The case was ordered to the provincial court, but never came up. Probably it was dropped, for Lumbrozo quickly silenced the main witness against him by marrying her.[67] It is worth noting that it was not necessarily the woman alleged to have had the abortion who was tried for the crime, but could be, as in these cases, the person accused of procuring it.

William Brooke was accused of killing his wife's (but apparently not his) unborn child by beating her with tongs. Rose Smith, a midwife, testified that she had delivered Mrs Brooke of a foetus about three months old which was badly bruised and black on one side, and that Mrs Brooke had told her the miscarriage had been caused by her husband's violent abuse. When the midwife challenged Brooke with this, he observed that his wife had also fallen out of a peach tree while pregnant, and Mrs Brooke admitted that this was so. Nevertheless, the case being sent to the provincial court, the judge 'Conceived that there is Cause of Suspition of Murther', and committed Brooke to provide security for his appearance at the next sessions. Six months later, Brooke appeared as required, and was discharged.[68]

Elizabeth Robins allegedly attempted to procure an abortion to hide her adultery. On being informed of this, the provincial court sent a jury of women to examine her. From as early as the fourteenth century, when English courts required an intimate examination it was usually carried out by a specially-impanelled jury of matrons, who from their own experience and knowledge were likely to be able to assess the woman's condition.[69] The women reported that Robins was

> in a very Sad Condition and in a Condition not like to other women, & confessed that She had twice taken Savin; once boyled in milk and the other time Strayned through a Cloath, and at the taking thereof not Supposing her self with Child as She Sayeth, takeing it for wormes not knowing the vertue thereof any other wayes, [and] farther Confessed that She Supposed her Self to have a dead Child within her, And if a Child, that the true begetter of it was her husband Robert Robins.[70]

Savin from *Juniper sabina*, a strong poison, was commonly used to produce abortions and was also an anthelmintic. Robins doubtless knew what she was doing, but the savin did not work and she gave birth to a live child. She was taken to court by her husband not for having attempted an abortion but for having committed adultery. There is no record of the outcome of the case.[71]

For mothers of unwanted children who did not attempt abortion, or whose efforts failed, there remained the possibility of infanticide. One of the earliest recorded inquests held in Maryland was to investigate the death of an infant, Anne Thomson, in 1642. The surgeon Robert Ellyson was a member of the jury of inquest, and he doubtless examined the body, possibly internally, but no details on this were recorded. The verdict given by the jury was that 'the said Anne came to a naturall death'.[72] Even where medical expertise was available, as in this case, it was extremely difficult to distinguish natural from unnatural death in the case of newborn children. Infant mortality in early Maryland was naturally very high – at least 30 per cent of infants died within a year of their birth – but in a society where, despite the severe penalties visited upon unmarried mothers, the incidence of illegitimate pregnancy was relatively high, there was often a suspicion of infanticide. An English statute of 1624 (21 Jac. 1 c.27) had rendered concealment of the death of a newborn bastard presumptive evidence of infanticide, punishable by death, unless one witness could prove that the child was stillborn.[73] In England many cases therefore hinged on whether the child had been born dead or alive. Remarkably, given that Maryland passed no law of its own on infanticide and therefore came under English law on this point, in none of the fourteen cases of suspected infanticide that came to light in Maryland between 1656 and 1680 does the question of live or still birth appear to have been considered. In all but one case, no body was actually found. Suspicions were aroused when there had been signs of pregnancy which suddenly disappeared, apparently without a birth taking place. The courts were concerned to find out whether a birth had occurred and, if so, what had happened to the child. Two cases were investigated by a 'Iury of able women', who gave the verdict that the suspects had not been pregnant.[74] Rose Smith was on one of these juries of matrons,[75] and although her midwifery skills are not mentioned in this case, she is clearly identified as a midwife in the Brooke case related above. Smith's participation in a pregnancy inquiry is another example of medical expertise being provided by impanelling a medical practitioner as an inquest juror. After one of these inquiries the suspect, Hannah Jenkins, immediately and successfully sued Isabella Head for slander, presumably for bringing the accusation.[76]

In five cases of alleged childmurder, the defendants were found guilty and condemned to be hanged. Elizabeth Green, accused of bearing a child and burning it, was examined by Grace Parker when the suspicion was first raised. Parker deposed that she 'did search her breast and the wench deny'd she was w[i]th child, but there was milke in her breasts And it was a goeing away being hard and curdled'; she therefore affirmed that Green 'had gone neer her full time and had had a Childe', despite the girl's insistence that she had borne a four-months foetus. Parker also swore that at this examination Elizabeth Green had eventually confessed to disposing of the body and burning it.[77] Grace Parker may have been a midwife, but she is not identified as one either in this case or in her other appearance in the Maryland court records.

Mary Marler was believed to have killed one of her newborn twins because she had 'cause[d] Hannah Lee [her mistress, also known as Price] ... to lay in the Cold' the male infant. The grand jury concluded:

> Though wee cannot by evidence finde Mary Marler guilty of the murder abovesaid according to the words of the Indictment yet by her flight wee finde the law makes her Guilty and ought to be indicted and prosecuted. Wee

alsoe finde Hannah Price by her Concealm[en]t of the murder of the Childe so many dayes to be accessary to the said murder.[78]

Marler was not captured. At the trial of Hannah Price no evidence was offered and she was cleared 'by Proclamation'.[79]

After Joan Colledge was convicted of infanticide, several people, including three of the witnesses against her, petitioned for her sentence to be suspended until the governor could review the case; she may have received a pardon.[80] In the remaining infanticide cases sent for trial at the provincial court the defendants were acquitted. The evidence against Mary Stevens was found to be unsatisfactory.[81] In other cases witnesses failed to appear at the provincial court, as happened in the trial of Jane Crisp in 1666. The non-appearing witnesses presumably included the local midwife fetched to examine her on first suspicion, to whom Crisp confessed that she had had a child and that it had been eaten by hogs.[82] There was strong circumstantial evidence that Elizabeth Harris was the mother of a dead child wrapped in rags found by the river but she was apparently saved by the evidence of a fellow servant (her bedfellow) who said that she had never appeared pregnant nor been sick at any time.[83] While there appears to have been a measure of sympathy for these women, suspected cases were nevertheless reported to the authorities and there was a moderate risk of the defendant being found guilty and hanged.

Legal proceedings sometimes arose from disputes about medical treatment, most often because a dissatisfied patient refused to pay, claiming that the fee was too high or that the treatment had been unsuccessful. In one case, a serious charge was laid by one surgeon against another: Peter Sharp accused Peter Godson of killing a patient by excessive bleeding. It may have been a defensive accusation, for Sharp's own treatment of the deceased was in question, and medical adjudication was thought to be necessary. The case was referred to the following session of the provincial court,

when men of Skill and ability Shall Iudge of the Action, what the Said Peter Sharp did Administer in Phisick or Chirurgery to Capt[ain] John Smith in the time of his Sickness, who is the party mentioned to have been killed as aforesaid.[84]

However, no further record of the case has been found.[85]

The evidence of medico-legal practice surveyed here shows that in early seventeenth-century Maryland defendants, jurors, and the authorities were aware that medical practitioners could provide relevant evidence in cases of suspicious death and in certain types of crime. In a number of cases, surgeons were actually directed to obtain this evidence. This awareness of the potential value of medical opinion presumably came from knowledge of its use in contemporary courts in England. This would seem to cast doubt upon the assertions usually made about the relative infrequency of medical evidence in inquests and criminal investigations within the jurisdiction of English common law before the eighteenth century. The fact that post-mortems were performed in early colonial Maryland to provide evidence for legal purposes suggests that the chronology of the medico-legal post-mortem in Anglo-Saxon jurisdictions needs to be revised.

Another significant finding of this study is that surgeons (and in at least one case, a midwife) were not infrequently called upon to serve on inquest juries. With so few people of education and standing in the colony, medical practitioners would inevitably find themselves impanelled as jurors from time to time. But since the instances where surgeons acted as jurors were all inquests into deaths that occurred after violent assaults, and in which medical skill was likely to be particularly valuable, it is probable that the coroner made a point of securing their participation in this way, making it unnecessary to appoint an investigating surgeon. This highlights an aspect of the history of legal medicine in the early modern period which has hitherto been almost completely overlooked.

Reading the records of the Maryland courts for the seventeenth century, one is left with the impression that the efforts of the authorities to administer justice were often frustrated. In small communities, the shortage of man-power may have promoted a reluctance to resort to capital punishment. Also, it has been suggested that the colonists may have reacted against the severity of English law.[86] Moreover, with a small population it must have been almost impossible to appoint a jury of persons who did not know the defendant, and with many freemen engaged at some time in litigation either as defendants, accusers or witnesses, there were bound to be grounds for hostilities. On the other hand, there may have been on juries men or women (in the case of juries of matrons) whose interests or sympathies lay in having the defendant acquitted. In such circumstances, it is likely that pressure was sometimes brought to bear on jurors and expert witnesses, and that medical evidence was sometimes made to serve ends other than the impartial administration of justice. Yet the Maryland records suggest that contemporaries were well aware of the potential importance of medical evidence, and that medical witnesses took their duties seriously.

NOTES

The authors would like to thank Michael Clark and Anne Goldgar for their help with this chapter.

1 William H. Browne et al., eds., *Archives of Maryland*, 72 vols. (Baltimore, MD, 1883–1965, hereafter cited as *AOM*), vol. III, pp. 49–55.

2 David W. Jordan, 'Maryland's privy council', in Aubrey C. Land, Lois Green Carr and Edward C. Papenfuse, eds., *Law, Society and Politics in Early Maryland* (Baltimore, MD, 1977), pp. 65–87.

3 Douglas Greenberg, 'Crime, law enforcement, and social control in colonial America', *American Journal of Legal History*, 26 (1982), 293–325, on p. 303.

4 Gust Skordas, *The Early Settlers of Maryland* (Baltimore, 1968).

5 Greenberg, 'Crime, law enforcement, and social control', p. 302.

6 For the provincial courts, see *AOM*, vols. IV, X, XLI, XLIX, LX, LXV, LXVI, LXVII, LXVIII, LXIX, LXX; for Kent County (1648–68), Talbot (1662–74) and Somerset (1665–8), see *AOM*, vol. LIV; for Charles County (1658–74), *AOM*, vols. LII, LIV.

7 Thomas R. Forbes, *Surgeons at the Bailey: English Forensic Medicine to 1878* (New Haven, 1985), pp. 45–6.

8 John Winthrop, *Winthrop's Journal 1630–1649*, ed. James Kendal Hosmer (New York, 1908), vol. I, p. 320; inquest on the body of an Indian shot by John Dandy (*AOM*, vol. IV, pp. 254–60), described below, p. 28.

9 For two other early English texts on forensic medicine, see below, p. 109, note 2.

10 *AOM*, vol. III, pp. 61, 91.

11 *AOM*, vol. IV, pp. 177, 180.

12 *AOM*, vol. IV, pp. 180, 181.

13 *AOM*, vol. IV, pp. 255, 260. The names of the other members of the coroner's jury are not recorded. Binx is elsewhere styled 'gent. Licentiate of Physic' (ibid., p. 72). For Ellyson's work as a medical practitioner, see ibid., pp. 240, 294; he also acted as sheriff for a time (ibid., p. 261).

14 *AOM*, vol. III, p. 146.

15 *AOM*, vol. V, p. 65.

16 *AOM*, vol. XLIX, pp. 11–12.

17 See Peter G. Yackel, 'Benefit of clergy in colonial Maryland', *Maryland Magazine of History*, 69 (1974), 383–97. In 1170 the Church won the right for men in holy orders to be tried for felonies in ecclesiastical courts. When brought before a crown court they could consequently be exempted from punishment by claiming 'benefit of clergy'. Gradually the privilege was extended to lay people, including women, provided they could read, and eventually even the reading requirement was dropped. Not all felonies were clergyable. A convicted felon, having claimed benefit of clergy successfully, was branded on the thumb, for he could only use this plea once. In 1717 branding was replaced by transportation for seven years, and benefit of clergy was finally abolished in 1827.

18 *AOM*, vol. XLIX, pp. 16–17.

19 *AOM*, vol. I, p. 18. For examples of such whippings by the courts, see *AOM*, vol. IV, p. 164; vol. LIV, pp. 184, 296; vol. LX, p. 196,

20 Darrett B. Rutman and Anita H. Rutman, 'Of agues and fevers: malaria in the early Chesapeake', *William and Mary Quarterly*, 3rd series, 33 (1976), 31–60, on p. 44.

21 *AOM*, vol. X, pp. 73–4.

22 *AOM*, vol. XIV, p. 9.

23 *AOM*, vol. LIV, p. 8.

24 *AOM*, vol. XLI, pp. 162, 172.

25 Robert P. Brittain, 'Cruentation in legal medicine and in literature', *Medical History*, 9 (1965), 82–8; Forbes, *Surgeons at the Bailey*, pp. 60–2.
26 *AOM*, vol. X, p. 525.
27 *AOM*, vol. X, pp. 534–40, 542–3, 544–5.
28 *AOM*, vol. XLI, pp. 500–2.
29 *AOM*, vol. XLI p. 504.
30 *AOM*, vol. XLI, p. 504.
31 *AOM*, vol. XLI, pp. 499–506.
32 Ibid., p. 385.
33 *AOM*, vol. LVII, p. 60. The verdict is recorded in slightly different wording in vol. LIV, p. 391.
34 Catherine Crawford, 'The emergence of English forensic medicine: medical evidence in common-law courts, 1730–1830', Ph.D thesis, University of Oxford, 1987, pp. 102–5.
35 *AOM*, vol. LIV, pp. 390–1; vol. LVII, pp. 59–65.
36 *AOM*, vol. XLIX, p. 307.
37 *AOM*, vol. XLIX, p. 308.
38 *AOM*, vol. XLIX, p. 312.
39 *AOM*, vol. XLIX, p. 166.
40 *AOM*, vol. XLIX, p. 235.
41 *AOM*, vol. XLIX, p. 303.
42 *AOM*, vol. XLIX, pp. 303, 312–13.
43 *AOM*, vol. XLIX, p. 351.
44 *AOM*, vol. XLIX, pp. 351, 401. Between 1665 and 1680 there were seven more instances in which masters were accused of the deaths of their servants. See *AOM*, vol. XLI, pp. 478–80; vol. XLIX, p. 453; vol. LVII, pp. 169, 568, 597, 601; vol. LXV, p. 1; vol. LXIX, pp. 413–14.
45 *AOM*, vol. XLI, pp. 190–1, 205–6.
46 *AOM*, vol. XIII, p. 457.
47 *AOM*, vol. LXV, pp. 2–8.
48 *AOM*, vol. XLIX, pp. 490–1.
49 *AOM*, vol. X, pp. 157–9.
50 *AOM*, vol. LIII, pp. 140–1.
51 *AOM*, vol. LIV, pp. 361–2.
52 *AOM*, vol. XLIX, p. 215.
53 *AOM*, vol. XLI, p. 452.
54 *AOM*, vol. XLIX, p. 113.
55 *AOM*, vol. XLIX, p. 88.
56 *AOM*, vol. XLIX, p. 114.
57 *AOM*, vol. LIV, p. 412.
58 *AOM*, vol. XLIX, pp. 113–14.
59 Lorena S. Walsh, 'Community networks in the early Chesapeake', in Lois Green Carr, Philip D. Morgan and Jean B. Russo, eds., *Colonial Chesapeake Society* (Chapel Hill, NC, 1988), pp. 200–41, see p. 237.
60 *AOM*, vol. LIII, pp. 356–7; vol. LIV, p. 69; vol. LVII, pp. 353, 597, 604; vol. LXV, pp. 12–14.
61 *AOM*, vol. I, p. 286; vol. X, p. 558.
62 *AOM*, vol. I, p. 373; Lois Green Carr and Lorena S. Walsh, 'The planter's wife:

the experience of white women in seventeenth-century Maryland', *William and Mary Quarterly*, 3rd series, 34 (1977), 542–71, see pp. 548–9 and 549n. Filiation proceedings in England are discussed by David Harley in chapter 2 of this volume.

63 *AOM*, vol. LIV, pp. 383, 386.

64 Lorena S. Walsh, '"Till death us do part": marriage and family in seventeenth-century Maryland', in Thad W. Tate and David L. Ammerman, eds., *The Chesapeake in the Seventeenth Century* (Chapel Hill, NC, 1979), pp. 126–52, on p. 132.

65 Angus McLaren, *Reproductive Rituals* (London and New York, 1984), pp. 115–29. For two seventeenth-century English abortion trials, see David Harley's chapter in this volume.

66 *AOM*, vol. X, pp. 183–5. In criminal cases heard in local (county) courts, the accused had the option of trial by jury or trial by judge (*AOM*, vol. LIII, p. xxi).

67 *AOM*, vol. LIII, pp. 387–91. Quotations: pp. 387, 389, 388.

68 *AOM*, vol. X, pp. 464–5, 488.

69 On the jury of matrons in Britain and America, see James C. Oldham, 'On pleading the belly: a history of the jury of matrons', *Criminal Justice History*, 6 (1985), 1–64, and Thomas R. Forbes, 'A jury of matrons', *Medical History*, 32 (1988), 23–33.

70 *AOM*, vol. XLI, p. 20.

71 *AOM*, vol. XLI, pp. 50–1, 79, 85.

72 *AOM*, vol. IV, p. 139.

73 See chapter 3, by Mark Jackson, in this volume.

74 *AOM*, vol. X, pp. 456–8; vol. LIV, p. 250.

75 *AOM*, vol. X, p. 457.

76 *AOM*, vol. LIV, p. 251.

77 *AOM*, vol. XLIX, pp. 218, 231–5.

78 *AOM*, vol. LVII, p. 74.

79 *AOM*, vol. LVII, p. 125.

80 *AOM*, vol. LVII, p. 599.

81 *AOM*, vol. LXV, pp. 13, 14, 20.

82 *AOM*, vol. LIV, pp. 394–5; vol. LVII, pp. 123–4.

83 *AOM*, vol. XLI, pp. 430, 432.

84 *AOM*, vol. X, p. 432 (1655).

85 This was not the only time that Godson's treatment was found wanting. He was taken to court by Thomas Ager who had paid him in advance for a cure that 'left him worse than he found him'. No medical evidence was called but Godson was 'Injoyned to make a Cure of Thomas Ager or else to Repay the Tobacco he had received in Satisfaction of his Cure', and he was judged not to have accomplished the cure (*AOM*, vol. X, pp. 434, 439).

86 Bradley Chapin, *Criminal Justice in Colonial America 1606–1660* (Athens, GA, 1983), pp. 3–5.

2

The scope of legal medicine in Lancashire and Cheshire, 1660–1760

DAVID HARLEY

Although there were no specialized treatises on legal medicine written in English before the later eighteenth century,[1] midwives and medical men had been called upon to give expert testimony for centuries before that. The work of the late Thomas Forbes suggests that the eighteenth-century explosion of professionally trained practitioners was accompanied by a corresponding increase in their use as experts in criminal trials.[2] His work has been taken to demonstrate that medical testimony did not have much authority until the nineteenth century, when coroners and assize courts increasingly relied upon autopsies to help them distinguish natural or accidental deaths from suicides and homicides.[3] Historians have only recently begun to explore crucial issues such as the impact of expert testimony and the extent to which medical practitioners mediated or modified ideas about the nature of criminal responsibility.[4]

Forbes's concentration on capital crimes gives the impression that such cases constituted the bulk of medical practitioners' expert testimony. This was far from being the case. Most of the occasions when midwives or medical men were required to testify on oath or provide written testimony were far more mundane. This essay is an attempt to sketch the broad range of medico-legal practice in provincial England in the early modern period. Such a study is necessarily limited by gaps in the records but nevertheless a sufficiently wide range of legal medicine can be portrayed to compensate for the impossibility of making statistical comparisons. For the purposes of this essay, medico-legal practice will be taken to include all testimony delivered by midwives and medical practitioners in their professional capacity, in cases where their specialized knowledge had some bearing. Evidence given in trials at the assizes is excluded because there is no record of what was said.

The commonest form of evidence required from both midwives and medical men in Lancashire and Cheshire during this period was probably the provision of testimonials for colleagues seeking ecclesiastical licences to practise. This system has been portrayed as almost pointless or farcical by historians who have applied anachronistic standards of comparison.[5] In fact, it worked reasonably well in areas where medical practitioners were willing to cooperate, although it did lay considerable stress on religious conformity.[6] The idea was that medical practitioners and midwives should present their testimonials of competence, good character and religious conformity and then be examined before a licence was issued. In practice, however, ecclesiastical courts touring the archdeaconry or diocese on visitation often issued licences to persons accused of unlicensed practice without first examining them. Nevertheless, the testimonials were not irrelevant to the task of assessing the technical competence of those seeking licences and it is hard to imagine what better evidence could have been provided in most of provincial England.[7]

When the Church of England was re-established in the early 1660s, the ecclesiastical courts faced a potentially huge burden of business and not all dioceses were able to reinstate the full range of court functions. Diocesan officials had perforce to start with their main priorities, namely the clergy and their tithes, nonconformists and fornicators.[8] In the vast Diocese of Chester, only the Archdeaconry of Chester was able to restore its court system in full. Consequently, most of the evidence for medical licensing comes from the populous southern archdeaconry.[9] These documents provide a glimpse of the practitioner at the moment of licensing, with some impression of the applicant's past, but in the context of legal medicine it is the referees who are of most interest.

In the Chester testimonials, there is some evidence of examination. Thus three leading Chester surgeons signed a statement in 1711 that 'upon examination of Mr Nath. Edgley [they] doe finde him a person quallified for a licence for the practice of surgery',[10] while in 1713, two physicians wrote that 'upon due Examinac'on we find Mr Robert Taylor of Blackburn apothecary rightly qualifyed for the Practise of Surgerie.'[11] The frequent presence of leading Chester surgeons as the referees for both local and rural practitioners suggests that there was some formal system of examination in the Chester court, but in the countryside the style of testimonial was more varied. Sometimes a country practitioner would append not only the endorsements of surgeons and physicians but also a copious catalogue of cures, as did Cornelius Smith of Nantwich in 1701 and Richard Davenport, a surgeon and bonesetter of Hanmer in Flint, in 1709.[12]

Just as those who applied for surgical licences tried to obtain endorsements from prominent surgeons, those who applied for medical licences tried to obtain the backing of graduate physicians. John Bruen produced a Latin certificate of examination signed by Henry Williamson MD (Leyden) and John Tylston MD (Aberdeen). Robert Oldfield of Chester was backed by Allan Pennington MD (Oxon) and Phineas Fowke MD FRCP, although Pennington himself had simply pestered the bishop when his own son needed a licence.[13] In the case of physicians of doubtful or obscure origins, more detailed references might be needed. Nathaniel Banne MD (Cantab.), a former minister of religion who had been excluded at the Restoration, provided a Latin testimonial and a covering letter for Guion Bosquet of Preston, a distressed French Protestant, in 1696. In his letter, Banne explained that Bosquet's father had been a physician and that Bosquet himself had studied medicine at the University of Montpellier.[14]

Testimonials on behalf of midwives tended to lay more stress on their good character than on their technical skills, since this was an important part of their qualification. Nevertheless, testimonials by the minister and churchwardens were often accompanied by tributes to their skill signed by satisfied patients and endorsements by other local midwives and medical practitioners. Thus Thomas Clayton, who had retired from his Manchester surgical practice on inheriting the family estate near Blackburn, signed testimonials for at least four midwives between 1722 and 1729, including one for Mrs Penelope Rishton who, according to the Rector of Blackburn, 'lays all Persons of the best rank'.[15] Sometimes the result could be a very impressive document, as in the case of Margery, wife of John Chorley of Manchester, whose 1704 testimonial was signed by forty women, two clergymen and two Cambridge MDs, Nathaniel Banne and Charles Leigh, FRS.[16]

Since a request for a licence often followed presentation before the ecclesiastical courts for unlicensed practice, testimonials were on occasion combined with another of the more routine forms of legal medicine, the sick note explaining the absence of a witness or accused person from court. This form of medical certification featured in a variety of contexts. In 1691, Silvester Richmond of Liverpool provided a note on behalf of Ellen Fletcher, the wife of a rich merchant, stating that she had been trained by her mother as a midwife, had practised for several years 'with great diligence and success; and I have been with her sev[era]l times on that occasion; and have Observ[e]d hir to be prudent in ye manadgm[en]t of those Concerns'. She was, however, pregnant and indisposed and was therefore unable to attend the visitation at Wigan. She was licensed *in absentia* the next day.[17] In 1727 John Barlowe, a Congleton surgeon, wrote on behalf of a man cited for adultery that he 'has been for a fortnight last past much visited with the Rheumatisme & neither able to walk or Ride'.[18] In the case of those accused of such offences before ecclesiastical courts, this was the only way to avoid excommunication for nonappearance.

Both accusers and accused had to sign substantial bonds to appear at the assizes, so it was important for them to prove their willingness yet inability to attend. A surgeon's note commonly served this purpose. Thus in 1696, a female relative of a defendant charged with vexatious litigation stressed on his behalf that a husbandman had offered 'to joyne with the Chyrurgeon in an Affid[avi]t of the def[endan]ts said indisposic[i]on in ord[e]r to putt off the said tryall for this assizes', but he was determined to attend in person. In 1737, a prosecutor's wife was unable to give evidence and a yeoman's wife put her mark to a statement

> that upon the seventh day of this Instant August she was sent for as a Midwife to Margery the Wife of the said Henry Pye and that on the Eighth day of August Instant she the said Joyce Brookes deliver[e]d the said Margery Pye of a female Child And that She the said Margery Pye then was and now is, in a deplorable weakly condition or ill state of health occasioned as this Deponent conceives and really believes by the Said Margery Pye's being delivered of a Child six weeks at least before her expected time.

Although the words are those of a clerk, the relevant expertise is clearly that of the midwife, assuring the court that her patient could not possibly travel in order to testify.[19]

A medical note excusing a witness took on a special significance when it concerned the victim of a crime of violence who might never be able to accuse his or her assailants in person. In 1744 a very formal deposition was sworn before a commissioner of the Court of Common Pleas by Richard Shepherd MB of Preston and a surgeon, John Walmesley. The husbandman whom they had attended had extensive internal and external bruising, stab wounds, and a broken jaw. They had found him 'very feverish Sick and almost insensible', having great difficulty breathing and in danger of losing his left eye. From the court's point of view, however, the most crucial aspect was probably Shepherd's prognosis: 'He continues stil Confined to his Bed languishing under all these Symptoms[.] And if his Life is saved, which is yet very doubtful, it is very uncertain whether he will recover all his Senses or not, by reason of the violent Concussion and Shake of his Brain.'[20]

Although the insanity defence in criminal trials was not fully developed until the nineteenth century, there had long been a need to provide diagnoses or prognoses of mental states. It had been a frequent feature of witchcraft trials, where the difference between natural and unnatural afflictions was central to the proceedings.[21] Although the records of Lancashire and Cheshire yield no examples of midwives or medical men being involved in witchcraft trials during the late seventeenth century, a controversial case of alleged demonic possession did involve several medical practitioners. Robert Whitaker, an extra-licentiate of the College of Physicians, committed himself in 1695 to a supernatural diagnosis of the strange condition of an afflicted boy: 'I do hereby testify, (as many more will, if there be Occasion) from my own Observation, as an Eye and Ear Witness, at the meeting concerning Richard Dugdale, that I verily believe he was then under a Diabolical Possession, or Obsession. I do also testify, that he is now delivered from that supernatural Malady.'[22]

In slightly less sensational circumstances, medical practitioners might be called upon to pronounce on mental states. Unfortunately, the records of the officials who assessed lunacy and supervised the administration of lunatics' estates for the Chancery Masters give little impression of the evidence presented but there are occasional traces of diagnoses in other courts.[23] When the Rector of Dodleston was cited before the Chester Consistory Court in 1697 for adultery and fornication, Henry Williamson MD and a Chester surgeon gave evidence of long-standing mental disorder, saving the Rector from losing his benefice, which was coveted by his accusers.[24] The Manchester surgeon-physician Thomas White and William Holbrooke, a surgeon-apothecary who had recently finished his apprenticeship with John Dicken of Manchester, signed a petition on behalf of a man gaoled for seditious words whose 'Extravigant Language' was said to be the product of his 'Natural Melancholy and Broken Constitution of Brain and Temper'. When drunk, he was 'like a Madman and not as other men are with the same Quantity'. The petitioners knew his father, '& as we have heard his Grandfather to be of such a Broken Crazy Temper, The same very prabably Comeing by Blood'.[25]

In the absence of professionally defended trials for criminal offences, probably the most evenly contested cases were disputes about wills. In such cases, evidence about a testator's state of mind was often crucial and medical attendants were increasingly coming to be recognized as the best witnesses to this. In 1723 James Guy, a Manchester apothecary who had attended Michael Pimlott in May 1713, testified on behalf of the plaintiffs that when witnessing the will in September 1714 he observed that the deceased 'was of a sound mind understood what he did and had a dispose-ing faculty', and he corroborated this opinion with circumstantial details. A much older Manchester apothecary, John Green, who had succeeded Guy as the deceased's attendant in July 1713, testified for the defendants that Pimlott was afflicted with a disease 'both Apoplectick & Convulsive in a very great degree and whereby his memory & understanding were very much affected & broken'. According to Green, Pimlott had had lucid 'Inervalls or Intermissions', but his memory was 'so weak & defective that he could not retain a Discourse tho' but for a short time upon any one subject'. Both he and a physician, Robert Maylin of Ashton upon Mersey, had refused the family's request to witness a deed signed by Pimlott. William Holbrooke MB (Cantab.) testified that he had refused to witness Pimlott's will when he found him unable to write more than his Christian name but he hesitated to say that Pimlott could never have been in a fit condition to dispose of his property.[26]

Medical witnesses were not always so readily available to appear for both sides in disputes about wills, since even affluent patients might only be attended by a single practitioner. Thus, in a Manchester case of 1729, only John Dicken was called to pronounce on the mental state of James Hilton, a bedridden patient whom he had attended two or three times every day for some fourteen weeks. Not only had be been weak, declining and incontinent but he had 'appeared in a Very Dull Heavy and Stupid posture and Condic[i]on and upon Questions askt him would give very Imperfect Answers and to the best of this Deponents apprehensions and belief was Uncapable to know or understand what he did'.[27] Nevertheless, even in relatively small communities, several practitioners could be involved with a dying man. When the death and alleged intestacy of John Windle of Cronton were the subject of a Chancery case, two Prescot apothecaries and a Liverpool physician were produced to say that the deceased had been of sound mind and had made a will disinheriting his brother.[28] When a dispute broke out between the guardians of the children of William Atherton in 1745, several medical witnesses appeared. The deceased had fluctuated somewhat in his state of mind, throwing himself into a well at one point. Thomas Clayton and William Prichard had witnessed the will, in company with a lawyer. Clayton, who 'had upon some Occasions before Attended sometimes as surgeon and at other times as phisician to the said William Atherton and others of his Family' was able to testify to the 'slight Fever which terminated in a collection of matter in his Upper Jaw', which abated and returned 'and in some degree affected his head and that in such condition he was better and worse by Intervals and in some of those intervalls very sensible'. Surprisingly perhaps, the concussion of his fall into the well did not 'impair his memory or understanding', Prichard had frequently attended him as his apothecary and agreed that his understanding varied but on the morning in question he had 'found him cool and in good order his head clear and he was very sensible'. Richard Shepherd of Preston also declared that the fever had affected Atherton but added that after the fall he had visited him several times a day 'and the Deceased talked and Discoursed in as rational a way as ever he had heard him'. The real fluctuations had not begun until after he had made his will. John Walmesley, the surgeon who had attended him after the well incident, agreed that his mind had been sound.[29]

By far the most common role of midwives in legal proceedings was their responsibility under the poor law to question mothers of bastard children during labour as to the identity of the putative father and then provide a deposition at the petty sessions which could form the basis for a maintenance order.[30] It was in the interest of the parish officers and all the ratepaying households that the father should be identified and, in some more populous parts of the north-west, it was not unknown for medical investigators to be called in at a much earlier stage, even before the diagnosis of pregnancy had been confirmed. When a Chester jeweller was accused of being the father of Elinor Hughes's bastard, he produced not only a petition on his behalf from the parish dignitaries and a statement by a barber-surgeon who had been falsely accused by the same woman but also a statement by Alderman Thomas Wilson of St John's parish that she had been searched by a surgeon and a midwife when suspected of being with child. They had failed to diagnose her as pregnant, she had denied it, and her mother had assisted her in an attempt to conceal the birth. No midwife or neighbour had been called in until the mother was unable to cope.[31]

Yet although an efficiently run parish or township would have attempted to secure a preliminary identification of the putative father from the mother-to-be, the statement to the midwife *in extremis* took precedence. When Hannah Jones of Nantwich, 'a common whore', falsely named a local miller in 1721, the magistrates refused to allow her to retract her sworn statement, so the midwife's evidence was crucial in clearing the man's name. The mother admitted 'in her greatest extremity' that her original statement 'was in prejudice to and to be revenged on Mr. Cook's wife with whom she had a Quarrel', so the magistrates revoked their order, the child was baptized as the son of the soldier she had named instead of the miller, and he escaped having to do penance for adultery.[32] Although mothers occasionally misled midwives, a midwife could be called upon to assess the truthfulness of the mothers' statements, as when an Ashton-under-Lyne midwife's statement of 1703 concerning two men named by the mother of a bastard was produced in court when the man whom the midwife thought innocent was accused of adultery.[33]

Even if the midwife arrived too late to deliver the child, she still might find the mother *in extremis*, in which case she could question her. In 1691, the Preston Quarter Sessions received a deposition concerning the bastard daughter of a woman who had died. The midwife 'who was sent for to the aboves[ai]d Grace Pollard att the birth of her said Bastard child (but could not come to her till after the birth thereof)' and the other women 'pr[e]sent att the tyme of her Extremity imediately after the birth of the s[ai]d child . . . (between the time of her deliverance & death, w[hi]ch was but short) asked who was the father of her s[ai]d bastard Child'.[34] Even women who did not practise midwifery regularly were well aware of what was required. Thus, in 1693, a Salford mother and the woman who delivered her signed a deposition, another woman who had been present merely making her mark: 'Mary Sutton of Salford afores[ai]d maketh oath that shee was by pr[e]sent when the s[ai]d Hannah Dickanson was in her utmost Extremity of Childbirth & that shee did officiate as midwife (for want of one att that time) to and for ye s[ai]d Hannah Dickanson and did demand of her who was the father of the Childe.'[35]

In this, as in all their functions, the integrity of the midwives was paramount. They were central figures in women's culture, acting as advisers and conciliators as well as organizing the rituals of lying-in and childbirth, but at times they also had to represent the wider interests of the town or village.[36] Midwives who failed to ensure the filiation of bastards might well fall foul of the ecclesiastical authorities since participation in the legal process was generally regarded as one of their principal duties. Ann Witter of Tarporley denied that she was a midwife when presented at the 1665 visitation but she was reported by the churchwardens as a midwife in the visitations of 1671 and 1674, and a few years later her widowed daughter was presented for failing to name the father of her bastard and Ann Witter was implicated as the midwife.[37] Jane King of Moor was cited by the curate of Daresbury in 1727 'for practiceing the Mistery of Midwifery without a License from the Ordinary and thereby makeing great gain to her Self and does not Cause the Naugty Women to filiate their Children, and telling the Minister to his face She neither wou'd take a License nor leave off the practice if She was Sent for to do ye office of a Midwife'.[38]

From the bastardy depositions which they signed and the evidence of both their wills and the occupations of their husbands, it is clear that, by the standards of their localities, midwives were generally upright, comparatively well-educated and affluent.[39] They were thus credible witnesses on behalf of couples accused of ante-nuptial fornication on the basis of the length of time between their marriage and the birth of a child. Sometimes the midwife would merely add her signature to a letter written by another to testify to the prematurity of a birth, as Mary Farmer of Manchester did in 1729.[40] On other occasions, the letter would be written by the midwife herself, as in the case of Elizabeth Walker of Radcliffe who wrote in 1724 that one of her patients 'wass cartinly brought in bed be fore har time[. B]oth I and ye rest of my nebouring womon Can and will make it to a pear[,] for ye Child when it was born had neither to[e] nele nor finger nele.' This letter, which goes on to plead poverty on behalf of the couple, is striking for its evocation of community support and traditional expertise.[41] The same factors are implicit in a letter of 1725: 'This is to satisfy this Honourable Court that I Mary Cheetham Midwife do fully believe that Elizabeth Daughter of Aaron Hilton was born before it's full time, Likewise severall other women att that time p[re]sent do believe the same as Witness my hand, Mary Cheetham.'[42]

If mistaken conviction for adultery or fornication could be a severe embarrassment, rape was a capital crime in which the midwife's evidence could be essential for the securing of a conviction. Since she would often know all the people involved and be called upon by interested parties to examine the alleged victim, it was vital that her moral probity be above suspicion.[43] Adam Martindale vividly recalled the behaviour of the jury of matrons when his young daughter had been a witness in a rape case: 'A midwife, being one of them, was much his friend, and talked hard for him; but when it came to swearing, she joyned with the rest, and tooke her oath, as all of them did, that (to the utmost of her judgement) the child was carnally known by some man.'[44]

The deliberations of juries of matrons are generally lost to history but midwives were also called in for preliminary investigations.[45] When a Chester barber-surgeon accused his two apprentices of raping his eight-year-old daughter in 1685, a midwife was called by the father of one of the accused to examine the child. She later deposed that she 'could not p[er]ceive or Finde any probabillity or signe or tocken in the least of any Rape'.[46] A Warrington midwife called in by the mother of an eleven-year-old girl in 1738 stated 'that she did this day Examine the private parts of the said Judith Henshaw and saith that some man hath lately Ravished or attempted to Ravish her the s[ai]d Judith, for that she had several marks of violence upon those parts'. The hesitancy of this evidence led to the man being charged with attempted rape only. Since this was not a capital crime, a conviction was relatively easy to secure and he was fined twenty shillings, sentenced to six months in gaol, and bound over for three years.[47]

In this period, there was no clear consensus as to how much evidence was required to prove rape. Yet despite very high standards of proof being applied, there were probably more convictions in Lancashire and Cheshire for rape than for infanticide, the other capital crime that involved the evidence of midwives. In theory, under the Act of 1624, the odds were stacked against an unmarried woman once she had been identified as having secretly borne a child subsequently found dead.[48] The normal presumption of innocence was supposed to be set aside in such cases and the onus of proof placed on the accused instead because of the difficulty of obtaining direct evidence of this furtive crime. In practice, it became increasingly hard to obtain convictions at the assizes, even when coroners' juries were convinced by the evidence; during the years 1730 to 1760, of twenty-two women tried for infanticide at the Lancaster assizes not one was found guilty. Apart from the sentiments of the trial jurors, the problem lay in providing convincing evidence that the child had been born alive, despite the law's stipulation that only secret birth need be shown.[49] In part, therefore, the onus of proof came to lie on the medical evidence. A respectable midwife could exonerate an accused mother simply by testifying that the child was still-born or premature, even if she had not herself been present at the birth. Thus Mary Trygorne, the wife of a Chester saddler, signed a deposition in 1678 that she could not have saved a bastard child born dead even if she had been present at its birth as she estimated it to have been about three months premature.[50]

The usual procedure when an infant's body had been discovered was for some respectable women of the neighbourhood, usually led by the midwife, to interrogate the most likely suspect, attempting to draw milk from her breasts if a confession was not forthcoming. By the time the coroner arrived, the identity of the mother had often been established. The midwife might also be required to examine a child's body to help determine whether it had been born alive or not, as in a case at Leyland in 1739 when Anne Elliott had to inspect a child that had been buried in the churchyard. She declared that it 'was come to its full Growth but cannot say whether the said Child was born alive'.[51] More than technical knowledge, however, the greatest asset of midwives in such investigations was probably their personal authority. When in 1696 a group of women went to question a Clayton-le-Dale spinster who was alleged to have thrown her child into the fire, the midwife 'said unto her can you looke me in ye face and say you have not borne a Child'.[52] By virtue of either their social status or their office, midwives in this period generally possessed considerable influence among the women in their localities.[53]

If a woman was believed to have given birth but there was no body for the coroner to examine, the justices would investigate the matter in petty sessions. Problems could arise when giving evidence before the gentry, as social conventions inhibited midwives' explicitness. Thus, when Sir Richard Standish of Duxbury, Baronet, and Sir Peter Brook of Astley, Knight, took evidence from the midwives of Chorley in a suspected infanticide case in 1684, the women stated that they 'do believe y[a]t the s[ai]d Mrs Ellin Ainsworth hath borne a Child but how lately they can none of them sweare and that they drew ye Brests of ye s[ai]d Mrs Ellin Ainsworth and found Milk therein; and likewise that there were other signes on her of haveing a Child but they cannot with modesty express it'.[54] In such cases, the decorum and reticence enjoined on midwives both by their oath of office and by social expectation tended to hamper their effectiveness as witnesses.

As male practitioners increasingly became involved in delivering even normal births, it is not surprising that they also started to figure in the investigation of infanticide. In 1736, an infanticide trial at Lancaster had to be postponed as the Cartmel apothecary who was due to appear for the prosecution 'cannot possibly now attend'. He was reported to have delivered the child in 1733 'for w[hi]ch trouble he rec[eive]d five Guineas & was p[ro]mis[e]d five Guineas more & s[ai]d he would not live but by such Businesse'.[55] Initially, coroners called surgeons as witnesses to supplement the evidence of the local midwife. In 1741, for example, Sir Henry Hoghton, Baronet, magistrate, and coroner for his own manor of Walton-le-Dale, called a Preston surgeon to examine the body of a child found dead. He 'found by various Circumstances that the s[ai]d Child was born alive and had been murdred'. Two days later, he watched Anne Elliott draw milk from the breasts of a suspect. The midwife deposed that she had never known a woman still to have milk five years after the birth of her last child.[56] At this stage, surgeons appear to have been used by coroners conducting infanticide investigations principally for their post-mortem expertise but without superseding the traditional expertise of the midwives.

There was no guarantee that the surgeon would be called at the trial. In his midwifery textbook of 1737, Henry Bracken complained that he had not been called to give evidence in an infanticide trial despite having viewed the body. He blamed the woman's acquittal on this, she being protected by 'good Friends'. Yet when Bracken himself sat as coroner *ex officio* as mayor of Lancaster in 1748, the only expert witness he called in a case of infanticide was Mrs Sarah Haresnape, probably because he trusted her judgement more than that of his professional rivals. The accused in that case was also found innocent.[57] Nevertheless, surgeons did gradually supplant midwives in court as autopsies became more routine in infanticide cases. In February 1755, a surgeon of New Church in the Forest of Rossendale opened an infant corpse and found its breast bone broken and, in the same month, a Liverpool surgeon examined a body found in a midden. Although he was certain it was born at its full term, he was unable to tell if it was born alive as it was decomposed.[58] Bracken's pupil, Ralph Holt of Liverpool, examined a dead child's body in 1761 'but cannot really tell whether it was born alive or not but it seems to have come to a proper time of Birth or nigh it tho he cannot be Exact as to that – that the said Child now seems to be disvigured by mice or Ratts'. Thus the introduction of surgeons does not seem to have brought about any immediate improvement in the quality of the evidence, and this defendant, like many others before her, was acquitted.[59] There is no suggestion, at this early date, of the use of such methods as 'swimming the lungs', which became a matter of heated controversy at the Lancaster assizes in the early nineteenth century.[60]

Physicians were not generally involved in investigations concerning the death of bastard infants unless a late abortion was involved. In November 1684, Thomas Worthington of Wigan was called to a woman who was straining and vomiting. He diagnosed poisoning and attributed the death of her premature infant to this cause. She blamed the child's father who 'with his own hands Gave her a Roasted Aple to Eate and also A peece of Marmalett in a white paper'.[61] Worthington's son Francis, also a physician, attended a similar case in 1700 when he too managed to save the mother but not the child.[62] Richard Stevenson made up and administered an antidote ordered by Dr Pennington to a pregnant Chester spinster in 1687, and told the inquest that he saw something like white arsenic in her vomit.[63] In this last case, it is striking that no opening of the body was performed. In the seventeenth century, clinical observation was generally relied upon at inquests despite what now seem to be the obvious advantages of internal examination to establish the cause of death. This is in marked contrast to the procedure followed in the case of a widow at Inglewhite in Goosnargh who died in 1751 after being given an abortifacient by a flax-dresser. He had tried to get hold of both pennyroyal and white mercury before an intermediary managed to buy some berries for him. A Preston surgeon opened the stomach of the deceased and decided that she had been poisoned. He estimated her to be two months pregnant.[64]

By this date, opening the body was fairly standard practice in cases of suspected poisoning, although the results were rarely as conclusive as evidence of the purchase or possession of poison. Nevertheless, there was a clear shift away from reliance on merely clinical evidence in such cases. When a Warrington woman gave poisoned gingerbread to her stepchildren, the apothecary whom her husband summoned to attend his vomiting sons 'did not rightly understand the Occasion of such Illness'. The surgeon called by the coroner found mortification in the upper part of the stomach and inflammation of the duodenum of one of the children but inspection of the stomach contents did not reveal any poison. Nevertheless, he believed that the symptoms had been caused 'by some voilent [sic] thing which was given to the Child (or which the Child had taken)'.[65] Not all poisons were immediately obvious to the naked eye, but coroners appear to have felt that an attempt should be made to detect them. In 1739 a Poulton apothecary was called to see the body of a bastard supposed to have been poisoned by the father. He deposed that 'he has since cut, open'd and view'd the Body of the said Child but cannot discover any marks of poison tho he says the same Child may have been poison'd and yet no Appearance thereof remain after it's death.' It is unclear whether the apothecary was searching for traces of poison or for the pathological effects on the internal organs.[66] Occasionally, with the spread of the surgeon-apothecary, the coroner was able to call on the practitioner on the spot to open the body and search for poison. In the 1758 case of a Salford labourer who confessed to poisoning his children with arsenic bought from Mrs Frodsham, a Manchester chemist and druggist, the bodies were opened by the surgeon who was attending their mother, who was also dying from the effects of the poison.[67]

In the investigation of other forms of violent death, seventeenth-century coroners called for the clinical evidence of medical practitioners rather than asking for autopsies.[68] In 1680, Richard Lathom, a surgeon of Maghull, attended a husbandman named Tildesley who had been assaulted by an Aintree husbandman and his servant. He deposed that he 'found him in a very high burning favor who continued therein w[i]th:out intermission untill hee died ... But the s[ai]d Tildesley had neither wound bruse nore fratture upon his bodye as this Informate verely beleives but dyed of a naturall sicknesse.' Nevertheless, the two Aintree men were tried for premeditated murder.[69] In 1695 Charles Leigh, a Manchester physician whose estate was near Preston, happened to see a traveller and his family accosted near the River Wyre. Later that night the assailant forced his way into the traveller's bedchamber and threatened the husband. The next morning, the husband, who was 'in a Malignant fev[e]r' from which he later died, told Leigh that 'he had been blooded ye weeke before at Preston by ye French Chirurgeon', presumably Guion Bosquet, for a pain in his limbs. However, Leigh would not commit himself concerning the fatal illness 'whether or no yt [i.e. that] was caused by ye fright, or by his great losses, and yt ill usage of a prison in France'. No autopsy was conducted.[70]

Even surgeons were in no hurry to introduce internal examinations, perhaps because they were not paid for their appearances at inquests, perhaps because popular opinion linked autopsies with the dissection of executed criminals.[71] In 1698, a Haigh joiner was under the care of an Aspull surgeon after he had been attacked on his way to church at Wigan. The surgeon told the inquest that the scalp had been loose, that there had been wounds as deep as the bone, 'but whether these wounds were the occasion of his death this Exam[inan]t knows not But the said Brocke for some time after was much out of health being frequently troubled with vomitting'.[72] A 1739 inquest at Cliviger into the death of a man struck over the head with a churn post after a drinking session was told by the Burnley apothecary who had attended him that, although there was a large wound, 'this Informant is not satisfied that the Skull of the said John Hindle was fractur'd or that the said wound was the cause of his death he being in his Lifetime so weak that it was not proper to make a diligent search.'[73] A Prescot surgeon-apothecary who was summoned to attend an innkeeper's wife in 1751 saw no wounds or bruises, although her husband admitted that there had been a quarrel, only an inflammation in her right breast. She died the next day 'but whether such Inflamation or fever was occasioned by such bruises or otherwise he cannot take upon him to determine.' The husband was later found guilty of manslaughter.[74]

Urban surgeons seem to have been as reluctant to display their post-mortem expertise as their rural colleagues. Thus Thomas Wilbraham of Chester does not appear to have made an internal examination before declaring that the blackened ears and bloody face of a boy believed by neighbours to have been killed by his drunken mother had been caused by convulsions. 'Visitation of God' was the verdict.[75] James Bromfield, a leading Liverpool surgeon, was called to attend a man injured during an argument at an inn in 1744. He drew water off him daily until he died, and told the inquest that 'this Examinant believes the s[ai]d Hanley's Illness Must proceed from a blow or some other external Cause'.[76] Even Charles White of Manchester, friend of William Hunter, does not appear to have conducted an internal examination in 1749 when he declared of a woman suspected of having been killed by her husband 'that the Blackness appearing upon the several parts of her Body might naturally be occasioned by the decay or Inflamation of the Intestines And saith that there does not appear to him any Bruises or Marks of Violence that might occasion her death'. Although the coroner's jury found a verdict of murder, the husband was acquitted at the assizes.[77]

In fact, the chief impetus for change in this respect appears to have come from the coroners themselves. They had, of course, been in the habit of asking surgeons to examine the bodies of victims of violence to measure the wounds and assess the likelihood of their having been fatal. Thus Edmund Darbishire summoned Thomas Orme of Ormskirk in 1695 to view the body of a Tarleton woman who had been murdered by a man who suspected her of having bewitched him. He found half-inch wide wounds on the front and back of her head and fingerprint bruises on her neck.[78] In the early eighteenth century, however, coroners appear to have started asking those practitioners whom they had summoned to be more thorough. Although internal examinations did not become routine until after the reform of the office of coroner in the 1830s, they did increase in frequency in the eighteenth century, especially after the remuneration of coroners was reformed in the 1750s.

When Sir Henry Hoghton held an inquest on the body of a man who died after a drunken scuffle in 1730, the apothecary who visited him while unconscious thought 'that he was seized with some thing of an appoplective fitt'. John Escolme, a Preston surgeon who had been apprenticed to Thomas Clayton in Manchester, removed the scalp and opened the brain. He found a small bruise, 'but from his observation of his scull and brain he does not apprehend his death Could proceed from any disorder in his head'.[79] When an Oldham man died in 1740 after being struck with a whip by one of a group of young horsemen, led by James Dawson of Manchester, the coroner had the head examined by the Oldham surgeon who had attended the deceased and a surgeon from Manchester. On scalping the corpse, they found extensive fractures.[80] At an inquest held by the mayor of Wigan in 1758, an apothecary was called to examine the body of a soldier's wife, thought to have been strangled by her husband. He found her face black, swollen and bloated, bloody foam coming from her right nostril, and a swelling on her neck, 'and that the said Swelling as well as the Bleeding or Foaming appeared to this Deponent to proceed from some Violence or Force used to the Deceased and not from any natural Cause'. However, following an order to open the body, he discovered 'That the said swelling was an Abcess containing Puss or Matter and that the same hath been growing or forming for some Months last past and was not occasioned by any force or violence offered to her at the time of her Death to the best of his knowledge.' The husband was acquitted at the assizes.[81]

It is difficult to assess the impact of changes in medico-legal practice on verdicts and trial procedures because of the lack of detailed reports of what took place in most English courts at this period. Nevertheless, it is clear that a wide variety of participants would have been aware of the potential importance of medical evidence through the dissemination of transcripts of sensational trials such as that of Mary Blandy in 1752 for murdering her father by poison at the instigation of her lover. The medical evidence at the inquest covered the front page of Chester's weekly newspaper and a Manchester newspaper carried coverage of the trial in seven successive issues.[82] Summoning surgeons became a fairly frequent recourse for more diligent coroners in the late eighteenth century. Edward Umfreville in his handbook for coroners of 1761 mentioned the need for surgeons' evidence and provided a sample form for summoning a surgeon.[83] By this date, there was throughout the country a well-established tradition of using the expert testimony of midwives and medical practitioners in a variety of legal actions. The use of autopsies, even in the provinces, began long before there was a body of literature on the subject. It is clear that the developments of the late eighteenth and early nineteenth centuries had their roots in older practices.

NOTES

I am grateful for helpful comments made at the seminars of Paul Slack in Oxford and Eric Evans in Lancaster and the 1990 conference of the American Society for Eighteenth Century Studies at Minneapolis.

1 Samuel Farr, *Elements of Medical Jurisprudence* (London, 1788); Thomas Percival, *Medical Ethics* (Manchester, 1803).

2 T. R. Forbes, 'Inquests into London and Middlesex homicides, 1673–1782', *Yale Journal of Biology and Medicine*, 50 (1977), 207–20; Forbes, 'Crowner's quest', *Transactions of the American Philosophical Society*, 68, pt. 1 (1978); Forbes, *Surgeons at the Bailey: English Forensic Medicine to 1878* (New Haven, 1985).

3 J. M. Beattie, *Crime and the Courts in England, 1660–1800* (Princeton, 1986), p. 91.

4 See Catherine Crawford, 'The emergence of English forensic medicine: medical evidence in common-law courts, 1730–1830', Ph.D. thesis, University of Oxford, 1987, and Joel Peter Eigen, 'Delusion in the courtroom: the role of partial insanity in early forensic testimony', *Medical History*, 35 (1991), 25–49.

5 T. R. Forbes, 'The regulation of English midwives in the sixteenth and seventeenth centuries', *Medical History*, 8 (1964), 235–44; Forbes, 'The regulation of English midwives in the eighteenth and nineteenth centuries', *Medical History*, 15 (1971), 352–62; J. R. Guy, 'The episcopal licensing of physicians, surgeons and midwives', *Bulletin of the History of Medicine*, 56 (1982), 528–42. Raw data from licensing material will be found in J. H. Bloom and R. R. James, *Medical Practitioners in the Diocese of London, 1529–1725* (Cambridge, 1935) and E. H. Carter, *The Norwich Subscription Books, 1637–1800* (London, 1937).

6 In recent times, totalitarian states have imposed far more draconian restrictions on dissent. Religious conformity was, of course, the aim of governments throughout Europe in the early modern period.

7 For contemporary criticism of the system, see J. Tristram, *The Ill State of Physick in Great Britain* (London, 1727), pp. 49–50. I discuss licensing in more detail in 'Licensed physicians in north-west England, 1660–1760', unpublished paper.

8 A. O. Whiteman, 'The re-establishment of the Church of England, 1660–1663', *Transactions of the Royal Historical Society*, 5th series, 5 (1955), 111–31; I. M. Green, *The Re-establishment of the Church of England, 1660–1663* (Oxford, 1978), pp. 117–42.

9 For example of visitations in this region, see W. Fergusson Irvine, 'Church discipline after the Restoration', *Transactions of the Historic Society of Lancashire and Cheshire*, 64 (1912), 43–71 and J. Brownbill, ed., 'List of clergymen, etc., in the Diocese of Chester, 1691', in *Chetham Miscellanies*, n.s., 3 (Chetham Society, n.s. 73, 1915). The surviving testimonials are mainly preserved in Cheshire Record Office: Diocesan Miscellany (Dioc. Misc.). The numbers given here relate to the sequence of the bundles and the approximate position of the document.

10 Cheshire Record Office (hereafter CRO): Dioc. Misc. 1/8.

11 CRO: Dioc. Misc. 1/4.

12 CRO: Dioc. Misc. 1/81, 1/75.

13 CRO: Dioc. Misc. 1/114; *The Diary of Dr. Thomas Cartwright, Bishop of Chester* (Camden Society, 1843), vol. XXII, 22, 39, 40.

14 CRO: EDC 6/1/1, nos. 13–14.

15 CRO: Dioc. Misc. 2/33, 2/62, 2/108, 2/110; EDC 6/1/7, no. 8.

16 CRO: Dioc. Misc. 1/41.

17 CRO: EDC 5/1691/30, testimonial for Ellen, wife of William Fletcher, 18/5/1691.

18 CRO: EDV 1/109, f. 10/1.

19 Public Record Office (PRO): PL 28/40/2: affidavit of Mary Cowband of Ashton on Ribble, 28/3/1696; affidavit of Joyce, wife of Charles Brooks of Halsall, 26/8/1737.

20 PRO: PL 28/40, deposition concerning James Howcroft of Preston, 10/8/1744. Shepherd was one of the few practitioners in Lancashire who might reasonably be expected to have known something of the best methods in legal medicine, since his extensive library included treatises on the subject by such authors as Paolo Zacchia. See *A Catalogue of Books in Various Languages Contained in the Library Collected by Richard Shepherd, Esq., M.B.* (Preston, 1839).

21 Michael Macdonald, ed., *Witchcraft and Hysteria in Elizabethan London: Edward Jorden and the Mary Glover Case* (London, 1991); Roger Smith, *Trial by Medicine: Insanity and Responsibility in Victorian Trials* (Edinburgh, 1981).

22 [Thomas Jolly and John Carrington], *The Surey Demoniack* (London, 1697), p. 64. For a full discussion of this case, see D. N. Harley, 'Mental illness, magical medicine and the Devil in northern England, 1650–1700', in R. French and A. Wear, eds., *The Medical Revolution of the Seventeenth Century* (Cambridge, 1989), pp. 114–44.

23 For Lancashire lunacy inquisitions, see PRO: PL 5. The Chancery jurisdiction in Lancashire was technically distinct from that in the rest of the country but similar problems arise with Chancery records as a whole.

24 CRO: EDC 5 (1697) no. 14; EDC 5 (1698) no. 10.

25 PRO: PL 28/1, f. 210, undated petition on behalf of Richard Shelmerdine of Salford; IR 1/48/136.

26 PRO: PL 10/151, *Dawson* v. *Pimlott*. Lancashire Chancery depositions will be referred to by bundle number and by the first named plaintiff and defendant.

27 PRO: PL 10/159, *Hilton* v. *Maude*; for a similar case in Preston, cf. PL 10/166, Hesketh v. Meredith.

28 PRO: PL 10/166, *Barron* v. *Windle*.

29 PRO: PL 10/176, *Atherton* v. *Atherton*.

30 For a discussion of the origins of this system and some early cases, see P. C. Hoffer and N. E. H. Hull, *Murdering Mothers: Infanticide in England and New England, 1558–1803* (New York, 1981), pp. 13–17.

31 CRO: EDC 6/1/9, statements on behalf of Robert Pont, 25/10/1728.

32 CRO: EDC 6/1/6; QJF 149/3/49, 78; QJB 3/7; Nantwich Parish Register, baptism on 29/8/1721.

33 CRO: EDC 5 (1704) no. 7.

34 Lancashire Record Office: QSP 697/10.

35 Lancashire Record Office: QSP 751/12.

36 For a discussion of the position of midwives within women's culture, see Adrian Wilson, 'The ceremony of childbirth and its interpretation', in Valerie Fildes, ed., *Women as Mothers in Pre-industrial England* (London, 1990), pp. 68–107.

37 CRO: EDV 1/34, f. 13; EDV 2/6, f. 4v; EDV 1/45, f. 5; EDV 1/51, f. 8.

38 CRO: EDV 1/109, f. 30v.

39 D. N. Harley, 'Provincial midwives in England: Lancashire and Cheshire, 1660–1760', in Hilary Marland, ed., *The Art of Midwifery: Early Modern Midwives in Europe* (London, 1993), pp. 27–48. See also the essays by Ann Hess and Doreen Evenden in the same volume.

40 CRO: EDC 6/1/12, letter on behalf of Abraham and Mary Barlow, 4/4/1729.
41 CRO: EDC 6/1/7, undated letter on behalf of Silence and Thomas Hardman.
42 CRO: EDC 6/1/8, letter on behalf of Aaron Hilton, 3/11/1725.
43 Recent historical studies of rape do not discuss this aspect of the process: N. Bashar, 'Rape in England between 1550 and 1700', in London Feminist History Group, *The Sexual Dynamics of History: Men's Power, Women's Resistance* (London, 1983), pp. 28–42; Roy Porter, 'Rape – does it have a historical meaning?', in Sylvana Tomaselli and Roy Porter, eds., *Rape* (Oxford, 1986), pp. 216–36, 270–9. See, however, J. M. Beattie, *Crime and the Courts in England 1660–1800* (Oxford, 1986), pp. 125–6.
44 *The Life of Adam Martindale*, ed. R. Parkinson (Chetham Society, 1845), vol. IV, pp. 206–7.
45 T. R. Forbes, 'A jury of matrons', *Medical History*, 32 (1988), 23–33.
46 Chester City Record Office: QSF/83/181–4, 219, 268.
47 PRO: PL 27/2, depositions re Judith Henshaw, 9/8/1738; PL 25/103.
48 James I, c. 27: 'An act to prevent the destroying and murthering of bastard children'.
49 See the essay by Mark Jackson in this volume (chapter 3).
50 Chester City Record Office: QCO/I/14/7.
51 PRO: PL 27/2, inquest on bastard of Margery Thornley, 15/11/1739.
52 PRO: PL 27/2, depositions re Elizabeth Boulton, 16 & 23/6/1696.
53 Harley, 'Provincial midwives in England'.
54 PRO: PL 27/1, depositions re bastard of Ellin Ainsworth, 28–29/4/1684.
55 PRO: PL 28/13, p. 5; PL 27/2, depositions re child of Margaret Lickbarrow, 12/5/1736 – 28/6/1736.
56 PRO: PL 27/2, inquest on infant found in millstream, 6–9/2/1741.
57 Henry Bracken, *The Midwife's Companion* (London, 1737), p. 38; PRO: PL 26/290, inquest on bastard of Mary Parker, 22/8/1748; PL 28/2, p. 73. For Bracken's unfavourable comparison of a graduate's diagnostic skills with those of Mrs Haresnape, see D. N. Harley, 'Honour and property: the structure of professional disputes in eighteenth-century English medicine', in Andrew Cunningham and Roger French, eds., *The Medical Enlightenment of the Eighteenth Century* (Cambridge, 1990), pp. 138–64, at p. 163.
58 PRO: PL 27/3, inquest on bastard of Mary Mather, 26/2/1755; inquest on bastard of Ann Kenion, 14/2/1755.
59 PRO: PL 27/2, inquest on the bastard of Martha Woods, 17/7/1761; PL 25/143.
60 P. A. O. Mahon, *An Essay on the Signs of Murder in New Born Children*, trans. Christopher Johnson (Lancaster, 1813), p. xii.
61 PRO: PL 27/1, statements concerning bastard child of Margaret Greene of Wrightington, 21/1/1685.
62 Lancashire Record Office: QSP 848/23.
63 Chester City Record Office: QCO/I/15/32.
64 PRO: PL 27/3, inquest on Margaret Brighouse, 20/7/1751.
65 PRO: PL 27/2, inquest on a child of Henry Lumix, 15–16/9/1728.
66 PRO: PL 27/2, inquest on child of Isabel Butler, 19/7/1739.
67 PRO: PL 27/3, inquest on Mary and Jane Grindrod, 15 & 19/9/1758.
68 Forensic autopsy had long been common in Europe, but not in England. For the rise and fall of private autopsies by physician-anatomists, see D. N. Harley,

'Political postmortems and morbid anatomy in seventeenth-century England' *Social History of Medicine* (forthcoming).

69 PRO: PL 26/23/3.

70 PRO: PL 27/2, deposition re Richard Greening, 22/6/1695.

71 For the argument that English trial procedure made expert witnessing in general unattractive to practitioners, see chapter 4, by Catherine Crawford, in this volume.

72 PRO: PL 27/2, inquest on Francis Brock, 29/12/1698.

73 PRO: PL 27/2, inquest on John Hindle, 23/8/1739.

74 PRO: PL 27/3, inquest on Phoebe Gill, 10/4/1751; PL 28/2, f. 119.

75 Chester City Record Office: QCO/I/21/10.

76 PRO: PL 26/290, inquest on Francis Hanley, 2/1/1744.

77 PRO: PL 27/2, inquest on Ann Hargreaves, 20/10/1749; PL 28/2, f. 86.

78 PRO: PL 27/2, inquest on Margaret Hollinhurst, 17/6/1695.

79 PRO: PL 27/2, inquest on William Boardman, 9/11/1730; IR 1/45/3.

80 PRO: PL 27/2, inquest on James Harrap, 2/4/1740.

81 PRO: PL 27/3, inquest on Mary Clarkson, 18/3/1758; PL 28/2, f. 223.

82 *Adams's Weekly Courant*, no. 971, Tuesday 19/11/1751; *Harrops's Manchester Mercury*, nos. 24–30 (1752). For the medico-legal significance of the case, see Forbes, *Surgeons at the Bailey*, pp. 133–4.

83 Edward Umfreville, *Lex Coronatoria: Or, the Office and Duty of Coroners* (London, 1761), pp. 510–13. For discussion of the changes of the 1750s, see R. F. Hunnisett, ed., *Wiltshire Coroners' Bills, 1752–1796* (Wiltshire Record Society, 1981), vol. XXXVI, and Hunnisett, 'The importance of eighteenth-century coroners' bills', in E. W. Ives and A. H. Manchester, eds., *Law, Litigants and the Legal Profession* (London, 1983), pp. 126–39.

3

Suspicious infant deaths: the statute of 1624 and medical evidence at coroners' inquests

MARK JACKSON

The investigation of sudden death in England during the seventeenth and eighteenth centuries was constrained by the equivocal status of the coroner and his inquest, and by the lack of provision for the regular admission of medical evidence in both pre-trial and trial procedures. When the office of coroner was established at the end of the twelfth century, coroners were required to act as keepers of the Crown pleas and to collect the revenue due to the Crown in connection with those pleas.[1] In the fourteenth and fifteenth centuries, changes in the local and central administration of justice, including the rise of the justices of the peace, combined to divest the coroners of much of their authority. By the seventeenth and eighteenth centuries, the coroners' loss of authority was accompanied in many cases by a lack of care and diligence in performing their remaining duties. In the seventeenth century, Sir Matthew Hale noted that most coroners' inquisitions were inadequate, and in 1761 Edward Umfreville, one of the coroners for Middlesex, was prompted by the disrepute into which the office had fallen to publish his own private notes in an attempt to encourage 'a general uniform Practice' amongst coroners.[2]

From a medico-legal perspective, one of the most significant features of the decline of the coroner's office is the fact that the coroner's jurisdiction to take inquisitions touching the death of a person *subito mortuis, super visum corporis* was restricted by the belief that only sudden deaths with manifest evidence of violence warranted inquiry. This view, given authoritative support by Hale,[3] rendered the presentation of medical evidence at inquests largely superfluous. When there were obvious marks of violence on a dead body, the cause of death was deemed to be evident even to those not medically trained; and when there were no marks of violence, an inquest was unnecessary.

The contribution of medical testimony to the investigation of sudden deaths was also limited by the general neglect of legal medicine in England, a neglect which has usually been unfavourably contrasted with the situation in Italy, France, and Germany.[4] The absence, before 1836, of any legislative provision for the payment of medical witnesses testifying at inquests discouraged coroners from calling medical evidence.[5] Furthermore, the lack of any substantial English texts or lecture courses on medical jurisprudence prior to the nineteenth century limited the forensic knowledge and skill of medical practitioners and restricted the value of their evidence in both coroners' and trial courts.[6]

Despite these limitations, coroners were not always deterred from holding inquests, and medical opinion as to cause of death was by no means disregarded during the seventeenth and eighteenth centuries. This is well illustrated by the large number of investigations held into the deaths of newborn children thought to have been murdered by their mothers.[7] Inquiries into the circumstances of these deaths were performed with a diligence which belies the low status of both coroners and medical evidence in this period. Although there were often no marks of violence on the children's bodies, and although some deaths might therefore have been attributed to natural causes, coroners were routinely notified of, and held inquests into, the deaths of newborn children throughout the eighteenth century. Indeed, by the turn of the nineteenth century, the coroner's inquest had become the major form of pre-trial investigation into these deaths, almost completely superseding inquiries by justices of the peace.

Medical testimony was a prominent feature of coroners' investigations into newborn-child murder and a regular part of trials for this offence. In the seventeenth century, and more so in the eighteenth, medical testimony as to cause of death and the possibility of still-birth made significant contributions to discussions of the crime both in and out of the courts. Indeed, medical writings on the problems of proof in such cases, and upon the validity of observations made on inspection and dissection of the body of a dead child, are among the earliest English works on legal medicine.

Some years ago, J. D. J. Havard suggested that medical interest in newborn-child murder stemmed from the passage of a statute of James I, 'An Act to prevent the Destroying and Murthering of Bastard Children', in 1624.[8] This certainly seems plausible, since the statute provided a focus for many discussions about the crime, discussions which revolved around issues that were increasingly acknowledged to fall within the cognizance of medical practitioners. However, the construction and interpretation of this statute were complex, and its impact on the development of legal medicine was not straightforward. Close analysis of the statute and of its application until its repeal in 1803 suggests that the statute influenced the development of medical evidence in two phases. At first, the statute's emphasis on still-birth encouraged the courts to focus on medical evidence that indicated that a child had been still-born. By the middle of the eighteenth century, however, opposition to the statute's severity and the proliferation of exceptions to it resulted in its virtual abrogation and a reversion to common-law rules of evidence. This led to a renewed emphasis on proof of live-birth and stimulated a prolonged and vigorous discussion of the validity of medical evidence on this point.

One of the consequences of Elizabethan and Jacobean legislation concerning the maintenance of bastards and the relief of the poor was that bearing a bastard that was chargeable to the parish became a shameful and punishable offence, and that the parents of such bastards were exposed to the hostility and accusations of ratepaying neighbours.[9] In an attempt to avoid the unpopularity, shame and punishment of unmarried motherhood, many single women attempted to conceal their pregnancies and give birth in secret. When the body of an infant was later found dead, neighbours and parish officers were quick to suspect that the child had been killed at birth.

Prior to 1624, all women and men suspected of murdering newborn children were tried according to common-law rules of evidence, which required the prosecution to prove that a dead child had been born alive before it could proceed to the question of murder. Direct evidence of live-birth, in the form of witnesses to the birth, was rare in such cases and the prosecution relied heavily upon circumstantial evidence: examination of the mother for signs of having gone to full term; estimates of the child's maturity and viability; signs of violence on the child's body; and the behaviour and reputation of the mother. In some instances, such evidence was sufficient to obtain a conviction for murder,[10] but in most cases converting the suspicions of neighbours and local officials into convictions in the courts proved singularly difficult.

The problems encountered by the prosecution, and the contemporary hostility towards bearers of bastards that were chargeable to the parish, eventually led to the provision of special evidential rules for the trials of women accused of murdering bastards.[11] After unsuccessful attempts to legislate on the subject in 1607 and 1610, an Act 'to prevent the Destroying and Murthering of Bastard Children' was passed in May 1624.[12] The text deserves careful reading:

> Whereas many lewd Women that have been delivered of Bastard Children, to avoid their Shame, and to escape Punishment, do secretly bury or conceal the Death of their Children, and after, if the Child be found dead, the said Women do alledge, that the said Child was born dead; whereas it falleth out sometimes (although hardly it is to be proved) that the said Child or Children were murthered by the said Women, their lewd Mothers, or by their Assent or Procurement:
>
> II For the Preventing therefore of this great Mischief, be it enacted by the Authority of this present Parliament, That if any Woman after one Month

> next ensuing the End of this Session of Parliament be delivered of any Issue of her Body, Male or Female, which being born alive, should by the Laws of this Realm be a Bastard, and that she endeavour privately, either by drowning or secret burying thereof, or any other Way, either by herself or the procuring of others, so to conceal the Death thereof, as that it may not come to Light, whether it were born alive or not, but be concealed: In every such Case the said Mother so offending shall suffer Death as in Case of Murther, except such Mother can make proof by one Witness at the least, that the Child (whose Death was by her so intended to be concealed) was born dead.

This statute marked a significant departure from common law for it created a legal presumption whereby a woman who had concealed the death of her bastard child was presumed to have murdered it. Although no longer obliged to prove live-birth, the prosecution still had to establish that the child's death had been concealed: 'Yet if Advantage be to be taken of this Statute *against* the Prisoner, the Concealment must then be proved by Evidence.'[13]

Although court records and contemporary writings sometimes misconstrued the statute by equating concealment of pregnancy, or concealment of the birth and body of a child, with murder, evidence on these issues was merely circumstantial. The legal presumption created by the statute only operated if the *death* of the child had been concealed.[14] Moreover, a mother's *intent* to conceal the death of her child was also material: 'whose Death was by her so intended to be concealed'. Circumstances implying a lack of intent to conceal, such as the preparation of clothes for the child, exempted a woman from the statutory presumption, leaving the case to stand at common law.[15]

The simplest way for a single woman to avoid the suspicions and accusations of her neighbours and, if necessary, to prove to a court that her child had been still-born, was to have an assistant at the delivery. Although, according to the seventeenth-century physician Percivall Willughby, a midwife was not absolutely necessary at delivery, her presence nevertheless served 'to avoid all future suspicions, and to free some of the looser sort from the danger of the statute-law, in case that the child should bee found dead'.[16] However, a single woman who had carefully concealed her pregnancy in order to preserve her reputation was unlikely to seek assistance at the birth, and most women tried for this crime had given birth alone.

In the absence of direct witnesses to the birth, the probability that a child had been still-born was usually determined by assessing the child's maturity and viability. In 1762, John Browne, a surgeon in Sheffield, told an inquest jury that the body he had examined 'appeared to this Informant to be of Maturity for Birth not only from its size but from the great quantity of Hair on its head, and from the Nails of its fingers and Toes'.[17] Such evidence testified to the child's maturity, but, in the absence of corroborating evidence, was not taken as proof that the child had been born alive. As the surgeon Stephen Cleasby testified at the inquest investigating the death of Ruth Peacock's child in 1793, 'the said Child appears to him to be or to have been at or near her full Time but whether the said Child had been born alive he does not pretend to say with certainty'.[18]

In contrast, evidence that a child had been born prematurely was regularly admitted as proof that the child had been still-born. Thus, for example, at a trial in 1725, a midwife deposed 'that to the best of her Judgment, the Prisoner did not go her full time, for the Toe-Nails of the Infant were not perfect'.[19] Prior to the middle of the eighteenth century, such evidence was usually presented by midwives. In the last half of the eighteenth century, however, as a result both of changes within the practice of midwifery and of increased medical interest in this crime, evidence was more frequently collected and presented by surgeons, man-midwives, and apothecaries.[20]

Medical evidence of prematurity and still-birth had some influence in the courts. In the north of England, a number of investigations into suspicious infant deaths did not proceed beyond the coroner's court because the inquest jury found that the child had been born prematurely and dead. At an inquest in Morpeth in 1790, for example, the jury echoed the opinion of the surgeon involved by concluding that 'the said Child was Born Dead; and that it appeared also to them not to have been Born at, or to have come to its full or due time of Birth'. No further legal action was taken against the mother.[21] Similar evidence contributed to acquittals at the trial courts. The *Old Bailey Sessions Papers* summed up the evidence at the trial of Jane Todd in 1727 in the following words:

> but no Marks appearing of any Violence offered, besides she did not go her full Time, the Child's Nails not being in their full Proportion, and she having made Provision for its Birth, it was the Opinion of the Court, from the strict Examination of the Evidences, that it was Still-born, (as she affirm'd) and that she flattered herself with concealing her Shame, by carrying it off with so much Privacy: Upon the whole the Jury acquitted her.[22]

At the beginning of the eighteenth century, Daniel Defoe warned that evidence about the prematurity of a child, even from a midwife present at the birth, was being admitted too readily by credulous jurors.[23] Although rare attempts to bribe midwives do appear in court records, there is little evidence to justify Defoe's concern. Most evidence presented by medical practitioners and midwives in the north of England in fact confirmed that the child had been born at full term, which, when corroborated by the presence of milk in the mother's breasts, served to dismiss her claim that premature delivery had caused her child to be still-born. Moreover, inquest juries sometimes ignored medical evidence that a child had been born prematurely when they felt that the circumstances merited a verdict of murder, such as when violence had been inflicted on the child's body.[24] It is true, however, that this type of evidence, whether in support of the prosecution or the defence, stimulated far less debate than other tests for live- and still-birth.

The regular, and largely unquestioned, admission of evidence concerning prematurity and still-birth in cases of newborn-child murder may have been due to two factors. First, the association between the growth of hair and nails, the degree of maturity and the probability of still-birth, had been used in the courts for many years prior to the passage of the 1624 statute.[25] Second, the admission of such evidence to exempt a woman from the 1624 statute had the unqualified, and influential, approval of Hale:

> If upon the view of the child it be testified by one witness by apparent probabilities, that the child was not come to its *debitum partus tempus*, as if it have no hair or nails, or other circumstances, this I have always taken to be a proof by one witness, that the child was born dead, so as to leave it nevertheless to the jury, as upon a common law evidence, whether she were guilty of the death of it or not.[26]

By emphasizing the importance of still-birth in the trials of women accused of murdering newborn bastard children, the 1624 statute focused attention on evidence relating to a child's viability. That evidence, largely the preserve of medical men and midwives, could only be gained from viewing dead bodies. The statute thus encouraged post-mortem inspections of dead newborn children and may have facilitated the development of more extensive examinations of dead bodies for forensic purposes in the eighteenth century. Furthermore, initial use of the statute created a space for medical testimony at both inquests and trials, which became increasingly important when changing attitudes further stimulated medical interest in the problems of proving the innocence, or guilt, of accused women.

In the middle decades of the seventeenth century, when the 1624 statute was much used, a high proportion of women accused of murdering their newborn children were convicted and hanged. In Essex, between 1620 and 1680, over 40 per cent of accused women were hanged for the crime, a figure well in excess of both execution and conviction rates for general homicide in the same courts.[27] The severity of the courts in the middle of the century was also commented on by Willughby, in his account of a 'naturall foole' who was sent for trial by the coroner's inquest. Concerned at the defendant's simplicity and her inability to plead for her life, Willughby asked the coroner to speak for her.

> Hee informed the judg, that it was a very small child, and the whole Bench saw that shee was a foole. It was in the Protector's dayes, and I feared that shee would have summum jus. The judg shewed the statute-Book to the jury. Neither judg, nor jury regarded her simplicity. They found her guilty, the judg condemned her, and shee was, afterwards, hanged for not having a woman by her, at her delivery.[28]

Interpretation and employment of the statute did not, however, remain static. In the early years of the eighteenth century, grumbling concerns at the number of acquittals for the crime and at some of the specious arguments used to exempt women from the legal presumption of the statute, reflected widespread problems in enforcing the statute's provisions. For example, in discussing the need for a foundling hospital, Defoe wrote:

> It is needless to run into a Declamation on this Head, since not a Sessions passes, but we see one or more merciless Mothers try'd for the Murder of their Bastard-Children; and to the Shame of good Government, generally escape the Vengeance due to shedders of Innocent Blood: ... I wonder so many Men of Sense, as have been on the Jury, have been so often impos'd upon by the stale Pretence of a Scrap or two of Child-Bed Linnen being found in the Murderer's Box, &c. when alas! perhaps it was ne'er put there till after the Murder was committed; or if it was, but with a view of saving themselves by that devilish Precaution; for so many have been acquitted on that Pretence, that 'tis but too common a Thing to provide Child-Bed-Linnen before-hand for a poor Innocent Babe they are determin'd to murder.[29]

Court records give some support to Defoe's concern. Conviction rates were lower in the eighteenth century than they had been one hundred years earlier. Although slightly over 20 per cent of women tried at the Old Bailey between 1730 and 1774 were convicted, elsewhere in the country the rate was much lower. In the north of England, only 3 per cent of women accused were convicted and an increasing number of women were discharged by the grand jury throughout the eighteenth century. In Staffordshire, not one of thirty-nine women tried between 1742 and 1802 was sentenced to death; and in Surrey, the conviction rate was much lower in the eighteenth than at the end of the seventeenth century.[30]

Although the conviction rate was low, however, prosecutions persisted. In the north of England two or three women were tried at the assize courts every year throughout the century. In 1743, a footnote in the *Old Bailey Sessions Papers* suggested that the frequency of such cases could be attributed to ignorance of the 1624 statute: ''Tis thought Cases of this Kind would not so frequently occur at the Old-Bailey, if the Law were more generally known, viz. 21 Jac. I. c.27'.[31] This comment was misguided. The provisions of both statute and common law appear to have been well known throughout the seventeenth and eighteenth centuries. Moreover, it was knowledge, rather than ignorance, of the statute that appears to have been the cause of its impotence.

Legal texts published in the seventeenth and eighteenth centuries, whether written for lawyers, justices of the peace, coroners, or parish officers, generally included an account of the statute.[32] Although these works occasionally misconstrued the statutory presumption, their coverage of the material points was comprehensive, and they provided judges and local officials with a detailed knowledge of the law relating to newborn-child murder. Abundant evidence of the statute's influence can be found in minute book or gaol calendar references to 'concealment'. More explicitly, several women were referred to as having murdered their children 'against peace and against Statute', and when Fletcher Rigge took over as clerk for the Northern Circuit assizes in 1772, he began to draw up indictments 'against the form of the Statute in such Case made and Provided', even though the legal authorities Kelyng, Hale and Hawkins had all expressed the opinion that this was not necessary for trial under the statute.[33]

Some coroners' inquisitions also made explicit reference to the statute, while others were drafted using its formal language. The inquisition taken on view of the dead child of Margaret Wanless in 1742, for example, concluded:

> as no Bruises were to be observed thereupon whether the said Child was born Alive or not or killed in her Labour for want of help the said Jurors know not But believe the said Child was so wrapt up by her that she might privately Bury the same to Conceal the Death thereof if the same was Born alive Contrary to the form of the Statute in that Case made and provided.[34]

It is clear that on occasions jurors were advised about the law by the coroner or his clerk, or by the clerk of assizes. In 1717, for example, at the trial of Ann Masie, the statute itself was read in court for 'the better Information of the Jury in this Case'.[35] And in 1741, when it appeared on evidence that the birth and body of Susannah Stephenson's newborn child had been concealed by Susannah and her mother, the inquest jury declared that:

> Susannah Stephenson ... had by some Means but by what Means does not appear to the Jurors Murder'd the said Male Child or at least the Law (*as the Jurors are advised*) deems it so it not Appearing to them by any Testimony that any Women or Others were Call'd in to the Birth of the aforesaid Child but on the Contrary it appears to them that its Birth was Intended to be Conceal'd.[36]

It is difficult to assess how much information about common and statute law filtered down from the courts to the general public. There is little direct evidence of 'lay' familiarity with the statute. The depositions of witnesses, which provide the best guide to local opinion, were taken down by the coroner or magistrate or by a clerk and reflect the knowledge of the examining official as much as that of the witness or suspect. However, the attendance of witnesses, jurors and on-lookers at the sessions, together with accounts of inquests and trials in the local newspapers, doubtless spread knowledge of the law beyond the confines of the courts. Indeed, on occasions, depositions contain details of the preliminary inquiries made in the neighbourhood before official intervention, and include accounts of the questioning of suspects by their neighbours. These fragments suggest that witnesses and suspects possessed a working knowledge of the main issues involved both at common law and under the statute, and that they were well aware of the significance of the signs of live- and still-birth, of the preparation of child's clothes, or of failing to call for help at the delivery.[37]

As attitudes to many aspects of the crime changed, awareness and discussion of the law led to a number of objections being raised against the statute, effectively limiting its application and scope. In the first place, certain circumstances were allowed to rebut the presumption laid down by the statute. For example, at the trial of Ann Davis in 1664, Sir John Kelyng and his associates on the bench adjudged that a woman who knocked for help during labour or who confessed that she was with child beforehand was not within the statute, 'because there was no intent to conceal it'.[38] As early as 1689, evidence that a woman had prepared clothes for a child was allowed to show that she had not intended to conceal the child's death.[39] And by the end of the eighteenth century, the presence of an accomplice (usually the child's father or the woman's mother) also took the case out of the statute, 'for if any person be present, although privy to the guilt, there can be no concealment by the mother within the statute, and the case stands as at common law'.[40] This last judgement shows how much legal opinion had changed since, according to the statute itself, the legal presumption applied to any woman who had concealed the death of her child 'by herself or the procuring of others'.[41]

The statute was also limited by the gradual rejection of the assumptions that pregnant, unmarried women were lewd and sinful, that only lewd and unnatural women would conceal and murder their children, and that concealment of the death of a child was sufficient evidence of intent to equate it with murder. During the course of the seventeenth and eighteenth centuries, the strength of these assumptions waned. While the crime of newborn-child murder was still described as barbaric and unnatural, the assumed connection between the nature of the crime and that of the criminal weakened. In the eighteenth century, suspects were more often described as modest, and sometimes virtuous, women than as lewd harlots. In *The Fable of the Bees*, published in 1714, Bernard Mandeville suggested that only modest women would feel the shame necessary to conceal or murder their children, and that 'Common Whores, whom all the World knows to be such, hardly ever destroy their Children ... not because they are less Cruel or more Virtuous, but because they have lost their Modesty to a greater degree, and the fear of Shame makes hardly any Impression upon them.'[42] This argument was repeated throughout the eighteenth century:

> The Women that have committed this most unnatural Crime, are real objects of our greatest Pity; their education has produced in them so much Modesty, or Sense of Shame, that this artificial Passion overturns the very Instincts of Nature! ... Hence the Cause of this most horrid Crime is an excess of what is really a Virtue, of the Sense of Shame, or Modesty.[43]

Although some writers, like the physician Thomas Percival, objected to the manner in which this argument 'exalted the sense of shame into the principle of virtue',[44] women accused of this crime were increasingly regarded as pitiable rather than punishable, a view complemented by the belief that men were also to some extent culpable:

> In most of these cases the father of the child is really criminal, often cruelly so; the mother is weak, credulous, and deluded. Having obtained gratification, he thinks no more of his promises; she finds herself abused, disappointed of his affection, attention, and support, and left to struggle as she can, with sickness, pains, poverty, infamy; in short, with compleat *ruin* for *life*![45]

The validity of equating concealment with murder was also questioned. Stripped of its connotations of moral depravity, separated from implications of sinfulness, and subjected to the scrutiny of lawyers who were increasingly concerned about the admission and weight of certain types of evidence, concealment came to be seen as no more than 'the lowest degree of presumptive evidence of felonious homicide',[46] and was interpreted as the natural response of any woman to a difficult situation. At the turn of the nineteenth century, just before the 1624 statute was repealed, Percival, who thought the statute to be humane in its attempt to protect bastards but too severe in its construction, wrote:

> The statute, indeed, which makes the concealment of the birth of a bastard child full proof of murder, confounds all distinctions of innocence and guilt, as such concealment, whenever practicable, would be the wish and act of all mothers, virtuous or vicious, under the same unhappy predicament.[47]

Of the attitudes embodied in the 1624 statute, the only one to survive with any force into the eighteenth century was the hostility towards the bearers of chargeable bastards. Locally, this attitude was responsible for the persistent accusation and prosecution of single women thought to have murdered their children but in the courts it was insufficient to justify convicting and hanging them: 'surely the only crime is the having been pregnant, which the law does not mean to punish with death'.[48]

Objections to the statute's severity prompted the courts to dispense with the statute and to try all women accused of murdering their newborn children according to common-law rules of evidence. The process was gradual but discussions of the offence in legal texts suggest that by the 1760s it was not common for women to be tried under the statute. Although texts published in the first half of the eighteenth century make no mention of the statute's severity nor of its replacement by common law, in 1766, Daines Barrington advised that 'no execution should be permitted, unless the criminal, convicted under this act, would have been guilty of murder by the common law'.[49] Two years later, William Blackstone suggested that the courts were by that time requiring evidence at common law that the child had been born alive and subsequently murdered before they would convict:

> it has of late been usual with us in England, upon trials for this offence, to require some sort of presumptive evidence that the child was born alive, before the other constrained presumption (that the child, whose death is concealed, was therefore killed by it's [*sic*] parent) is admitted to convict the prisoner.[50]

Clear indications as to whether cases were being tried according to the evidentiary standards of the statute or the common law are rare in the court records. The fact that very few women were convicted of child murder in the north of England during the eighteenth century supports the suggestion that the statute had fallen into disuse, and that the acquittal rate was due both to the leniency of judges and juries, and to the difficulties of proving the crime at common law. Given the general attitude to the statute by this time, and the high acquittal rate from these courts, it is likely that even those women who were explicitly indicted 'against the form of the Statute' were in fact tried at common law.

By the early 1770s, the statute's demise appears to have been complete. During the course of that decade, members of Parliament made four unsuccessful attempts to repeal the statute, arguing, on one occasion, 'that nothing could more strongly prove the absurdity and inexpediency of the law, than the impossibility of putting it in execution, under which the judges found themselves; that the laws were made to be executed, not dispensed with'.[51] The practice of dispensing with the statute was, however, welcomed by the jurist William Eden: 'The modern exposition of this statute is a good instance, that cruel laws have a natural tendency to their own dissolution in the abhorrence of mankind . . . These humane deviations from the harsh injunction of the statute have nearly amounted to a tacit abrogation of it.'[52]

By the 1760s and 1770s, therefore, the prosecution was once more having to demonstrate to the court's satisfaction that a child had been born alive before it could hope to prove that it had been murdered. It was precisely in these decades that medical testimony began to flourish, both at inquests and at trials. Although there had been discussions of medical evidence about still-birth, about marks of violence on the child's body, and about the various tests for live-birth for many years prior to the 1760s, it was in this period that medical evidence became a prominent issue both in and out of the courts. From this time onwards, the testimony of medical men played an increasingly critical role in investigations into newborn-child murder.

Of course, factors other than the decline of the statute encouraged medical involvement in the investigation of suspected child murders in the middle of the eighteenth century, perhaps the most important of which was the growing emphasis that was placed on the body generally as a source of knowledge during the course of the century.[53] However, it is noticeable that the blossoming of medical evidence in the courts, and the expansion of medical literature on tests for live-birth, coincided with the vigorous discussion, and decisive rejection, of the statute, and with a return to 'the Wisdom and Experience' of the common law.[54]

In trials at common law, the most important question was whether a supposedly murdered child had been born alive or dead. A number of signs indicating live-birth received some attention in both coroners' and trial courts: a child's cry; the clenched, or sometimes unclenched, state of a child's hands; the passage of meconium (the distinctive first bowel motion of a newborn infant); and the warmth of a child's body. But the test that attracted the most interest, and stimulated the most heated discussions, was the removal of a child's lungs to see if they floated in water. Although used occasionally in the courts in the early decades of the eighteenth century, the hydrostatic lung test came to prominence in the middle years of the century precisely when the courts were returning to common-law rules of evidence. As well as illustrating the extent of medical interest in this crime and the medico-legal problems faced by the courts, this test exemplifies the novel concern with the body as a source of evidence.

The differences between foetal and adult lungs had been known since Galen's comments in *De Usu Partium*.[55] The possible application of such differences to distinguish between live- and still-births was pointed out by William Harvey in 1653: 'And by this observation of the different complexion, you may discover whether a Mother brought her Childe alive or dead into the world; for instantly after inspiration the Lungs change colour:

which colour remains, though the fetus dye immediately after.'[56] In 1668, an English translation of Bartholin's work on anatomy included the observation that the substance of foetal lungs was 'compact and thick; so that in being cast into Water it sinks, which the Lungs of grown persons will not do'.[57] However, the sinking or swimming of the lungs in water does not appear to have been used in the courts in England until the early eighteenth century. There is no mention of the test in the first edition of William Cheselden's *The Anatomy of the Humane Body*, published in 1713, but the second edition of 1722 includes the following discussion:

> The Lungs of Animals before they have been dilated with Air, are specifically heavier than Water, but upon inflation they become specifically lighter and swim in Water; which experiment may be made to discover whether a Dead Child was Still Born or not; but if the Child has Breath'd but a little, and the experiment is made long after, the Lungs may be Collaps'd, and grow heavier than Water, as I have experimented, which may lead a Man to give a wrong Judgment in a Court of Judicature; but then it will be on the Charitable side of the Question.[58]

The origins of the forensic use of the test in England in Cheselden's time are unclear. The courts and medical practitioners may have been influenced by the extensive employment of the test in continental courts from the end of the seventeenth century,[59] or they may have been prompted to pursue the suggestions of Harvey and Bartholin as common-law trials became more frequent. By the 1730s, the test was commonly performed and presented in evidence at the Old Bailey: in 1737, a surgeon testified in court that 'The Coroner desired me to try the Experiment on the Lungs, which is commonly done on such Occasions.'[60] There is, however, no record of the test being used in the northern courts until the 1760s. In that decade and the next, the test was employed by nearly 50 per cent of medical practitioners, but thereafter it appears less frequently in the court records. But in spite of Bartholomew Parr's opinion, in 1809, that 'The English courts do not admit this experiment as evidence',[61] the lung test was performed at inquests and discussed in trials throughout the late eighteenth and nineteenth centuries, and it remains a topic of debate in modern textbooks of forensic medicine.[62]

Opinions differed with regard to the conclusions that could be drawn from the test. Some surgeons were convinced that the swimming of the lungs in water was certain proof of live-birth. In 1765, Richard Ferrly, giving evidence at an inquest in Westminster, stated that 'the lungs of the said child were inflated, and floated entirely upon the surface of the water, which is an incontestable proof that the child was born alive'.[63] Similarly, sinking of the lungs was interpreted by some surgeons as proof that the child had died before birth. An inquisition from 1775 stated that 'Mr

William Robinson Surgeon in Otley opened the Body of the said Child and took out the Lungs which immediately Sunk in Water from which Circumstance together with the Putrified appearance of Body he believes that the said Child had been dead some time before it was born.'[64]

In spite of the certainty expressed by some witnesses, the nature of the test and the validity of its conclusions were always subject to controversy. Even Cheselden's early discussion of the test was qualified by a warning about circumstances that could lead to error. When the statute lost its force, and the lung test became more widely used, an increasing number of medical practitioners expressed the opinion that it should be interpreted with caution. In 1774, a correspondent to *The Gentleman's Magazine* quoted a lecturer's opinion that although the test 'may sometimes prove true, upon the whole it should be regarded no other ways than as a very uncertain and precarious proof of the fact in question'.[65] At an inquest in Newcastle in 1775, William Smith testified that 'though he agrees with the general opinion of the Lungs swimming in Water as a sign of Air having been inflated into the Lungs and consequently that the Child was borne alive yet declares that he does not look upon this as an infallable [*sic*] Criterion'.[66]

Although Giovanni Battista Morgagni (whose work was published in English in 1769) and Samuel Farr, in 1788, both discussed circumstances in which the lungs of a live-born infant might sink in water,[67] concern about a mistake of this nature was limited by the knowledge that such an error would, as Cheselden had indicated, 'be on the Charitable side of the Question'. In an atmosphere of increasing leniency towards accused women, far more effort was expended in debating 'the material question, viz. in suspicious cases, how far may we conclude that the child was born alive, and probably murdered by its mother if the lungs swim in water?'[68]

All writers on the subject accepted that if the lungs swam, they must contain air. However, the presence of air in the lungs need not imply that the child had respired. The lungs could have been inflated by respiration, by putrefaction, or by efforts to resuscitate the child by blowing air into its mouth. Provided the test was confined to normal lungs, putrefaction need not pose a problem; close inspection and dissection of the corpse would determine whether the lungs or the rest of the body had undergone any decomposition and would distinguish between inspired air and the large collections of gas found in putrefied lungs. This principle was recognized at several inquests. In 1771, in a case in which the lungs floated, the coroner's jury commented that 'as the Body is turned into a State of Putrifaction the experiment is very Uncertain and not to be depended upon'.[69] In 1795, James Shaw, another Otley surgeon, deposed that 'Upon Opening the Body and taking out the Lungs they floated in Water, from all which

Appearances (the Child being perfectly fresh without the smallest Appearance of Putrefaction) It is my Opinion the said Child was born alive.'[70]

In his dissertation on drowning, published in 1746, the physician Rowland Jackson suggested that: 'The last Method of restoring still-born Children to Life is, to blow into their Mouths.'[71] In 1752, William Smellie agreed that the lungs of a still-born child could be expanded by blowing into its mouth with a cannula, having successfully resuscitated a child himself by that method.[72] Although a number of eighteenth-century writers were convinced that the lungs of a still-born child would swim in water if the child's mother had attempted to resuscitate it,[73] in the early years of the nineteenth century there was some reluctance to accept that resuscitation attempts could inflate the lungs sufficiently to cause them to float.[74] To a large extent, the question was academic. The matter appears only once in the northern court records, when, in 1764, a surgeon, finding that the lungs of Jane Stuart's child swam in water, concluded that the child had been born alive. Jane testified to the magistrate that 'so soon as she was able after the birth of the said Child which might be two or three Minutes she Blew into the Mouth of the said Child but could not perceive any signs of Life in it'.[75]

In the absence of putrefaction, and of any attempt to resuscitate the child, many surgeons inferred that a child whose lungs floated in water had been born alive. This conclusion was complicated, however, by the fact that in English law a child was not deemed to have been born until its body (excluding the umbilical cord and placenta) had been completely expelled from its mother. In the context of newborn-child murder this had two important implications. First, it meant that a mother who killed her child during birth could not be indicted for murder. Second, it followed that a child that had breathed during birth and died before complete expulsion had legally been born dead. It was, therefore, feasible that a child whose lungs were found to float in water could nevertheless have been still-born. At the trial of Mary Wilson in 1737, a surgeon testified that:

> On trying the Experiment upon the Lungs of this Child, they floated on the Water: But I think the Certainty of this Experiment may have Objections to it. As for instance, where a Child hath stuck in the Birth a few Minutes, if it comes in the natural Way, it may respire and breath a little; which Respiration may make the Lungs specifically lighter than the Water, yet the Child may die before 'tis born.[76]

This aspect of the lung test was extensively discussed in the trial courts, particularly in the middle decades of the century. It led some witnesses to limit their conclusions to the opinion that the child had breathed, without affirming that this constituted live-birth. In the early years of the nineteenth century, the idea that a child might be strong enough to breathe during birth yet die before complete expulsion was regarded by Parr as 'a fancy within the verge of possibility only, but too improbable to induce us to enlarge on it'.[77] But in the middle of the eighteenth century, medical witnesses, examined by the courts, acknowledged the possibility and were reluctant to conclude that a child had been born alive purely on the basis of the lung test.

William Hunter also doubted whether even evidence of live-birth should be accepted as evidence of murder. In his paper 'On the Uncertainty of the Signs of Murder, in the Case of Bastard Children', published in 1784, he suggested that many newborn children 'from circumstances in their constitution, or in the nature of the labour, are but barely alive; and after breathing a minute or two, or an hour or two, die in spite of all our attention. And why may not that misfortune happen to a woman who is brought to bed by herself?'[78] Inquest juries in the north of England often returned verdicts of natural death or still-birth at the end of the eighteenth century, and the possibility of a child dying naturally during birth or soon afterwards further weakened the force of the lung test.

In general, the courts' handling of the medical evidence, and the caution advised by medical writers, demonstrate a reluctance to accept the lung test as conclusive when the life of an accused woman was in the balance. At the trial of Mary Wilson in 1737, for example, a surgeon testified that 'without some other Circumstances to corroborate this Experiment, I should be loth to determine thereby positively. I think the Experiment (where a Person's Life is at Stake) too slight to be built upon.'[79] Although some medical witnesses did express the opinion that swimming of the lungs indicated live-birth, and although some writers, particularly at the end of the century, were critical of the arguments put forward against the test, the test was never established as anything more than 'very inconclusive evidence'.[80] In 1755, one surgeon even refused to perform the test at an inquest because the coroner expected a 'final answer' from it:

> The coroner asked me whether I thought the child was born alive? I said it was very difficult to distinguish that. After that he said, will you try the experiment upon the lungs? And there was water brought up. I asked him what he did expect upon that? He said, for me to give a final answer, whether it was born alive or not. Then I declined it, as looking upon it not conclusive.[81]

To a large extent, the lung test's inability to provide the courts with sufficient certainty about live- and still-birth stemmed from the sentiments that had encouraged its use in the first place. Dissatisfaction with the severity of the 1624 statute, and growing leniency towards accused women, had prompted the courts to require common-law standards of evidence before convicting for murder. The same leniency prompted medical practitioners to object to swimming of the lungs being taken as certain proof of live-birth when a capital sentence might depend upon it. Letters and books arguing for cautious use of the lung test in the 1760s, 1770s and 1780s, were written from the same viewpoint as those arguing for cautious use, or repeal, of the 1624 statute. Although inspired by the prosecution's need to prove live-birth, the lung test almost invariably assisted the defence by increasing the court's doubts about live-birth, and by providing some justification for juries' reluctance to convict accused women on the basis of circumstantial evidence alone.

It would be a mistake, however, to ascribe the test's inability to clarify the issue of live-birth solely to leniency, on the part of either medical practitioners or the courts. Doubts about the test's conclusiveness were also generated by the legal problems inherent in establishing guilt at common law. Legal definitions of birth, live-birth, and still-birth, and the absence of any legal protection of a child during birth, rendered even the clearest medical evidence doubtful.[82] It is interesting that medical witnesses expressed more doubts about the test in the trial courts than in the coroners' courts, especially when they were examined by the court or by counsel. While this caution may have reflected an awareness of the punishment that could be imposed by the trial courts, it is also possible that the assize judges' greater awareness of the evidential problems involved rapidly exposed any uncertainty or indecision on the part of medical witnesses.

Acceptance of the test was also hampered by the lack of a standard procedure for its performance. Different surgeons performed the test in different ways, each of which could lead to errors of judgement. While some surgeons immersed the whole lungs in water, sometimes with the heart attached, others immersed them separately, or divided them into lobes or smaller sections before testing them. Although the advantages and disadvantages of performing the test in different ways were discussed in various works by continental authors, some of which were available in English,[83] no attempts were made to develop a standard procedure for the test during the eighteenth century and it is not surprising that practitioners differed in their assessment of the test's certainty and fallibility.

In spite of doubts about the lung test's validity, both coroners' and trial courts regularly employed medical witnesses to perform the test and to interpret its results. In addition, the test was acknowledged and discussed by legal writers. In 1766, Daines Barrington, then Recorder of Bristol, referred to the test in a footnote to his comments on the 1624 statute.[84] And in the 1791 edition of Gilbert's *Law of Evidence*, Capel Lofft, a barrister, discussed surgical opinion on the lung test as an example of 'Proof by Experts'.[85] Although Lofft recognized that the test was unable to establish with certainty that a child had been born live, his comments highlight the extent to which the lung test, and medical testimony, had become accepted by the courts.

Awareness of the importance of medical evidence in cases of newborn-child murder contributed to, and was in turn enhanced by, the resurgence of the inquest as the major form of pre-trial inquiry in these cases. When medical evidence derived from the examination of the bodies of dead children became prominent in a new way in the middle of the eighteenth century, the coroner's remit to investigate suspicious deaths only 'upon view of a body' made the inquest the obvious forum for the initial presentation of this evidence. The inquest, however, provided more than a simple forum. By specifically requesting that the lung test be performed, and by examining medical witnesses, the coroner and his jury also encouraged debate about the validity of medical evidence and assisted in the dissemination of medico-legal knowledge.

The effect of this process on the status of the inquest is evident. Inquests were held, and dissections performed, even when the infants' bodies exhibited no marks of violence and when the probability of natural death might have deterred further inquiry. In addition, an increasing number of inquest verdicts of still-birth and natural death were no longer overruled by magistrates. During the first half of the eighteenth century, it was usual for magistrates to direct inquiries into cases of suspected child murder and it was not uncommon for them to bring cases to trial despite an inquest verdict of 'still-birth'. The court records, however, show a definite decline in their activities in these cases from the 1760s, and by the end of the eighteenth century investigations into suspicious infant deaths were carried out far more frequently by coroners and their juries than by justices of the peace.[86] It is significant that the declining involvement of justices of the peace in such cases, and the rise of the inquest, became most apparent in the 1760s, precisely when the need for medical evidence became prominent. After this date, magistrates' inquiries were usually confined to cases in which there was no body, and where the coroner therefore had no jurisdiction.

By the end of the eighteenth century, medical evidence and coroners' inquests were both established as essential components of investigations into the suspected murders of newborn children. In 1803, when Lord Ellenborough introduced the repeal of the 1624 statute, he suggested that the problems involved in prosecuting women for murdering their newborn bastard children were due to the fact that 'the judges were obliged to strain the law for the sake of lenity, and to admit the slightest suggestion that the child was still-born as evidence of the fact'. His solution was to repeal the law as it then stood and to enact 'that evidence should first be duly admitted, that such bastard child was, or was not, born living, previous to the final decision upon any trial'.[87] By authorizing a return to common law, and by establishing an official requirement for evidence about live- and still-birth, the 1803 Act was simply endorsing the evidential rules and procedures, including the routine admission of medical testimony, that had been adopted in both coroners' and trial courts since the middle of the eighteenth century.

NOTES

1 See, for example, J. D. J. Havard, *The Detection of Secret Homicide: A Study of the Medico-Legal Investigation of Sudden Death* (London, 1960), pp. 11–36.
2 Matthew Hale, *History of the Pleas of the Crown* (1736), vol. II, p. 222; Edward Umfreville, *Lex Coronatoria: Or, the Office and Duty of Coroners* (London, 1761), p. v.
3 On Hale's influence, see Havard, *Secret Homicide*, pp. 39–42.
4 Ibid., pp. 1–10.
5 'An Act for the Attendance and Remuneration of Medical Witnesses at Coroners' Inquests', 1836 (6 & 7 Will. IV c. 29).
6 On these issues, see T. R. Forbes, *Surgeons at the Bailey: English Forensic Medicine to 1878* (New Haven and London, 1985), pp. 1–48.
7 The term 'infanticide', frequently used by historians, does not appear in seventeenth- and eighteenth-century court records, which refer instead to 'the murder of a bastard child', 'the murder of a new-born infant bastard', or a similar phrase.
8 Havard, *Secret Homicide*, pp. 6–7. For the text of the statute, see below, pp. 66–7.
9 For the punishments that could be inflicted on bastard-bearers, see 18 Eliz. c. 3 (1576) and 7 Jac.I c. 4 (1610); for the relevant poor-law legislation, see 39 Eliz. c. 3 (1597) and 43 Eliz. c. 2 (1601).
10 In 1580, sentence of death was passed for an infant's murder even though 'it was not directly proved the child was in life' (a clerk's note). Quoted by J. S. Cockburn in 'Trial by the book? Fact and theory in the criminal process, 1558–1625', in J. H. Baker, ed., *Legal Records and the Historian* (London, 1978), pp. 60–79.
11 The 1624 statute was applicable only to the mothers of bastards. By virtue of the strong presumption of legitimacy concerning children born in lawful wedlock, the majority of women tried under the statute were single women. The mothers of legitimate children, and the few men accused of the crime, were still tried at common law.
12 *House of Commons Journal* [*HCJ*], 1 (1607), pp. 368, 370, 1040, 1042; *HCJ*, 1 (1610), p. 421; *HCJ*, 1 (1624), pp. 769, 778, 786, 793, 796. The 1624 statute was continued by 3 Car.I c. 4 and 16 Car.I c. 4 until its repeal in 1803. For comments on the possible origins of the statute, see Daines Barrington, *Observations on the Statutes, Chiefly the More Ancient* (London, 1766), p. 427; Thomas Percival, *Medical Ethics* (Manchester, 1803), p. 80; and P. C. Hoffer and N. E. H. Hull, *Murdering Mothers: Infanticide in England and New England 1558–1803* (New York, 1981), ch. 1.

13 Umfreville, *Lex Coronatoria*, p. 45.
14 Zachary Babington was insistent on this point in *Advice to Grand Jurors in Cases of Blood* (1677), p. 173. But see the misconstruction in, for example, Thomas Wood, *An Institute of the Laws of England*, 5th edn (London, 1734), p. 355, and R. W. Malcomson, 'Infanticide in the eighteenth century', in J. S. Cockburn, ed., *Crime in England 1550–1800* (Princeton, 1977), pp. 187–209.
15 Umfreville, *Lex Coronatoria*, p. 46; E. H. East, *A Treatise of the Pleas of the Crown* (London, 1803), vol. I, p. 228.
16 Percivall Willughby, *Observations in Midwifery*, ed. H. Blenkinsop, (Warwick, 1972; 1st edn 1863), pp. 11–12.
17 The case of Hannah Frost, 1762; the depositions of the surgeon and other witnesses are in the Northern Circuit court records in the Public Record Office (hereafter PRO), ASSI 45 26/6/22–3.
18 Ruth Peacock, 1793, PRO/ASSI 45 38/1/141–2.
19 Deborah Greening, *Old Bailey Sessions Papers* (hereafter, *OBSP*), Feb. 1725, p. 1. For an account of the *OBSP*, see p. 170 below.
20 For a discussion of the intrusion of men into the practice of midwifery in this period, see Jean Donnison, *Midwives and Medical Men, A History of Inter-Professional Rivalries and Women's Rights* (London, 1977), chs. 1 and 2. The rise of man-midwifery is evident in the records of child murder investigations.
21 PRO/ASSI 44/106iii.
22 Jane Todd, *OBSP*, July 1727, p. 2.
23 'Old-Bedlams [*sc*: beldams], or pretended Midwives', Defoe pointed out, had 'got the ready rote of swearing the Child was not at its full Growth, for which they have a hidden Reserve, that is to say, the Child was not at Man's or Woman's Growth'. Daniel Defoe, *The Generous Protector, or a Friendly Proposal to prevent Murder and other enormous Abuses, By erecting an Hospital for Foundlings and Bastard-Children* (London, 1731), p. 9.
24 In 1789, a surgeon testified that a child had been born in about the sixth month of gestation, a degree of prematurity usually accepted as proving still-birth. But the jury, perhaps influenced by marks of violence, found that the child had been born alive and wilfully murdered; Dorothy Henderson, 1789, PRO/ASSI 45 36/3/84 and ASSI 44/104ii.
25 For an example of the recognized association between hair, nails and prematurity in 1574, see Alan Macfarlane, 'Illegitimacy and illegitimates in English history', in P. Laslett, K. Oosterveen, and R. Smith, eds., *Bastardy and its Comparative History* (London, 1980), pp. 71–85.
26 Hale, *Pleas of the Crown*, vol. II, p. 289.
27 J. A. Sharpe, *Crime in Seventeenth-Century England: A County Study* (Cambridge, 1983), pp. 134–7.
28 Willughby, *Observations in Midwifery*, p. 274.
29 Defoe, *Generous Protector*, pp. 9–10.
30 Figures for the north of England are taken from the Northern Circuit records between 1720 and 1799. For a discussion of the conviction rates at the Old Bailey and in Staffordshire, see Malcolmson, 'Infanticide in the eighteenth century'; for Surrey, J. M. Beattie, *Crime and the Courts in England 1660–1800* (Oxford, 1986), pp. 117–19.
31 A footnote to the trial report of Elizabeth Shudrick, *OBSP*, Oct. 1743, pp. 276–7.

32 Hale, *Pleas of the Crown*, vol. II, pp. 288–9; William Hawkins, *A Treatise of the Pleas of the Crown* (London, 1716–21), vol. II, pp. 438–9; Richard Burn, *The Justice of the Peace, and Parish Officer*, 3rd edn (London, 1756), p. 90; Umfreville, *Lex Coronatoria*, pp. 44–7.

33 Sir John Kelyng, *A Report of divers cases in Pleas of the Crown, adjudged and determined in the reign of . . . Charles II* (London, 1708), pp. 32–3; Hale, *Pleas of the Crown*, vol. II, p. 289; Hawkins, *Treatise of the Pleas of the Crown*, vol. II, p. 438.

34 Margaret Wanless, 1742, in PRO/ASSI 44/57.

35 Ann Masie, *OBSP*, July 1717, p. 4. The statute was also read at the trial of Ann Price at the Old Bailey in 1681 (*OBSP*, April 1681): 'but the concealing of the Child being a material Point of Evidence against her; upon the reciting the Statute, she was found guilty of Murther.'

36 Susannah Stephenson, 1741, in PRO/ASSI 44/56 (my italics).

37 See, for example, the questions asked of Martha Gleadhill by Grace Ditch, a midwife, in 1749, in PRO/ASSI 45 24/1/38A; and the deposition of Catherine Coulson taken before a magistrate investigating the death of Rebecca Stephenson's child, in PRO/ASSI 45 24/2/105–8.

38 Kelyng, *Report of divers cases*, pp. 32–3.

39 East, *Pleas of the Crown*, vol. I, p. 228, referring to a case at the Old Bailey in 1689.

40 Ibid., p. 229, referring to the trial of Jane Peat at Exeter in 1793.

41 It remains unclear to what extent widespread awareness of these exceptions enabled women to exploit the statute's limitations. Evidence concerning the preparation of linen, often instrumental in securing acquittal, was clearly open to abuse.

42 Bernard Mandeville, *The Fable of the Bees: Or, Private Vices, Publick Benefits*, 6th edn (London, 1732), reprinted with commentary by F. B. Kaye (Oxford, 1924), vol. I, pp. 74–6.

43 Letter from Erasmus Darwin, 1767, reproduced in D. King-Hele, ed., *The Letters of Erasmus Darwin* (Cambridge, 1981), pp. 41–2.

44 Percival, *Medical Ethics*, p. 84.

45 William Hunter, 'On the uncertainty of the signs of murder, in the case of bastard children', *Medical Observations and Inquiries*, 6 (1784), 269–70.

46 Percival, *Medical Ethics*, p. 81.

47 Ibid., pp. 84–5.

48 Hunter, 'On the uncertainty of the signs', p. 286.

49 Barrington, *Observations on the Statutes*, p. 424.

50 William Blackstone, *Commentaries on the Laws of England* (Oxford, 1769), vol. IV, p. 198.

51 *Hansard's Parliamentary History*, vol. XVII, col. 453.

52 William Eden, *Principles of Penal Law*, 2nd edn (London, 1771), pp. 15–16.

53 The bodies of both dead infants and suspects were increasingly exposed to the view of medical practitioners. For wider perspectives on this, particularly relating to gender, see L. J. Jordanova, 'Gender, generation and science: William Hunter's obstetrical atlas', in W. F. Bynum and Roy Porter, eds., *William Hunter and the Eighteenth-Century Medical World* (Cambridge, 1985),

pp. 385–412; Jordanova, *Sexual Visions: Images of Gender in Science and Medicine Between the Eighteenth and Twentieth Centuries* (Hemel Hempstead, 1989).

54 See Michael Foster's comments in 1762 on the superiority of the common law over 'Penal Statutes made upon special and pressing Occasions, and savouring rankly of the Times': *A Report of Some Proceedings on the Commission of Oyer and Terminer . . . to which are added Discourses upon a Few Branches of the Crown Law* (Oxford, 1762), pp. 299–300.

55 Galen, *De Usu Partium*, trans. Margaret Tallmadge May (New York, 1968), vol. II, bk 15, p. 670. Galen's comments were referred to by Giovanni Battista Morgagni in his discussion of the lung test in *The Seats and Causes of Diseases*, trans. Benjamin Alexander (London, 1769), vol. I, bk 2, p. 536.

56 William Harvey, *Anatomical Exercitations, Concerning the Generation of Living Creatures* (London, 1653), p. 435.

57 *Bartholinus Anatomy; made from the Precepts of his Father*, (London, 1668), p. 117.

58 William Cheselden, *The Anatomy of the Humane Body* (London, 1722), p. 156. This passage was repeated in subsequent editions of the work in the eighteenth century.

59 R. P. Brittain, 'The hydrostatic and similar tests of live birth: a historical review', *Medico-Legal Journal*, 31 (1963), 189–94.

60 Mary Wilson, *OBSP*, April 1737, p. 90.

61 Bartholomew Parr, *The London Medicinal Dictionary* (London, 1809), vol. II, p. 181.

62 See, for example, Alan A. Watson, *Forensic Medicine: A Handbook for Professionals* (Aldershot, 1989), pp. 273–4.

63 Quoted in G. I. Greenwald and M. W. Greenwald, 'Medicolegal progress in inquests of felonious deaths, Westminster, 1761–1866', *Journal of Legal Medicine*, 2 (1981), 193–264.

64 From an inquisition taken before Thomas Parkinson at Leathley in Yorkshire, 6 November 1775, in PRO/ASSI 44/91i.

65 *The Gentleman's Magazine*, October 1774, pp. 462–3.

66 Mary Hills, 1775, PRO/ASSI 45 32/1/121. William Smith gave the same opinion at another inquest that year: Elizabeth Bryson, 1775, PRO/ASSI 45 32/1/38.

67 Morgagni, *Seats and Causes of Diseases*, vol. I, bk 2, pp. 536–7; Samuel Farr, *Elements of Medical Jurisprudence* (London, 1788), p. 59.

68 Hunter, 'On the uncertainty of the signs', p. 284.

69 From an inquisition taken in Yorkshire, before Thomas Parkinson, in PRO/ASSI 44/86ii.

70 Ann Gibson, 1795, PRO/ASSI 45 38/3/45–6.

71 Rowland Jackson, *A Physical Dissertation on Drowning* (London, 1746), p. 79.

72 William Smellie, *A Treatise on the Theory and Practice of Midwifery* (London, 1752), p. 226; ibid., 1764 edn, vol. II, p. 384.

73 Hunter, 'On the uncertainty of the signs', p. 285; Morgagni, *Seats and Causes of Diseases*, vol. I, bk 2, p. 538; Farr, *Elements of Medical Jurisprudence*, p. 59.

74 Parr, *London Medicinal Dictionary*, vol. II, p. 181.

75 Jane Stuart, 1764, PRO/ASSI 45 27/2/142–4.

76 Mary Wilson, *OBSP*, April 1737, pp. 90–1.

77 Parr, *London Medicinal Dictionary*, vol. II, p. 181.
78 Hunter, 'On the uncertainty of the signs', pp. 287–8.
79 Mary Wilson, *OBSP*, April 1737, p. 91.
80 Mary Robinson, *OBSP*, Feb.–March 1768, p. 107.
81 Frances Palser, *OBSP*, July 1755, p. 239.
82 For discussions of these problems, see Stanley B. Atkinson, 'Life, birth, and live-birth', *Law Quarterly Review*, 78 (1904), 134–59; D. Seaborne Davies, 'Child-killing in English law', *Modern Law Review*, 1 (1937), 203–23.
83 Morgagni, *Seats and Causes of Diseases*, vol. I, bk 2, p. 537; review of M. Portal, *Mémoire dans lequel on démontre l'action du Poumon sur l'Aorte, pendant le temps de la Respiration; et ou l'on prouve que dans l'Enfant qui vient de naître, le Poumon droit respire avant le gauche* (1769), *Medical and Philosophical Commentaries*, 1 (1773), 409–12.
84 Barrington, *Observations on the Statutes*, p. 424.
85 Lord Chief Baron Gilbert, *The Law of Evidence*, 'considerably enlarged by Capel Lofft' (London, 1791), vol. I, p. 301.
86 The relative importance of the inquest over the magistrate's inquiry cannot be attributed simply to the improved survival of coroners' records following the 1752 'Act for giving a proper Reward to Coroners' (25 Geo.II, c. 29). The number of suspected child murder cases in which coroners were involved was already increasing before that date, and the records of justices of the peace, which were unaffected by the 1752 statute, show a definite decline in magistrates' inquiries from the 1760s. See M. A. Jackson, 'New-born child murder: a study of suspicion, evidence, and proof in eighteenth-century England', Ph.D thesis, University of Leeds, 1992, ch. 4 and app. C.
87 *Hansard, The Parliamentary History of England from the Earliest Period to the Year 1803* (London, 1820), vol. XXXVI, col. 1246. The repealing Act was 43 Geo.III c. 58.

II

The growth of a science

4

Legalizing medicine: early modern legal systems and the growth of medico-legal knowledge

CATHERINE CRAWFORD

It has long been remarked that Britain lagged nearly two centuries behind continental Europe in developing a science of forensic medicine. In his 'Early history of legal medicine' (1950–1), Erwin Ackerknecht cited more than a dozen monographs on medico-legal problems published in France and Italy during the late sixteenth and early seventeenth centuries. Thereafter, German publications began to multiply, and 'there was in Germany during the 18th century an almost uninterrupted production of treatises on legal medicine'. By contrast, wrote Ackerknecht, the English contribution to the science of forensic medicine before 1800 was 'practically nil'.[1] Subsequent research has identified a few more English writings on the subject,[2] but the paucity of English medico-legal literature in the early modern period in comparison with that of the Continent remains striking.[3]

England did not lack medico-legal activity. Between 1730 and 1760, medical testimony was heard at more than half the homicide trials at the Old Bailey, the main criminal court for London and Middlesex.[4] It was also not uncommon in America and northern England in the seventeenth and eighteenth centuries, as the first three chapters of this book show. The medical questions that arose in legal proceedings were rather different from those encountered in private practice, yet English medical and legal literature provided practitioners and magistrates with very little guidance on the subject. This chapter attempts to account for both the rarity of medico-legal studies in early modern England and the relative abundance of such publications in Italy, France and especially Germany. I shall argue that differences between legal systems were a crucial factor. Roman-canon law fostered the development of medico-legal science, whereas English common law tended to discourage it.

In the past decade or so, revisionist historiography has shown that English law was never quite so peculiar or insular as lawyers and legal historians have tended to portray it.[5] Moreover, work on continental trial records of the seventeenth and eighteenth centuries has revealed that differences in trial procedure between England and the rest of Europe did not in practice produce such dissimilar outcomes in criminal trials as was previously thought.[6] One clearly differing outcome, however, is the development of a substantial medico-legal literature in one context and not in the other. By tracing the relations between legal systems and the science of forensic medicine in early modern Europe, I hope to show that a comparative approach can enhance our understanding of particular medico-legal cultures, as well as of the development of forensic medicine as a body of knowledge. I shall focus on four aspects of legal procedure in the Roman-canon tradition: the official status given to medical experts; the law of proof and the extensive literature on evidence that it produced; the French system of judicial review and appeal; and the German procedure of *Aktenversendung*, whereby university medical faculties were consulted directly by the courts.

The status of medical experts

On one level, the dearth of English texts on forensic medicine before 1800 can be understood as reflecting a lack of enthusiasm among English medical practitioners for this type of practice. For example, at an Old Bailey trial in 1740, a surgeon of St Bartholemew's Hospital told the court how he came to testify. He had returned home one day to find a crowd of people waiting outside his door. He suspected that there had been a violent quarrel, 'and so I would have passed by, but some People in the Croud knew me, and would not let me'; he was therefore obliged to treat the injured man and to give evidence when the wounds proved fatal and the matter came to trial.[7] A similar attempt at evasion was acknowledged at a murder trial in 1678. The London physician Richard Lower testified that he had declined to attend an autopsy in the hope of avoiding an appearance in court:

> LOWER: [W]hen I came I found him dying, and seeing no hopes of his recovery, left him; I was desired to be present at the dissection, but because of the rumour of this business, I said it would be a troublesome matter, and therefore would purposely avoid it.
> L.H.ST [judge]: So you did not see him dissected?
> LOWER: No, my lord. I did fear being troubled, and would have avoided it, but could not, it seems, for I am here come to testify this.[8]

Elizabeth Mayle, a London midwife, was equally candid about having refused to examine a suspected rape victim lest she become involved in criminal proceedings. Mayle testified at the trial of Elizabeth Canning for perjury in 1754:

> I left her mother an order to give her a glyster: she said, Will you examine her body, to see if she has been hurted? I said, No; I never was before the face of a judge in the Old-Bailey in my life, and I did not care to be in dirty work.[9]

According to Thomas Percival, writing in 1794, such disobliging attitudes on the part of medical practitioners were a common cause of complaint among magistrates, coroners and judges.[10] Percival's claim seems to be borne out by the fact that in Edward Umfreville's handbook for coroners, published in 1761, the sample warrant 'against a Witness for Contempt of Summons' is for the purpose of compelling a surgeon to attend an inquest.[11]

In Percival's experience, medico-legal investigations were 'generally painful, always inconvenient, and occasion[ed] an interruption to business of a nature not to be easily appreciated or compensated.'[12] Merely testifying could be onerous. Even when trials were heard in a specified order, which was not always the case, the rate at which the court would get through the list could not be predicted and a witness could be kept waiting for a long time.[13] In 1780, the physician John Monro spent several days at the Old Bailey waiting for a case to come up, 'at great inconvenience'.[14] Monro was waiting to testify on behalf of a defendant, and at the trial only; witnesses for the prosecution usually had to appear before two separate tribunals (an inquest and a grand jury hearing) before the trial itself. As the surgeon John Foot observed after taking part in a homicide trial in 1768, 'the coroner's jury, the grand jury, and the petit jury at the Old-Bailey were accompanied with disagreeable circumstances enough to make anyone wish to decline such sort of attendance.'[15] Foot went on to say that William Bromfield, the St George's Hospital surgeon who had treated the victim in this case before the man's death, freely admitted that he had refused to come to the post-mortem when summoned by the coroner 'because he apprehended it might be an *Old Bailey* business'.[16] Bromfield had sent two pupils in his place. However, the fact that all these practitioners, including Bromfield, did eventually testify shows that they were unable to avoid appearing in court. Like any other witness, a medical practitioner with firsthand knowledge of a case could be subpoenaed, and the penalties for not appearing were considerable – often as much as £20 at the Old Bailey in the mid-eighteenth century.[17]

While English medical witnesses could thus be fined for not obeying a summons, until the Medical Witnesses' Act of 1836 there was no legal provision for paying them for testifying.[18] An Elizabethan statute stated that witnesses living at a distance could not be penalized for non-appearance unless they were paid reasonable expenses beforehand, and statutes enacted in 1751 and 1753 empowered judges to compensate very poor witnesses at felony trials, but medical practitioners residing locally would not have qualified for these small sums.[19] Dudley Ryder's personal notes on the trials he presided over in the 1750s describe a case of medical resistance to the perceived injustice of the medical witness's position. It was a trial for assault and battery in which a surgeon, who had treated the victim and been summoned for the prosecution, made a determined attempt to withhold his evidence until he had been paid for attending the trial. However, Ryder was having none of it, and the surgeon was eventually obliged to capitulate.[20] A medical man brought in to assist the defence, like the alienist Monro in the trial mentioned above, was probably paid by the defendant or his family, but most medical witnesses were subpoenaed and were therefore in no position to demand any payment for attending trials.

Little is known about the terms on which practitioners who had no previous involvement with a case were commissioned to conduct medico-legal investigations. A comment in Umfreville's guide for coroners indicates that surgeons with parish contracts for treating the sick poor might be expected to assist at inquests as part of their duties, but that this was an area of contention:

> If the Parish Surgeon shall refuse to attend without being paid, (and this I have known objected) you may then direct your Warrant to the Church Wardens and Overseers of the Parish where the Inquest is taking [place], to procure and send one.[21]

Joan Lane's research on medical practice in eighteenth-century Warwickshire confirms that local overseers of the poor did sometimes hire medical practitioners to do medico-legal work.[22] In 1766 the parish of Allesley paid a Dr Gibbons £4 for 'attending Inquest at Warwick', a sum which would have included his travel expenses and perhaps overnight accommodation. The Aston Cantlow overseers paid a Dr Burman 10s 6d for his part in an inquest in 1794; the overseers of Bedworth paid Richard Brown a guinea in 1800 for 'attending and inspecting the body of Jacques and attending the Inquest'. These sums are not derisory: they compare favourably with the fees laid down by Parliament in 1836.[23] It is likely, though, that the willingness of parish officers to commission and pay for medico-legal work varied greatly according to individual overseers, changing local financial circumstances, and the perceived importance of particular corpses. Remuneration of this kind was in any case completely discretionary, and may well have been seen as an uncertainty rather than a routine procedure. It was Percival's opinion that medico-legal tasks should be 'regarded as appropriate debts to the community, which neither equity nor patriotism will allow to be cancelled', and many early modern practitioners doubtless performed them in this spirit. It seems reasonable to conclude, however, that English medical practitioners did not consider forensic medicine a very attractive or lucrative area of professional practice.

In continental Europe, by contrast, medico-legal work appears to have been actively sought after as a privilege. It was performed by practitioners whose qualifications, duties and emoluments were typically regulated by statute, and was frequently restricted to a designated elite. Laws enacted in Bologna as early as 1292 limited medico-legal reporting to a named group of doctors over the age of thirty who were 'wisest and most worthy in the sciences of surgery and medicine'; in 1298 Magister Bonnesegna, who was under thirty, petitioned for the age requirement to be waived in his case on account of his exceptional knowledge and skill.[24] In fourteenth-century Barcelona, when Francesc de Pla was named as the sole physician authorized to accompany surgeons in their legal investigations of wounds, the other physicians in Barcelona protested that his monopoly was against their interests.[25] The desirability of medico-legal employment is also attested by the wording of a Venetian ruling in fourteenth-century Crete, where Officers of the Night were permitted to hire only the official town doctors for wound investigations; the ruling observed that hiring ordinary physicians to examine wounds for legal purposes was 'at the expense of the benefit and dignity of the paid [official] physicians'.[26]

French edicts and decrees also indicate that practitioners considered medico-legal work to be well worth having. As early as 1311, officially appointed surgeons were given exclusive rights to perform medico-legal investigations in Paris,[27] while an edict of 1603/1606 expressly prohibited all but sworn surgeons (*chirurgiens jurés*) from making legal reports in other French towns.[28] It is clear from subsequent legislation that other practitioners wanted the right to make official reports. The criminal code of 1670 relaxed the earlier prohibitions by allowing ordinary surgeons to make official reports on the living wounded, though not post-mortem or other legal reports; however, a further decree of 1692 withdrew this concession. According to the preamble to the 1692 legislation, both laws were occasioned by complaints and conflicts among surgeons over the right to make medico-legal assessments.[29] The 1670 code also referred to reports by physicians, but because a permanent office of sworn physician did not exist outside Paris at the time, no provincial physicians possessed special authority to make reports. This evidently led to problems, for the edict of 1692, which created the office of sworn physician (*médecin juré*) in each town, announced that it was necessary to do so in order 'to stop the conflicts which occur daily' over the medico-legal work of physicians.[30] Wrangling over the right to make statutory reports nevertheless continued.[31]

The key to all this enthusiasm seems to have been the fact that medico-legal work was relatively well paid. It was at least as remunerative as normal private practice in fifteenth-century Florence.[32] A French scale of obligatory payments for specific tasks, laid down in 1671, also compared favourably with what could be earned in ordinary practice; a royal edict of 1742 increased these rates because, according to the edict, the prescribed fees had depreciated and actual payments had come to vary considerably.[33] Furthermore, payment for medico-legal work could apparently be relied upon. A ruling in thirteenth-century Bologna, which specified statutory fees for medico-legal reports, directed that they were to be paid by the offender or, if that source were not forthcoming, by the city treasury.[34] French medical reports of the eighteenth century are sometimes accompanied by a magistrate's order for payment.[35] In most continental jurisdictions, medical reports had to be made on all suspected homicides and, in France, on all cases of drowning and wounding, including accidents, so there was potentially a lot of work to be had by those fortunate enough to be nominated to a medico-legal office.[36]

The official, well-paid position of continental medical experts was certainly more favourable to the growth of medico-legal knowledge than were the more informal, *ad hoc* arrangements that existed in England.[37] But the importance of this factor in fostering a science of legal medicine in continental countries should not be overstated. The fact that medico-legal work was lucrative, fairly plentiful, and much sought after in Roman-canon jurisdictions did not necessarily lead to research and publication on medico-legal matters. Moreover, the fact that the qualifications of experts were formally regulated by no means guaranteed the quality of their work, for complaints that surgeons' reports were superficial and faulty were not uncommon in seventeenth- and eighteenth-century France.[38] The development of forensic medicine as a body of knowledge was encouraged far more directly by other features of Roman-canon legal systems. The following sections outline the differences between Roman-canon law and common law in matters of proof and trial procedure, tracing their implications for medico-legal practice and for the production of works on medico-legal science.

Modes of proof

In early medieval Europe, including Britain, the disputed facts in a criminal trial were usually decided by ordeal or combat. Divine intervention was thought to ensure that the truth would be revealed by the outcome of battle, submersion in water (the innocent sank), or exposure to fire (the flesh of the innocent healed quickly).[39] During the twelfth century, however, the Church became increasingly sceptical about these methods of proof, and in 1215 the Fourth Lateran Council effectively abolished ordeals by forbidding priests to participate in them.[40] In England, trial by jury, which was already in limited use in the form of the jury of accusation, was extended to replace ordeals. The statement of twelve local men under oath thus came to be accepted in England as the authoritative judgment on questions of fact.[41]

Early English jurors combined the functions of witness and arbiter of fact. Being from the neighbourhood, they were expected to have personal knowledge of the circumstances surrounding an alleged crime and to decide on the basis of that knowledge. It is probable that jurors also obtained information privately from people whom they trusted.[42] Like the judgment by ordeal, the verdict of a trial jury was a simple pronouncement, for which no rationale was given. Then as now, juries deliberated in private, and the reasoning they employed was not ordinarily disclosed to anyone.[43] In the words of Frederic Maitland, the common law accepted 'the rough verdict of the countryside, without caring to investigate the logical processes, if logical they were, of which that verdict was the outcome'.[44] The English standard of proof was thus in effect lay consensus; jurors' unanimous opinion in favour of one party or the other was thought to provide an acceptable level of certainty.

Between the twelfth and fifteenth centuries, trial jurors largely ceased to be self-informing and came to base their decisions on the evidence of witnesses whom they heard only in formal proceedings. Little is known about how or when this change occurred.[45] But belief in the jury's special access to the truth nevertheless persisted. Gabriel Tarde suggested that religious belief enabled a 'presumption of oracular infallibility' to become attached to jury decisions;[46] Barbara Shapiro's impression is that juries were believed to possess a kind of divine spark.[47] These religious allusions are apt, for long after it ceased to be usual for jurors to have personal knowledge of the people and events on which they returned verdicts, faith in juries remained an article of belief within English national mythology. Only in the late seventeenth century did epistemological developments begin to provide a rational justification for relying on the decisions of passively informed juries.[48]

In continental Europe, on the other hand, trial by ordeal was replaced by inquisitorial methods of investigation and proof derived from the learned traditions of Roman and canon law, in which fact-finding was a skilled function. A hybrid Roman-canon procedure developed in Italy during the twelfth century, and by 1300 was in use in Paris as well as in the Italian states.[49] Its reception elsewhere was gradual and incomplete, and in many regions local customary laws remained important, but a recognizably Roman-canon procedure was in place in France by the fifteenth century and in Germany by about 1550, particularly in courts that dealt with serious crimes like homicide.[50]

The essential features of Roman-canon procedure were that the state did the prosecuting and professional judges did all the adjudicating. There were no juries. Judges interrogated witnesses privately, established the facts of a case, and decided the verdict. The power this gave to judges was supposed to be controlled by a law of proof which minimized the role of subjective judgement in the process of adjudication, for a judge's personal convictions were not considered a sufficient basis for a decision that entailed capital punishment.[51] The aim of Roman-canon legal procedure was to guarantee the certainty of judgements by requiring proof that came close to a demonstration.[52] Whereas the English standard of proof was that jurors should be persuaded in their 'conscience' or (from the eighteenth century) convinced 'beyond reasonable doubt',[53] the Roman-canon idea was that proof should be 'as clear as the sun at noon' or 'clearer than day'.[54] Continental judges were consequently supposed to be constrained in serious criminal cases by rules that specified what evidence and how much of it justified what conclusions.[55] The theory of proof assigned numerical values to different types of evidence, which were combined arithmetically. Two good eyewitnesses constituted a full proof, as did a confession; one unobjectionable witness made a half-proof. Less reliable types of evidence, such as the testimony of women, children and paupers, and various indications (*indicia*) such as physiognomy, common repute and circumstantial evidence, were held to provide lesser fractions of proof which might, in combination, amount to a half-proof.[56] The two-witness standard was often impossible to meet in criminal cases, but a half-proof (one mature male witness or sufficient *indicia*) warranted torturing the suspect in order to extract a confession, which *was* a legally sufficient basis for capital conviction.

In recent years, historians investigating the actual practice of continental courts have shown that these exacting standards of proof were applied much less frequently in early modern legal practice than had been assumed. They were circumvented mainly by recourse to *poena extraordinaria* (exceptional punishment), whereby very strong evidence that amounted to less than a full legal proof or even a half-proof could justify, without torture and without confession, a sentence short of death, such as banishment, imprisonment, galley service or corporal punishment.[57] Capital punishment required full proof, but a 'violent presumption' allowed punishment that could be almost as severe.

What needs to be emphasized, however, is that, in either case, continental judges were meant to justify decisions on matters of fact by reference to doctrine about how to investigate and decide factual questions. Authoritative doctrine on this came in several forms. Basic components of the theory of legal proof were enacted as statutes. The Carolina, the criminal code of the Holy Roman Empire promulgated by Charles V in 1532, consists of 230 articles, most of which are concerned with procedure and proof: what evidence must be sought and the manner in which it must be obtained and weighed, as well as the rules to be followed after various contingencies in the process of investigation.[58] Article 21, for example, forbids the investigation of suspicions raised by soothsayers. Article 33 describes the indications of unwitnessed homicide:

> When the person suspected and accused of the murder was seen in a suspicious manner at the time the murder occurred with bloody clothes or weapon; or when he has taken, sold, given away, or still retained property of the murder victim; that may be deemed legally sufficient indication upon which examination under torture may be employed, unless he can contradict such suspicion with credible indication or proof (which shall be heard before any examination under torture).

Article 54 orders judges to verify confessions by independently investigating some of the circumstances admitted under torture; Article 71 states that a judge must pay 'particular attention to whether the witness is found inconsistent and shifting in his testimony; and he shall transcribe such circumstances, and how he observes the demeanour of the witness in the proceeding'. The French codes of criminal procedure of 1539 and 1670 make less detailed prescriptions, but they nevertheless reflect the same goal of ensuring rational decisions through the regulation of the judicial process. Thus, for example, the 1670 ordinance forbids judges to decide capital cases in the afternoon, on the assumption that their reasoning powers would be less acute after lunch.[59]

A code of law could not provide a prescription for every set of circumstances that might arise, but additional guidance was provided by the writings of learned jurists. This vast body of literature originated with twelfth-century Italian canon lawyers and was still being refined and added to in the eighteenth century. Treatises and commentaries worked out the particulars of the theory of proof, specifying the many circumstances that amounted to legal presumptions of varying strengths.[60] An excerpt from Muyart du Vouglans's exposition of the indications of the crime of sorcery illustrates the level of specificity to be found in such texts:

> If there have been found in the accused's house books or instruments relating to magic, such as sacrifices, human limbs, waxen images transfixed by needles, the bark of trees, bones, nails, locks of human hair, feathers intertwined in the form of a circle or nearly so, pins, embers, parcels of embers found at the head of children's beds ..., 2d, If he has been seen placing anything in a stable, and the cattle therein have soon afterwards died, 3d, If a document has been found upon him containing a compact with the devil ..., 7th, If those living in intimacy with the accused have been seen to change

> their abode immediately after his arrest . . ., 8th If he has the name of the devil constantly upon his lips, and if he is in the habit of calling his own children or those of other people by that name.

A sufficient quantity of indications of this kind warranted examining the suspect under torture. Muyart went on to give detailed guidance on how to assemble evidence in such cases, stressing the necessity of proceeding cautiously on account of the 'inordinate credulity of the common people' and the need to screen out superstition.[61]

The writings of legal scholars had great authority in the courts and were in effect part of the law itself.[62] Continental judges needed to ground their factual judgments in doctrine about proof and procedure, and where the law code was not specific enough, guidance was to be found in scholarly works on the theory of legal proof. Treatises on legal proof thus had an important place in continental jurisprudence and, in theory at least, in legal practice.

This approach to legal decision-making fostered a science of forensic medicine in several ways. The fact that all decisions in Roman-canon proceedings were made by judges meant that technical evidence could be incorporated more fully into the process of adjudication than was possible in common-law trials, where the use of juries tended to discourage testimony that ordinary laymen could not readily comprehend.[63] Furthermore, the existence and role of scholarly proof doctrine meant that there was an obvious place for medico-legal learning in Roman-canon jurisdictions.

On this point it is worth noting the formal and methodological similarities between early modern medical doctrine and the Roman-canon doctrine of legal proof, which reflect their common intellectual heritage and the applied character of both sciences. Proof theory, like medical theory, was a body of principles and rules that prescribed how the evidence of particular cases should be collected and interpreted, and what actions should be taken (by judge or physician) in different circumstances. Both traditions were conservative: a continental judge could, in the seventeenth century, draw on the authority of Durandus or Bartolus in the same way that a medical practitioner might appeal to the teachings of Hippocrates or Galen. Furthermore, legal presumptions, like medical ones, were established with reference to current experience as well as to ancient authorities, for continental legal scholars were closely connected with the daily practice of the courts, which presented new problems and suggested new inferences.[64] The textual forms of medical doctrine and proof doctrine were also similar. They included treatises, in which the principles of medical and legal theory were expounded; medical consultations and case histories (legal *consilia* and *decisiones*), which served as examplars; and aphorisms (statutes), which were concise statements of principle. The parallel between statutes and medical aphorisms is clear in the case of the Carolina. The articles of this code which lay down statutory presumptions are analogous to the many Hippocratic aphorisms about how to interpret appearances – in both cases the basic structure is 'signs x and y indicate z'. And the Carolina articles that specify the judicial actions called for by particular circumstances resemble the prescriptive medical aphorisms, the form of each being essentially 'in the case of x and y, take action z'.[65]

If early modern medical doctrine was analogous to the literature on legal proof, forensic medicine was even more so. Early works on forensic medicine gave instructions on how medico-legal inspections should be conducted, what observations should be made, and what conclusions might be drawn from various bodily signs. Medico-legal texts on wounds, for example, explained the effects of different kinds of wounds in various parts of the body in diverse circumstances. Wounds were classified as mortal, not mortal or contingently mortal, and attempts to construct reliable doctrine on this complex matter produced lengthy expositions of bodily signs that were similar to the delineations of *indicia* in general treatises on proof.[66] The purposes of medico-legal scholarship and legal-proof scholarship were in fact the same: to provide authoritative guidance on legal decision-making.

Indeed, continental writings on forensic medicine can be considered a subspecies of the legal literature on proof and procedure. This relationship is illustrated by doctrine about the investigation of childmurder. Article 36 of the Carolina prescribes the basic procedures and lays down a presumption of fact:

> [In cases of suspected infanticide, when] the baby was killed only such a short time before that the milk in the breasts of the mother has not yet gone away, then she may be milked in the breasts; and when mother's milk is found in the breasts, there is in consequence a strong presumption for the use of examination under torture. Since, however, some [state] physicians [*leibmedici*] say that for several natural reasons a woman who has not borne a child may have milk in the breasts, when, therefore, a girl exculpates herself in this way, she shall be further investigated by the midwife or other.[67]

This is an example of medico-legal doctrine contained in a code of law. It explains the significance of milk in the breasts of a suspect, affirms – on medical authority – the possibility of exceptions, and indicates the procedures to be followed in special cases. It is a kind of aphoristic version of what can be found in a medico-legal text on infanticide. The childmurder statute of the Carolina thus bears the same relation to a medical text about infanticide as other statutes of the Carolina bear to legal commentaries. In other words, just like legal treatises, texts on forensic medicine were commentaries on law. Just as the Carolina article about proving unwitnessed homicide (the 'bloody weapon' presumption, quoted above) was elaborated and qualified in legal treatises, so the content of the statute on childmurder was treated in detail by appropriate authorities – in medico-legal treatises.[68]

A final illustration of how forensic medicine formed part of the genre of legal-proof doctrine can be seen in the continuity between the three levels of written authority in France that governed the medico-legal examination and assessment of wounds: statute, legal treatise, and medico-legal treatise. At the level of statute, an order of January 1652 by the Parlement of Paris forbids conviction for homicide if the death occurs more than forty days after the assault (thereby laying down a medico-legal presumption about the lethality of wounds),[69] while the criminal ordinance of 1670 describes, briefly, the procedures to be followed in medical inspections of wounds.[70] At the level of legal treatise, Guy du Rousseaud de la Combe's *Treatise on Criminal Subjects* (1741) contains several pages describing the appropriate legal procedures in more detail. It states that the forty-day rule is no longer considered sound doctrine and should not be rigidly applied, and gives a list of questions that wound reports should address.[71] Another relevant legal treatise is *Principles of Jurisprudence Concerning the Judicial Visits and Reports of Physicians, Apothecaries and Midwives* (1753), by the jurisconsult Claude-Joseph Prévost.[72] Finally, medico-legal texts by medical men, such as René Gendry's *How to Report Well in Justice the Indispositions and Changes that Occur in Men's Health* (1650) and Jean Devaux's *The Art of Making Reports in Surgery* (1703), provide even more comprehensive instruction on how to investigate and interpret wounds for the courts.[73] Like the works of the jurists Rousseaud de la Combe and Prévost, those of the surgeons Gendry and Devaux were specialized contributions to the doctrine of legal procedure and proof.

From the perspective of Roman-canon law, then, the development of medico-legal scholarship did not represent much of an innovation. There was a place within legal learning for a specialized literature on medico-legal questions, as well as a pre-existing model for its application in legal proceedings. Indeed, there was an implicit demand in the Roman-canon context for learned guides to investigation and adjudication, including the investigation and adjudication of medico-legal questions.

English law did not generate a corresponding demand for medico-legal texts, for it needed much less in the way of proof doctrine of any kind. There was little scope for bringing textual authority to bear on factual questions in common-law trials because facts were determined by juries. Judges could to some extent control what jurors heard, and they might exert considerable influence over juries during trials, but the processes by which juries determined facts were not scrutinized.[74] A very few English statutes prescribed evidentiary standards, notably the law of 1547 which required two witnesses for a conviction of treason, and that of 1624 (frequently disregarded from the late seventeenth century), which stated that concealment of an infant's death was proof of infanticide.[75] On other matters of fact, however, jurors were free to satisfy their consciences as they saw fit.

Some fragmentary discussion of evidence and inference did appear in English handbooks for magistrates such as Michael Dalton's *The Countrey Justice* (1618). This concerned the decisions a magistrate had to make before a case reached the grand-jury stage, such as whether arrest or bail were justified – pre-trial decisions which correspond to the early stages of a Roman-canon trial. As Barbara Shapiro has shown, evidentiary guidelines on such matters resembled Roman-canon *indicia*, and in fact represented unacknowledged English borrowing from European civil law traditions.[76] But these rules for English magistrates were never presented in any detail, and their relevance largely ended when a case reached the grand jury; grand-jury verdicts of *ignoramus* (dismissal of the case) or *billa vera* (authorization to proceed to trial) were, like all jury verdicts, arrived at privately on the basis of oral testimony and did not need to be explained.[77] In England, the authority to try as well as to convict was provided by jury verdicts, and, mainly for this reason, there was little occasion for English lawyers to create an extensive learned literature on proof.

The English counterpart to the Roman-canon law of proof was a rather different law of *evidence*, but this could not really regulate jury decision-making except by excluding certain kinds of evidence as inadmissible.[78] In any case, the English law of evidence was negligible in the early modern period compared to what it later became, and 'before 1800 lengthy treatments of evidence as a distinct subject were almost unknown'.[79] Since there were few publications on evidence and proof in general in England before the later eighteenth century, it is not surprising that there was scarcely any literature on *medical* evidence and proof before that date.[80]

Trial procedure and expertise

Who wrote these early continental treatises on forensic medicine, how did they come to write them, and how did they acquire special expertise in the subject? On these matters, too, the facilitative role of Roman-canon law is clear. Leading medical practitioners in continental countries were encouraged to formulate and improve knowledge about medico-legal questions by the legal practices of review and consultation.

Provision for review of judgments was one of the safeguards of justice in Roman-canon jurisprudence. The most elaborate system for reviewing legal decisions developed in France, where, from as early as the thirteenth century, persons found guilty of serious crimes had a right to have their cases deliberated a second time by a superior court.[81] But even trials of first instance involved a considerable amount of judicial review in France. Various decisions had to be made at different stages of a Roman-canon trial, and French royal justice allowed both prosecutor and defendant to appeal against the important ones, such as decisions on whether to order torture and whether to admit proof of any exonerative facts claimed. A comprehensive written record of all the evidence and proceedings was kept for each case, from the initial suspicion through to final judgment. During the course of a trial, which might take months, this dossier repeatedly changed hands so that a hierarchy of judges could either approve the interim judgments, thus allowing the trial to proceed to the next stage, or challenge them and perhaps order further inquiries. This continual process of review gave enormous importance to the dossier. Final judgment depended solely on its contents. Consequently, all the evidence considered by inferior judges had to be spelled out to allow its re-evaluation by higher courts. The grounds of factual decision-making had to be such that they could be communicated in writing.

Medical judgments were no exception to this principle of review. After a statutory medical investigation had been made by a local sworn surgeon, French judges were free to order additional examinations by other medical practitioners in whom they had more confidence. As the eighteenth-century jurist François Serpillon explained, when additional reports were thus obtained, judges based their decisions 'on the reputation of these second experts'. He cited the authority of sixteenth-century legal theorists to the effect that when medical men disagree, the most worthy and experienced are to be believed.[82] Alternatively, highly respected medical men might be commissioned to evaluate the written reports of other practitioners. A pair of reports on a suspicious death in seventeenth-century Brittany illustrates this practice. The first, signed by five rural medical practitioners, consists of a list of observations from the autopsy they conducted, the various inferences they drew from them, and their conclusion that death was caused by blows to the head. The second report, prepared by three master surgeons of Rennes, consists of a critical evaluation of the first. Taking the rural practitioners' observations point by point, it explains why particular inferences are not warranted, discusses several omissions and possible errors in the dissection and gives reasons for concluding that the most probable cause of death was apoplexy.[83]

In difficult or important cases a judge could apply to the highest medical authorities of the realm. To quote Serpillon, 'if the case is important, the judge can name the King's physician and the King's surgeons, or such other physicians and surgeons of the place, or from neighbouring cities, as he judges appropriate'.[84] This meant that the most problematic medico-legal decisions were systematically referred to the elite of the medical profession, who produced written opinions on them. French legal procedure thus tended to create a group of superior medico-legal experts, who were not necessarily legal officials. Ambroise Paré, for example, author of the earliest European guide to medico-legal practice (*Treatise on Reports*, 1575), was, between 1552 and 1590, Surgeon to Henri II, First Surgeon to Charles IX, and First Surgeon and Counsellor to Henri III. These positions entailed advising on a variety of medical matters of state concern, including medico-legal problems.[85] Jean Devaux, whose medico-legal textbook *The Art of Making Reports in Surgery* was published in 1703, was also well connected, having been the apprentice of Claude David, who later became First Surgeon to the Queen. Devaux was twice elected Provost of the Company of Master Surgeons in Paris, in which position he would have been an obvious choice as medico-legal consultant.[86] His text implies familiarity with the common faults of surgeons' work in this area,[87] and reproduces dozens of medico-legal reports by Parisian surgeons from the 1670s to the 1690s. It seems likely, then, that specialized work on forensic medicine was facilitated, even encouraged, in France by the legal practice of review by higher authority – usually legal, but medical where appropriate.

The Italian and German systems of legal consultation allowed medico-legal problems to be referred to the medical elite even more effectively. A practice whereby judges consulted scholars learned in the law became common in medieval and Renaissance Italy.[88] Church courts began to refer doubtful legal questions to expert canonists, and the practice grew in secular Italian courts along with the use of learned jurisprudence. Some Italian cities sent disputes to the new universities for resolution; others created local institutions of learned justice to provide legal expertise. The need for expert legal opinions expanded with proof-scholarship itself because the growing number of authorities and the evolution of doctrine multiplied the ambiguities and inconsistencies contained in it. The decisions of commissioned legal scholars were effectively, and in some places legally, binding.[89] Leading legal scholars of the fourteenth and fifteenth centuries spent much of their time preparing judgments for the courts, and collections of their *consilia* formed a considerable part of the growing legal literature.

The Italian system of expert consultation was not reproduced in France, in part because the large stationary judiciary and the comprehensive system of hierarchical review meant that advice from learned outsiders was less needed.[90] However, a similar system of recourse to legal scholars developed on a massive scale in Germany, where well into the seventeenth century most courts were staffed by judges who were not trained in Roman-canon law. A persistent theme of the Carolina (1532) is the duty of judges to consult higher authority in all doubtful matters. Article 219 states that legal guidance should be obtained from 'a nearby academy, city or town, or from other learned scholars', and there is abundant evidence that this injunction was followed.[91] The procedure that developed under this directive was called *Aktenversendung* (despatch of the record) because rather than formulating specific questions, German courts forwarded entire dossiers to law faculties for appraisal. Decisions for the courts were rendered by individual professors or by faculty committees; professors of law also dispensed opinions to private clients on a wide range of legal matters. By the end of the sixteenth century the volume of paid consultation was so great that it constituted a major source of income for academic lawyers in Germany.[92] James Whitman has noted that this Roman-canon practice of deferring to legal scholars lay behind the dramatic rise in power and prestige of German law professors in the late sixteenth century. It produced a new form of academic legal culture in which adjudication became the job of law professors, who largely displaced the traditional lay judges (*Schöffen*).[93] Collections of law faculty *consilia* were published because, as in Italy, such decisions were authoritative, and printed collections of them provided useful precedents and exemplars. The first German compilation of legal consultations appeared five years after *Aktenversendung* was authorized by the Carolina, and by 1600 forty-one such volumes had been published.[94]

Among the questions that German judges had to deal with were those arising from medical examinations. By 1600 it was common practice for courts to refer these sorts of questions to the universities as well, to be resolved by the medical faculties.[95] German medical professors were consulted in the same way as law professors. Expert judgements were supplied by medical academics individually and collectively, to private applicants as well as to the courts.[96] Medico-legal problems in Germany were thus resolved on a regular basis by medical academics at leading centres of medical teaching and research.

The assessment of trial proceedings by professors of medicine in seventeenth-century Germany meant that these scholars had firsthand experience of medico-legal adjudication and were well informed about the shortcomings of contemporary medico-legal knowledge in relation to the needs of criminal justice. The system of official, paid, written consultations also made forensic medicine a rewarding activity within an academic medical career. These factors go a long way towards accounting for the dominance of German publications in the field of forensic medicine in the seventeenth and eighteenth centuries. They also help to explain the extremely scholarly character of German medico-legal literature in this period.

A medico-legal consultation was a written account of the evidence, reasoning and medical authorities on which the consultant based his opinion. The Roman physician Paulo Zacchia drew on unequalled experience of preparing such consulations to write his *Quaestiones Medico-legales*, published in eleven volumes between 1621 and 1661, which is considered an important landmark in the history of forensic medicine. This massive work is mainly a collation of the medical doctrine and opinions that were relevant to the medico-legal problems that Zacchia dealt with during his long career as personal physician to the Pope, Protomedicus to the Church State, and medical consultant to the Rota Romana, the high court of appeal in canon law.[97] Many of Zacchia's own consultations are printed in full in this work, and medico-legal decisions make up the entire content of the final two volumes.[98] Several early German publications on legal medicine are little more than collections of consultations. Paul Ammann's *Medicina Critica* (1670) and Johann Friedrich Zittmann's *Medicina Forensis* (1706) are annotated compilations of medico-legal cases decided by the medical faculty at Leipzig.[99] The 'earliest serial devoted wholly to forensic medicine', *Der medicinische Richter* (*The Medical Jurist*, 1755–9), consists of reports of the decisions of the medical faculty at Ansbach.[100] The Roman-canon system of legal consultation clearly played an important part in bringing these works into existence. The practice of *Aktenversendung* meant that German courts did not so much stimulate medico-legal studies as commission them.

By comparison, English common-law procedure was inhospitable to the development of forensic medicine as a learned science. In English criminal trials, all evidence, including medical testimony and opinion, was elicited by oral examination before the jury (grand and petty); jurors did not study dossiers. The evidence on which a criminal conviction was based was therefore only partially documented, for use when a witness died or was too ill to travel.[101] Moreover, English criminal convictions could not be appealed. An application could be made for a royal pardon, but this did not involve an actual review of the evidence heard, and a pardon did not alter the verdict.[102] It was in any case not really feasible to review common-law decisions on factual matters, for the verdict of a jury was not normally accompanied by even oral justification. If a judge was uncertain about a difficult question of *law*, he could postpone pronouncing judgment until he had consulted his colleagues. But in such cases the jury still had to reach a verdict about the *facts* of the case as soon as the evidence had been heard, and any medical questions were necessarily resolved in this factual decision, known as a special verdict. In non-criminal cases appeals were more common, but they, too, were grounded on doubtful points of law; the finding of a jury with respect to the facts of a dispute was quite final.[103] Common-law procedures thus did not encourage the written presentation or review of medico-legal opinions.

Furthermore, a criminal trial in England could not normally be adjourned for the purpose of obtaining more evidence or resolving difficulties. A decision had to be made on the basis of whatever testimony the parties could present on the day. If a medical witness was uncertain and could not give a firm opinion, or if medical witnesses contradicted each other, there was no procedure by which the trial could be interrupted to allow another medical opinion to be procured. The medical evidence of a case was assessed by a leading practitioner only when the prosecution or the defence had retained one in advance and produced him at the trial. Even then, however, the process of critical evaluation could be hampered by common-law procedure.

These points can be illustrated by the trial of John Donellan at Warwick assizes in 1780 for poisoning his brother-in-law, Sir Theodosius Boughton. Although this trial took place at the very end of the long period considered in this essay, and was exceptional in being a *cause célèbre* involving a titled victim, a large inheritance and several distinguished medical witnesses, it shows clearly the potential effects of common-law procedures. The defence employed the London anatomist, teacher and hospital surgeon John Hunter. Hunter was provided in advance with a description of Boughton's symptoms and death and a brief account of the post-mortem examination, obtained from a medical witness for the prosecution who had attended the dissection.[104] There was no legal provision for supplying Hunter with this information; without this fairly informal communication he could have remained unaware, until the actual trial, of all but the general conclusion drawn from the autopsy. Hunter made notes in the margins of the dissection report which appeared to demolish the prosecution's medical case: the head was not opened, the intestines were not examined, external appearances usual in a dead body were wrongly interpreted as signs of poison, and similar errors were made respecting the internal appearances, which indicated nothing but death and putrefaction. In Hunter's pre-trial opinion the medical evidence made apoplexy a more likely cause of death than poison.[105]

However, Hunter had no opportunity to raise most of these points at the trial because the questions put to him focused on new evidence which was presented by the prosecution medical witnesses in the course of the oral proceedings. This consisted of an account of the experimental poisoning of a dog, a cat and two horses with laurel water (the specific poison thought to have killed Boughton) and the comparison of Boughton's symptoms with the symptoms produced in these animals before they died. This was the first

Hunter had heard of laurel water in connection with the case; the poison talked of at the inquest had been arsenic. Although Hunter was able to assure the court that he had 'poisoned some thousands of animals' and had performed many dissections on humans, including hundreds on the bodies of persons who had died by apoplexy, and could draw on extensive personal research on the processes of death by poisoning, he had little to say about the physiological effects of the particular poison in question.[106] In short, Hunter had not foreseen the kind of medical evidence that the prosecution would present and was not well prepared to testify about laurel water. It is said that Hunter often regretted afterwards that he had not been better prepared at this trial.[107]

Hunter can reasonably be considered an English counterpart to what I have described as a superior medical expert in Roman-canon contexts. But, whatever the rights and wrongs of the Donellan case may have been, the procedure by which Hunter was 'consulted' did not permit him to evaluate the medical issues fully. The information he received beforehand was incomplete, he had no opportunity to research recorded cases of poisoning by laurel water or to conduct experiments with it, he had to justify his opinions on the spot, and he had to testify on the same footing as other witnesses – under the constraints of adversarial examination and cross-examination. Unlike the continental medico-legal consultant who deliberated over a dossier in his study, Hunter had to travel from London to Warwick to face the fray of the assizes and, as it turned out, suffer public embarrassment, for the judge's comments on Hunter's testimony in his summing-up were not complimentary. Finally, of course, the medical disagreement was resolved by a jury of laymen, not by a panel of medical professors.

English criminal trial practices thus did not much facilitate the consultation of leading medical men in difficult medico-legal cases. Adversarial procedure and the role of the jury as the arbiter of fact militated strongly against the establishment of a hierarchy of medico-legal authority and expertise. Since even when a knowledgeable medical man like Hunter was consulted he testified orally, interpreting evidence he had only just heard, nothing about the process encouraged a scholarly approach to medico-legal work or the production of written opinions on particular cases. English procedures arguably had some beneficial effects on medico-legal practice insofar as they favoured medical witnesses with relevant personal experience and empowered lay scepticism about medical claims. But they did little to encourage highly qualified practitioners to take a special interest in medico-legal work.[108]

Neither common-law nor Roman-canon procedures for employing medical expertise reflected medical priorities. Rather, medico-legal culture in each context acquired its distinctive character from the procedural framework that governed legal inquiries into facts of all kinds. Roman-canon trials nurtured medico-legal science through their use of professional fact-finders, their emphasis on written evidence, and their provision for hierarchical review. Because the entire system was built on the principle of deference to expertise, medical expertise occupied a more formally privileged place in continental trials than it did in English ones. Furthermore, the rationalist law of proof from which continental practices derived, entailed the elaboration of a body of scholarly commentary on legal procedure and proof, of which medico-legal commentary formed a part. A learned literature to guide medico-legal practice developed naturally in a legal system where inquiries into facts in general were conducted with reference to doctrine. The judicial consultation of experts was especially conducive to medico-legal scholarship, and German pre-eminence in forensic medicine from the late seventeenth century owed much to this legal practice.

Common-law trials, with their adversarial methods, their limited scope for reviewing decisions, and, above all, their use of juries to ascertain facts, exerted pressure in the opposite direction: towards the oral presentation of evidence and a reluctance to give much authority to any sort of expert. The relative lack of incentives for English medical practitioners to collate and distil medico-legal opinions into a systematic body of doctrine that could be consulted by others did not reflect a national lack of respect for medical expertise. On the contrary, the fact that English coroners, magistrates and trial participants often sought medical testimony though it was not required by law shows that medical evidence was valued. English slowness to create an indigenous literature on forensic medicine ultimately reflected the common-law method of proof by jury.

While forensic medicine in the early modern period needs to be understood in relation to particular legal systems, legal factors arguably have less relative importance in the later history of medico-legal science. Admittedly, the eventual creation of an indigenous medico-legal literature in England closely paralleled the growth of an English legal literature on evidence, and both these developments reflected, among other things, changes in legal practice. But English legal procedure did not become markedly more hospitable to medical expertise in the early nineteenth century. On the contrary, the increased participation of defence counsel in English criminal trials from the late eighteenth century seems to have heightened the unfavourable circumstances under which medical witnesses testified. What changed in England around 1800 was the matter of incentives. In the context of the strong contemporary drive to reform the medical profession and enhance its public status, the improvement of medico-legal knowledge and practice came to be viewed as an important priority for the medical profession as a whole, and medical reformers actively promoted the field. The growth of general medical interest in pathological anatomy at this time also played a part in stimulating interest in forensic medicine. It was non-legal developments such as these that produced an effusion of publications on legal medicine in England after 1800, and led to legislation to ensure the payment of medical witnesses (1836) and to provide a legal supply of corpses for teaching relevant anatomical skills (1832). Before about 1800, however, the contrasting state of medico-legal scholarship in England and continental Europe reflected nothing so much as the logic of their legal systems.

NOTES

This paper has benefited greatly from the comments and advice of Peter Bartlett, Michael Clark, Anne Goldgar, Ludmilla Jordanova, Joan Lane, Harvey Mitchell, James Oldham, Roger Smith, and Andrew Wear.

1 Erwin H. Ackerknecht, 'Early history of legal medicine', *Ciba Symposia*, 11 (1950–1), 1288–1304, 1313–16, at pp. 1296, 1298. See also J. D. J. Havard, *The Detection of Secret Homicide: A Study of the Medico-legal System of Investigation of Sudden and Unexplained Deaths* (London: Macmillan, 1960), ch. 1: 'The belated reception of legal medicine in England'.

2 For example, [Richard Hawes,] *The Poore-Man's Plaster-Box ... Whereunto is added certaine directions, whereby a man may know by what means a person (being found dead) came by his Death* (London, 1634), containing four pages on forensic medicine; Thomas Brugis, *Vade Mecum: or, a Companion for a Chyrurgion. ... To which is added the maner of making Reports before a Judge of Assize, of any one that hath come to an untimely end* (London, 1652), containing fifteen pages on forensic medicine which are heavily indebted to Ambroise Paré, *Traité des rapports*, first published in *Les Oeuvres de M. Ambroise Paré* (Paris, 1575), pp. 931–44.

3 For bibliographies of continental publications in the early modern period, see Christian-Friedrich Daniel, *Entwurf einer Bibliothek der Staats-Arzneikunde oder der gerichtlichen Arzneikunde und medicinischen Polizey von ihrem Anfange bis auf das Jahr 1784* (Halle, 1784); Christian Friedrich Ludwig Wildberg, *Bibliotheca medicinae publicae*, 2 vols. (Berlin, 1819); R. P. Brittain, A. Saury and M.-R. Guidet, *Bibliographie des travaux français de médecine légale* (Paris: Masson, 1970). Valuable accounts of early writings on forensic medicine are to be found in Jaroslav Nemec, *International Bibliography of Medicolegal Serials, 1736–1967* (Bethesda, MD: National Library of Medicine, 1969), pp. 2–9 and Esther Fischer-Homberger, *Medizin vor Gericht: Gerichtsmedizin von der Renaissance bis zur Aufklärung* (Berne: Huber, 1983), passim.

4 Thomas R. Forbes, *Surgeons at the Bailey: English Forensic Medicine to 1878* (New Haven: Yale University Press, 1985), p. 21.

5 Gino Gorla and Luigi Moccia, 'A "revisiting" of the comparison between "continental law" and "English law" (16th–19th century)', *Journal of Legal History*, 2 (1981), 143–56; Barbara Shapiro, *'Beyond Reasonable Doubt' and 'Probable Cause': Historical Perspectives on the Anglo-American Law of Evidence* (Berkeley and Oxford: University of California Press, 1991), chs. 3 and 4, especially pp. 120–4.

6 Alfred Soman, 'Criminal jurisprudence in ancien-régime France: the Parlement of Paris in the sixteenth and seventeenth centuries', in Louis A. Knafla, ed., *Crime and Criminal Justice in Europe and Canada* (Waterloo, Ontario, 1981), pp. 43–75; Mirjan R. Damaska, 'The death of legal torture', *Yale Law Journal*, 87 (1978), 860–84.

7 *The Proceedings at the Sessions of Peace, Oyer and Terminer, for the City of London, and County of Middlesex*, 1739–40, p. 124. For a brief account of this source (known as the *Old Bailey Sessions Papers*), see p. 170 below.

8 'The trial of Philip Earl of Pembroke and Montgomery, at Westminster, for the murder of Nathanael Cony . . . 1678', in Thomas Bayley Howell, ed., *A Complete Collection of State Trials*, 33 vols. (London, 1816–26), vol. VI, cols. 1309–50, at col. 1340.

9 'The trial of Elizabeth Canning for wilful and corrupt perjury', in Howell, *State Trials*, vol. XIX (1816), cols. 283–679, at col. 427.

10 Thomas Percival, *Medical Jurisprudence; or a Code of Ethics and Institutes, Adapted to the Professions of Physic and Surgery* [Manchester, 1794], p. 89. An expanded version of this book was published in 1803 as *Medical Ethics*.

11 Edward Umfreville, *Lex Coronatoria: or, the Office and Duty of Coroners*, 2 vols. (London, 1761), pp. 512–13.

12 Percival, *Medical Jurisprudence*, p. 89.

13 See J. M. Beattie, *Crime and the Courts in England 1660–1800* (Princeton: Princeton University Press, 1986), p. 334n.

14 *OBSP*, 1779–80, p. 612.

15 J. Foot, *An Appeal to the Public, Touching the Death of Mr. George Clarke*, 2nd edn (London, 1769), p. 7.

16 Foot, *Appeal to the Public*, p. 9.

17 John H. Langbein, 'Albion's fatal flaws', *Past and Present*, 98 (1983), p. 103. Legislation compelling the attendance of witnesses was enacted in 1563 (Shapiro, *'Beyond Reasonable Doubt'*, p. 6).

18 6 and 7 Will. IV, c. 89.

19 Richard Burn, *The Justice of the Peace and Parish Officer*, 2nd edn (London, 1756), vol. II, pp. 311–13.

20 Lincoln's Inn Library, shorthand notes of Sir Dudley Ryder (Chief Justice of King's Bench 1754–56), transcribed by K. L. Perrin, Document 13, p. 24.

21 Umfreville, *Lex Coronatoria*, pp. 295–6.

22 Personal communication. I am grateful to Dr Lane for allowing me to cite the following examples from her research.

23 The Medical Witnesses Act 1836 specified the fee of one guinea for attending an inquest, two if a post-mortem examination was required (6 and 7 Will. IV, c. 89, Schedule B).

24 Alessandro Simili, 'The beginnings of forensic medicine in Bologna', in Heinrich Karplus, ed., *International Symposium on Society, Medicine and Law*,

Jerusalem, March 1972 (Amsterdam: Elsevier, 1973), pp. 91–100, p. 94 (statute); Eugenio Dall'Osso, *L'organizzazione medico-legale a Bologna e a Venzia nei secoli XII–XIV* (Cesena: Orfanelli Addolorata, 1956), pp. 33–4n (petition).

25 Michael R. McVaugh, *Medicine before the Plague: Practitioners and their Patients in the Crown of Aragon, 1285–1345* (Cambridge: Cambridge University Press, 1993), p. 238.

26 G. Pentogalos, G. A. Stathopoulos and N. Kapanidis, 'Deontological arrangements in the capitularia of Crete during its occupation by Venice in the 15th Century', *6th Mediterranean Conference of Legal Medicine, Halkidiki 24–27 May 1984*, pp. 45–56, at p. 46. See also Peter Volk and Hans Jurgen Warlo, 'The role of medical experts in court proceedings in the medieval town', in Karplus, *International Symposium on Society, Medicine and Law*, pp. 101–16.

27 M. Guérin, *Le Médecin et la justice du XVII au XVIII siècle en France et en Lorraine* (Verdun, 1929–30), p. 19.

28 Jean Devaux, *Edit du Roy portant création de médecins & chirurgiens jurez*, appended to Devaux, *L'Art de faire les rapports en chirurgie* (Paris, 1703), p. 3; Edmond Locard, *Le XVIIIe Siècle médico-judiciaire* (Lyon, 1902), p. 70.

29 Devaux, *Edit du Roy*, pp. 4–5, 8, 32.

30 Ibid., pp. 12–13.

31 François Serpillon, *Code criminel, ou commentaire sur l'ordonnance de 1670* (Paris, 1784), vol. I, p. 406. For competition among surgeons, physicians, midwives and apothecaries for medico-legal authority in early modern Germany, see Fischer-Homberger, *Medizin vor Gericht*, pp. 43–50, 55–60, 74–9.

32 Katherine Park, *Doctors and Medicine in Early Renaissance Florence* (Princeton: Princeton University Press, 1985), pp. 86, 96, 99.

33 Locard, *XVIIIe Siècle médico-judiciaire*, pp. 80–1; Serpillon, *Code criminel*, vol. I, pp. 469–70.

34 Alessandro Simili, 'Forensic medicine in Bologna', pp. 91–100, at p. 93.

35 See Charles Desmaze, *Histoire de la médecine légale en France* (Paris, 1880), pp. 216, 220; Armand Corre and Paul Aubry, *Documents de criminologie rétrospective. Bretagne, XVIIe et XVIIIe siècles* (Lyon, 1895), p. 70.

36 Achille Geerts, *L'Indemnisation des lésions corporelles à travers les siècles* (Paris: Librairies Techniques, 1962), ch. 9; Catherine Crawford, 'Medicine and the law', in W. F. Bynum and Roy Porter, eds., *Encyclopedia of the History of Medicine* (London: Routledge, 1993), pp. 1619–40, at pp. 1622–3.

37 This point has been made by J. B. Speer in an essay review of 'Crowner's Quest' by Thomas R. Forbes, *Annals of Science*, 37 (1980), 353–6.

38 See, for example, Devaux, *L'Art de faire les rapports*, pp. 23–4; Serpillon, *Code criminel*, vol. I, p. 409n.

39 Paul R. Hyams, 'Trial by ordeal: the key to proof in the early common law', in Morris S. Arnold, Thomas A. Green, Sally A. Scully and Stephen D. White, eds., *On the Laws and Customs of England* (Chapel Hill: University of North Carolina Press, 1981), pp. 90–126.

40 Shapiro, '*Beyond Reasonable Doubt*', pp. 3, 118; John H. Langbein, *Prosecuting Crime in the Renaissance: England, Germany, France* (Cambridge, MA: Cambridge University Press, 1974), pp. 134–7.

41 John H. Langbein, *Torture and the Law of Proof: Europe and England in the*

Ancien Régime (Chicago: Chicago University Press, 1977), pp. 75, 77–8; Thomas A. Green, *Verdict According to Conscience: Perspectives on the English Trial Jury, 1200–1800* (Chicago, 1985), ch. 1.

42 James Bradley Thayer, *A Preliminary Treatise on Evidence at the Common Law* (Boston, 1898), pp. 90–2, 120–3, 168–70; Shapiro, *'Beyond Reasonable Doubt'*, pp. 4–5.

43 Langbein, *Torture and the Law of Proof*, pp. 75, 77–8.

44 *The History of English Law*, 2nd edn (Cambridge, 1898), vol. II, pp. 660–1, quoted in Langbein, *Torture and the Law of Proof*, p. 78.

45 See J. B. Post, 'Jury lists and juries in the late fourteenth century', and Edward Powell, 'Jury trial at gaol delivery in the late Middle Ages: the Midland Circuit, 1400–1429', in J. S. Cockburn and Thomas A. Green, eds., *Twelve Good Men and True: The Criminal Trial Jury in England, 1200–1800* (Princeton: Princeton University Press, 1988), pp. 65–77 and 78–116; Langbein, *Torture and the Law of Proof*, p. 79; Shapiro, *'Beyond Reasonable Doubt'*, pp. 4–6.

46 Cited in Adhémar Esmein, *A History of Continental Criminal Procedure with Specific Reference to France*, trans. J. Simpson (London: J. Murray, 1914), p. 629n.

47 Shapiro, *'Beyond Reasonable Doubt'*, p. 241.

48 Ibid., ch. 1, pp. 242–3.

49 Langbein, *Prosecuting Crime in the Renaissance*, pp. 137, 220; J. Dawson, *The Oracles of the Law* (Ann Arbor: University of Michigan Law School, 1968), p. 193.

50 Dawson, *Oracles of the Law*, p. 193.

51 An eighteenth-century defender of this 'objective' mode or proof, the jurist Augustin-Marie Poullain du Parc, explained:

> It is not enough that the judge is as thoroughly convinced as any reasonable man could be by a collection of presumptions and facts leading to presumptions. This is a most erroneous way of judging, and is really nothing but the expression of a more or less [well-] based opinion.

(*Principes du droit françois*, Rennes, 1767–71, vol. X1, p. 112, quoted in Esmein, *Continental Criminal Procedure*, p. 251n).

52 Peter Stein, *Legal Institutions: The Development of Dispute Settlement* (London: Butterworths, 1984), pp. 57–8.

53 Shapiro, *'Beyond Reasonable Doubt'*, pp. 13–25.

54 Esmein, *Continental Criminal Procedure*, pp. 133, 270.

55 See Esmein, *Continental Criminal Procedure*, pp. 251–71; Jean P. Levy, *L'hiérarchie des preuves dans le droit savant du moyen âge depuis la renaissance du droit romain jusqu'à la fin du XIV siècle* (Paris, 1939); R. C. Van Caenegem, 'La Preuve dans le droit du moyen âge occidental', in *Recueils de la Société Jean Bodin, pour l'histoire comparative des institutions*, 17 (1965), 691–740.

56 Esmein, *Continental Criminal Procedure*, pp. 626 (physiognomy), 259–69 (others).

57 See Alfred Soman, 'Deviance and criminal justice in western Europe, 1300–1800: an essay in structure', *Criminal Justice History*, 1 (1980), 1–28; Richard Fraher, 'Conviction according to conscience: the medieval jurists' debate concerning judicial discretion and the law of proof', *Law and History Review*, 7 (1989), 23–88; Langbein, *Torture and the Law of Proof*.

58 A translation of two-thirds of the articles of the Carolina, including all the ones cited in this essay, can be found in Langbein, *Prosecuting Crime in the Renaissance*, Appendix B, pp. 259–308.

59 Title XXX, Article IX. The complete ordinance is printed in Serpillon, *Code criminel*, passim. Serpillon notes that judges could decide such cases after noon if they postponed the midday break to do so. English juries were forbidden food and drink altogether until they agreed on a verdict, apparently to encourage unanimity. See John H. Baker, *An Introduction to English Legal History*, 3rd edn (London: Butterworths, 1990), pp. 89–90.

60 See Dawson, *Oracles of the Law*, pp. 124–48; Shapiro, *'Beyond Reasonable Doubt'*, pp. 118–20, 200–6; O. F. Robinson, T. D. Fergus and W. M. Gordon, *An Introduction to European Legal History* (Abingdon: Professional, 1985), chs. 3 and 4.

61 Muyart de Vouglans, *Instituts du droit criminel* (1757), quoted in Esmein, *Continental Criminal Procedure*, p. 267.

62 See James Q. Whitman, *The Legacy of Roman Law in the German Romantic Era: Historical Vision and Legal Change* (Princeton: Princeton University Press, 1990), pp. 29–31.

63 Stein, *Legal Institutions*, p. 41–4.

64 Dawson, *Oracles of the Law*, pp. 142–3.

65 For example: 'IV.39. Should one part of the body be hotter or colder than the rest, disease is present in that part'; 'VII.56. Distress, yawning and shuddering are cured by a draught of wine mixed with an equal quantity of water'. See G. E. R. Lloyd, ed., *Hippocratic Writings* (Harmondsworth: Penguin, 1978), pp. 206–36.

66 For an account of early modern medico-legal doctrine about wounds see Fischer-Homberger, *Medizin vor Gericht*, pp. 311–21.

67 From the translation of the Carolina in Langbein, *Prosecuting Crime in the Renaissance*, Appendix B.

68 Such as Michael Berhard Valentini, *Corpus Juris Medico-legale* (Frankfurt-on-Main, 1722), pp. 490–528.

69 Serpillon, *Code criminel*, vol. I, p. 416.

70 Title V, Articles I, II, III.

71 Guy du Rousseaud de la Combe, *Traité des matières criminelles, suivant l'ordonnance du mois d'août 1670 et les édits, déclarations du Roi, arrêts et règlemens intervenus jusqu'à présent* (Paris, 1741), pp. 297–301.

72 Claude-Joseph Prévost, *Principes de jurisprudence sur les visites et rapports judiciaires des médecins, chirurgiens, apothicaires et sages-femmes* (Paris, 1753).

73 René Gendry, *Les Moyens de bien rapporter à Iustice les indispositions et changements qui arrivent à la santé des hommes* (Angers, 1650); Jean Devaux, *L'Art de faire les rapports en chirurgie, où l'on enseigne la pratique, les formules & le stile le plus en usage parmi les chirurgiens commis au reports* (Paris, 1703).

74 Arthur Engelmann, *A History of Continental Civil Procedure*, trans. Robert W. Millar (Boston, 1927), p. 48; Stein, *Legal Institutions*, pp. 33–4, 41–2.

75 John H. Wigmore, 'Required numbers of witnesses; a brief history of the numerical system in England', *Harvard Law Review*, 15 (1901), 83–108, pp. 100–6. On the infanticide statute, see the chapter in this volume by Mark Jackson.

76 Shapiro, *'Beyond Reasonable Doubt'*, pp. 129–70.

77 Like petty juries, grand juries did not normally view the records of magistrates' pre-trial examinations; witnesses had to appear personally and testify before them. See Shapiro, *'Beyond Reasonable Doubt'*, p. 50; Beattie, *Crime and the Courts*, p. 334.

78 Stein, *Legal Institutions*, p. 37; Langbein, *Torture and the Law of Proof*, p. 80.

79 William Twining, 'The rationalist tradition of evidence scholarship', in Enid Campbell and Louis Waller, eds., *Well and Truly Tried: Essays on Evidence in Honour of Sir Richard Eggleston* (Sydney: Law Book Company, 1982), pp. 211–49, at p. 214. See also Beattie, *Crime and the Courts*, pp. 362–3, 363n.

80 The crime of witchcraft provides an interesting exception, for it is 'one of the few instances where discussion of early modern evidence is to be found' in English sources (Shapiro, *'Beyond Reasonable Doubt'*, p. 164). English legal writings on witchcraft borrow a great deal from Roman-canon sources and recommend the consultation of medical experts on certain questions. Further research on the role of medical testimony in witchcraft prosecutions is clearly desirable, although, as Shapiro cautions, it is unclear whether or not witchcraft offers a window into the normal operations of the criminal law (p. 165).

81 This paragraph is based on Esmein, *Continental Criminal Procedure*, pp. 218–41 and Langbein, *Prosecuting Crime in the Renaissance*, pp. 223–51.

82 *Code criminel*, vol. I, pp. 409–10.

83 The first report and a précis of the second are printed in Locard, *XVIIIe Siècle médico-judiciaire*, pp. 148–50. No additional information about the case is given.

84 '[S]i le cas est important, le Juge peut nommer le Médecin du Roi, ou tels autres Médecins & Chirurgiens du lieu, ou des villes voisines qu'il jugera à propos' (*Code criminel*, vol. I, p. 410).

85 Wallace B. Hamby, *Ambroise Paré, Surgeon of the Renaissance* (St Louis, MO: Green, 1967).

86 See Pierre Suë, *Eloge historique de M. Devaux* (Paris, 1722); *Nouvelle Biographie Générale* (Copenhagen, 1855).

87 See Devaux, *L'Art de faire les rapports*, pp. 20–5.

88 This paragraph is based on Dawson, *Oracles of the Law*, pp. 138–43 and Whitman, *Legacy of Roman Law*, pp. 5–8.

89 Whitman, *Legacy of Roman Law*, pp. 29–30.

90 This paragraph is based on Dawson, *Oracles of the Law*, pp. 196–205 and Langbein, *Prosecuting Crime in the Renaissance*, pp. 198–201. See also G. Dahm, 'On the reception of Roman and Italian law in Germany', in Gerald Strauss, ed., *Pre-Reformation Germany* (New York: Harper & Row, 1972), pp. 282–315.

91 The translation of this article is taken from Whitman, *Legacy of Roman Law*, p. 31.

92 Dawson, *Oracles of the Law*, p. 205.

93 Whitman, *Legacy of Roman Law*, pp. 29–34.

94 Dawson, *Oracles of the Law*, p. 196.

95 Detailed summaries of thirty-five selected medico-legal *consilia* written by German and Danish university medical professors in the late sixteenth and early seventeenth centuries are printed in Fischer-Homberger, *Medizin vor Gericht*, passim. See also Wolfgang Nachtmann, *Die gerichtsmedizinischen Gutachten der*

Tübinger medizinischen Fakultät (1600–1923) (Institut für Gerichtliche Medizin: Tübingen, 1978).

96 The operation of this system in eighteenth-century Württemberg is discussed in Mary Wessling's chapter in this book.

97 Ackerknecht, 'Early history', p. 1292; Nemec, *International Bibliography of Medicolegal Serials*, p. 5.

98 Emile Mahier, *Les questions médico-légales de Paul Zacchias, médecin romain; études bibliographiques* (Paris, 1872); Heinrich Karplus, 'Medical ethics in Paolo Zacchia's Quaestiones Medico-legales', in Karplus, *International Symposium on Society, Medicine and Law*, pp. 125–33.

99 *Medicina Critica; sive Decisoria, Centuriâ Casuum Medicinalium in Concilio Facult. Lips. Antehàc Resolutorum* (Erfurt, 1670); *Medicina Forensis, h.e. Responsa Facultatis Medicae Lipsiensis ab Anno MDCL usque MDCC* (Frankfurt, 1706). It was not unusual for earlier collections of medical consultations to include medico-legal ones: see, for example, Hieronymus Mercurialis, *Consultationes Medicinales*, Vol. II, consultation 66.

100 Jaroslav Nemec, *Highlights in Medicolegal Relations* (Bethesda, MD: US Department of Health and Welfare, 1976), p. 60; Johann Georg Hasenest, *Der medicinische Richter, oder Acta physico-medico-forensia Collegii medici Onoldini, von Anno 1735 biss auf dermalige Zeiten zusammen getragen.*

101 Beattie, *Crime and the Courts*, pp. 21–2, 270–1.

102 A notorious exception, in which medical evidence was reviewed after a verdict, occurred after the conviction of Edward M'Quirk for murder after an election skirmish in 1768. He had allegedly been hired by the government to create trouble at the hustings, and the subsequent intervention of government ministers, which led to a review of the medical evidence by a committee of the College of Surgeons and a royal pardon for M'Quirk, certainly supports the allegation. There was a considerable outcry against these irregular proceedings, which were seen as a blatant misuse of political power. See Catherine Crawford, 'The emergence of English forensic medicine: medical evidence in common-law courts, 1730–1830', Ph.D thesis, University of Oxford, 1987, pp. 103–5.

103 On the procedures discussed in this paragraph see Peter Stein, 'The procedural models of the sixteenth century', *Juridical Review*, 1982, pp. 188–9; Baker, *Introduction to English Legal History*, pp. 116–21, 420–1; Beattie, *Crime and the Courts*, pp. 395–415.

104 'Statement of Sir Theos. Boughton's case with notes by John Hunter', London, Royal College of Surgeons, MS 49.d.11; *The Trial of John Donellan ... Taken in Short-Hand, by Joseph Gurney*, 2nd edn (London, 1781), p. 49.

105 'Statement of Sir Theos. Boughton's case'.

106 *Trial of Donellan*, pp. 49–51.

107 John Kobler, *The Reluctant Surgeon: A Biography of John Hunter* (New York: Doubleday, 1960), p. 219.

108 This trial was extremely unusual for the period before 1800 in benefiting from special medical preparation and it did, in fact, result in a publication, by one of the local medical witnesses: Bradford Wilmer, *Observations on Poisonous Vegetables which are either Indigenous to Great Britain or Cultivated for Ornament* (London, 1781). This is a short account of the various toxic plants,

based on Richard Mead's *A Mechanical Account of Poisons* (1702), several continental authorities, cases reported in the *Philosophical Transactions of the Royal Society* and Wilmer's own experiments on the physiological effects of laurel. The book is dedicated to Sir William Wheler (Sir Theodosius Boughton's guardian, mentioned in the text as having witnessed one of Wilmer's experiments and the accompanying dissection), and clearly represents the research Wilmer did for the Donellan trial, but it makes no reference to the trial or to any potential medico-legal applications. See the discussion in Joan Lane, 'Eighteenth-century medical practice: a case study of Bradford Wilmer, Surgeon of Coventry, 1737–1813', *Social History of Medicine*, 3 (1990), 369–86.

5

Infanticide trials and forensic medicine: Württembergs 1757–93

MARY NAGLE WESSLING

Introduction

It is no accident that infanticide has emerged as a topic of intense debate in recent historical writing. Research on criminality generally has grown out of social historians' broad interest in the less-than-privileged, while cultural historians have looked beyond descriptions of offences and offenders into the social and cultural origins of 'criminal' activities.[1] However, much of the current interest in infanticide doubtless responds to the feeling that the last great battle of feminism is being fought over the control of women's bodies. At one political extreme, abortion is seen as the modern version of infanticide; on the other, as the final step in woman's emancipation from biological and legal bondage.[2]

Common as infanticides were in later medieval times, they were not prosecuted with any intensity in the German-speaking lands until after the Protestant Reformation.[3] In the communes of seventeenth-century and eighteenth-century Germany, where the supernatural order penetrated the natural, infanticide was regarded as a sign of *Übel*, Satan's work made manifest. It was the duty of the magistracy to see that God's wrath be expiated by punishing the guilty person. The act itself set off a perturbing chain of events in community life: suspicion, accusation, investigation. The crime of infanticide was thus highly disruptive both socially and morally, calling into question the nature of the individual, the relative claims of individual and community, and the proper relationship between gender and social role.

Public execution was a matter for complex deliberations. The method of punishment and the level of defilement of the body of the convicted criminal were carefully chosen for their religious connotations and representational power. The accusers had the moral duty and legal authority to ensure that the criminal suffered enough earthly pain to cleanse the soul and ensure penitence before the community and God.[4] At the same time, punishment was construed for most of the early modern period as a method of deterrence, a view increasingly challenged in the later eighteenth century. In 1780, the Mannheim jurist and administrator Ferdinand von Lamezan proposed a prize question in the best Enlightenment academic tradition: 'What are the best workable means to prevent infanticide?' More than four hundred answers were published, compared to the usual twenty to fifty. Infanticide was clearly a pressing issue among intellectuals. At the same time, questions of the morality of judicial torture and the efficacy of severe punishment were moving to the forefront of enlightened debate.[5]

Within the states forming the Holy Roman Empire, infanticides were punished under the stipulations of a three-century-old code of penal practice, the *Constitutio Criminalis Carolina.* The Carolina, as it is usually referred to, was based on scholarly glosses on the Roman *Corpus iuris civilis* of the first century AD.[6] Two articles of the Carolina, which served as the basis for German criminal law until 1900, are of particular importance for the present study. Article 35 made it an offence for women to conceal pregnancy and the delivery of a child. That provision covered not only the mother, but also any other woman who knew of the pregnancy, and had the effect of placing a barrier between an unwed mother and those who might be sympathetic to her plight. Article 131 made a woman convicted of killing her child with premeditated intention to do so liable to the death penalty. The form of execution was decided by the territorial high court, and varied considerably with time and place. Women convicted of infanticide were usually beheaded, but those whose offence was judged especially heinous were placed in sacks (sometimes with animals) and drowned, or buried alive.

The Carolina prescribed that where any doubt about the criminal charge existed, the case should be decided through consultation with the sovereign and with the expert witnesses (*Rechtverständigen*). It mandated expert medical advice in three kinds of crimes, all punishable by death: cases of violent death by undetermined cause (possible homicide), cases where death resulted from attempts to heal (*Kunstfehler* or malpractice), and infanticide. The task of the physician, or surgeon, as medical expert, was to establish a causal relationship between any physical evidence of injury and the death. In 1658 these provisions of the Carolina were incorporated into the legal code of Württemberg, the duchy with which this paper is concerned.[7]

The involvement of physicians as advisers in infanticide trials represented only one example of the manifold interactions between medicine and law in early modern German society. As Esther Fischer-Homberger has shown, the intertwining of official, professional duty and moral issues has a long history.[8] As medico-legal advisers, official physicians were deeply involved in the processes that preserved the unity and moral tone that the commune perceived as essential to its social and economic integrity. Between the sixteenth and early nineteenth centuries, the official physician (*Physicus*) combined forensic duties with his other responsibilities to the district, that is, treating the sick poor, warning of approaching epidemics, enforcing quarantines, and observing local environmental influences upon public health. His education prepared him to take his place among the *Gelehrtenstand*, roughly translated as 'the society of learned persons'.[9] His position in the commune was a difficult one: his mandate came from the ducal medical establishment but he was beholden to local elites for his appointment and salary.[10]

The first section of this paper is based on records of infanticide trials, and begins with a detailed analysis of four trials that took place in the mid-1770s, when judicial torture became an especially divisive issue. It examines the political context within which the infanticide trials occurred and the way that power contests between the duke and bureaucratic elites impinged on legal medicine. The built-in strife between physicians and jurists, for centuries expressed as competition for rank,[11] surfaced in the legal criteria for acceptable medical evidence. As the argument surrounding judicial torture continued, it split the upper judiciary into factions. I shall argue that in later eighteenth-century Württemberg, medical opinions served to bolster the arguments of progressive jurists against the use of judicial torture, and made successful prosecution of the most serious level of infanticide almost impossible.

In the second section, I describe briefly the mid-eighteenth-century attempts by the high medical administration to seize power over local health appointments, and how physicians on the Tübingen medical faculty tried to provide better training in legal medicine. An increasingly self-critical attitude within the medical profession mandated a more scientific approach to cause and effect reasoning.[12] In particular, I will discuss four progressive physicians on the Tübingen medical faculty who developed the tradition of teaching legal medicine at the university. Only at the end of the eighteenth century did forensic medicine begin to emerge as a separate, regular course of study, during a crucial period of re-examination of both traditional medical education and the appointment of official physicians.[13] The way that expert medico-legal opinion, particularly in infanticide trials, gave added impulse to that re-evaluation, is the story this paper tells.

Medical evidence and infanticide

Trial procedure

In its larger outlines, infanticide conviction followed the bipartite procedure common to German criminal trials. Initially, the judiciary attempted to establish that a punishable crime had been committed by assembling facts derived from the circumstances of the case (*indicia*) into a body of legally indisputable evidence, the *corpus delicti*. Then, the judiciary councils and the ruler came to an agreement concerning suitable punishment. The Carolina standardized the first part of the procedure for the lands of the Holy Roman Empire; punishments, however, were subject to the specifications of territorial statute law, and here the ruler had the final word.

A schematization of the flow of evidence in an infanticide investigation in Württemberg is presented in Figure 1. The inquisitory process began when a local criminal court (*Malefiz Gericht*) initiated formal inquiry into an infant's death under suspicious circumstances, or even presumed infant death without a corpse – when a woman suspected of pregnancy underwent a sudden change in physical appearance or indulged in unusual behaviour. In Württemberg, the initial medico-legal report (*Inspectione legale* or *Visum repertum*) was done by the official physician and/or surgeon in the locality (*Physicus, Chirurgus juratus*), accompanied by the city clerk (*Stadtschreiber*), and two members of the magistracy (*Gerichts- und Raths-Personen*).[14] The medico-legal inspection (*Visum repertum*) and other local trial records (*Acta*) were then studied by members of the law faculty of the university at Tübingen. Articles 20 and 22 of the Carolina specified that 'legally sufficient' evidence, the so-called 'half-proof,' had to be present before torture could be initiated. Articles 35 and 36 offered criteria: change of body size and milk in the breasts were indications that a woman 'of whom such a suspected crime could be believed' might be a candidate. The medico-legal inspection, if it supported live-birth and death by wilful application of force, weighed heavily at this point. In light of the opinion (*Gutachten*) of the academic jurists, the high court (*Regierungsrat*) would authorize or disallow the local court to attempt to extract a confession from the suspect by means of judicial torture. If the high court had difficulty making a decision on torture, for instance if the issues of live-birth and cause of death seemed insufficiently clear, they could request an additional opinion from the medical faculty at Tübingen.[15]

If the accused confessed, the confession was only valid if repeated without torture after an interval of twenty-four hours (*Besiebnung*). The second part of the proceedings, the decision concerning punishment, began

INQUISITION
(*Peinliche Prozess*)

Malefiz Gericht: (local court)
Legal inspection (*Visum repertum*, autopsy)
Suspicion (*Verdacht*)
Visitation by midwife, medical officers
Questioning (*Inquisition*)

Regierungsrat: (high court)
Consideration of *corpus delicti*
Judicial faculty opinion (*Gutachten*)

If half-proof criterion satisfied: Judicial torture (*Peinliche Frage*)

Confession: Waiting period (*Besiebnung*)
Repetition of confession

REVIEW AND SENTENCING
(*Strafprozess*)

Resubmission of documents to central judicial authorities

Regierungsrat (high court)
Acta, *Amtsprotocol* considered
Perhaps *Gutachten* requested of medical faculty

corpus delicti: *Materiale* (live birth of viable child) (unnatural death)
Formale (intent to kill)

Geheimerrat (privy council to the duke)

Protocol: Summary of all documentation and process
Recommendation for sentence

Duke (final decision-making authority)

Comments appended to *Protocol*

Figure 1 Criminal proceedings in Württemberg, 1757–1817

with a reading of all the accumulated documentation (*Acta*). The high court first discussed two categories of evidence in the *corpus delicti*, to determine the legally supportable level of guilt. Live birth of a viable infant and conclusive argument for unnatural death constituted the material evidence (*materiale*); it was supplied primarily by the testimony of local medical officials, but could be supplemented by further investigations by other medical experts. Evidence for intent (*formale*) included wilful concealment of pregnancy and failure to seek assistance in childbirth. The gravest form, intentional childmurder (*infanticida dolosa*) was punishable by death; but conviction could only be supported when both material and formal parts of the *corpus delicti* were complete and unambiguous.[16] It was theoretically impossible to justify an *infanticida dolosa* conviction without a confession by the accused. Causing the child's death through neglectful or careless behaviour (*infanticida culposa*) was not a capital crime, and the court resorted to such a charge where wilful imposition of violence could not be proven or live-birth was doubtful. If the foetus was too premature to be viable, or showed deformities that would preclude survival, the accused was punished for fornication, adultery, or procuring abortion. The decision of the high court was then examined by the duke's privy council and finally, after consideration of the council's position paper, the *Protocol*, by the duke himelf. Negotiation between the high judiciary and the duke decided the fate of the accused.

The protocols, the documents that provide the major basis for the present analysis, are at once a condensation of the entire judicial process, and its culmination. Written by men in the innermost circle of the duke's advisers, his privy councillors, the protocols can be conceptualized as an archaeological record, where the original character of each stratum has been distorted, but by a process that is itself comprehensible. Thus we are aware that the city clerk, in transcribing the answers of the accused at the local inquisition, necessarily captured a version of the testimony in language that differed from the actual words spoken by the accused. We are also aware that few traces of the local persons who first pointed the finger of suspicion remain in the protocols. The opinions of the legal and medical faculties, on the other hand, were written by identifiable individuals acting as representatives of their colleagues and speaking in their own voices.[17] And the privy councillors who affixed their signatures to the protocols thereby certified that the documents constituted a fair representation of their proceedings. The duke, whose words are appended in the generous margin of the front page of each protocol, signed for himself but as one responsible to God for the moral well-being of his subjects.

Close reading of the protocols suggests fascinating aspects of the infanticide problem that need to be explored through deeper research in local archives. The voice of the accused is heard faintly, her individuality penetrating dispassionate official language. Also, positions are not identified as held by individuals but by groups (with the exception of the duke). The protocols, nevertheless, faithfully preserve elite perceptions of crime and its punishment, though those perceptions were by no means monolithic. Each group – local officials, faculty members, high court judges, ducal confidants – had its own interests to defend and viewed infanticide, even as they all agreed on its horror, through a different lens.

Justice and infanticide, 1757–92

In December 1757, Maria Barbara Lenzin of Tübingen was condemned to death by the sword. She had confessed to delivering in secret and then murdering her illegitimate child. Four months later, Anna Magdalena Maijerhöferin received the same sentence. In this case, however, the newborn child had been hideously abused, ostensibly by the mother, and therefore the ducal council made the additional demand that Maijerhöferin's severed head be impaled on a post and publicly displayed. This sentence was intended not only to punish the woman but to cast the taint of her unnatural and ungodly act over her entire family. The public display of her severed head was a grotesque warning to any others who might be tempted to commit the heinous crime of infanticide.[18]

Such brutal punishment was increasingly being called into question, however, not only in Germany but in most countries influenced by Enlightenment ideas. The executioner and his block were being replaced by the workhouse, previously a quasi-charitable place for housing the indigent unemployed. Moreover, the evidence that convicted Lenzin and Maijerhöferin was obtained by judicial torture, where the suspect was pressed to confess under verbal threat (first level), sight of instruments of torture (second level), or their application (third level). In Württemberg as in other areas whose criminal codes were based on the Carolina, this procedure was being challenged by humanitarian reformers. The 'enlightened' in the later eighteenth century found painful death, the mutilation of the human body, public shame, and physical or psychological torture all contrary to their belief in a humanity infinitely educable and perfectible.

Modern historians of law differ about the motivation and progress of the eighteenth-century judicial reformers. Wilhelm Wächtershäuser sees Enlightenment ideals emanating most prominently from Frederick II himself and from Prussian legal thinkers.[19] John Langbein argues to the contrary, that the legal reform movement was 'neither publicistic nor political, but juristic'.[20] Württemberg documents, however, point to an undeniable influence of the campaign for reform of judicial procedures upon jurists and indeed upon the duke himself. Increasingly often, they refer to the 'newer judicial thinking' that found public expression in the writings of Voltaire and Beccaria, as well as in learned commentaries on the Carolina.[21]

The same intellectual atmosphere that nurtured ideals of judicial reform also emphasized the role of the woman as mother and moral guardian of society.[22] Conversely, the treatment of women by society could stand allegorically for the level of moral responsibility the society itself was willing to accept – as Montesquieu argued in his *Persian Letters*.[23] Moreover, Cameralistic thinking, which saw population growth as a primary determinant of economic strength, heavily influenced government policymaking in later eighteenth-century Germany, in Württemberg as elsewhere.[24] Although Württemberg's population was in fact increasing, the perception of the duke and his advisers was that it was declining. In the neighbouring territory of the Palatinate, the physician and political writer Franz Anton May – himself a contributor to the Mannheim prize contest – decried the wretched conditions of the poor, especially the peasantry, and stressed their adverse effects on population growth. He blamed social ills on poverty and poorly thought-out use of charitable resources. His arguments were representative of thinkers on medical policy in the later eighteenth century. They raised the question: could a fertile young woman, who killed her child only as a last desperate act prompted by visions of a future of poverty and ignominy, be saved, be regenerated in the workhouse, where she would be instructed by the pastor in the joys of a Christian life well led?[25] For all these reasons, infanticide took on a heightened importance in comparison with other capital crimes during this period. In the world of Württemberg's educated administrators and professionals, opinions on infanticide were varied and complex. Positions on legal issues represented a mixture of philosophical principle, deeply held moral conviction, and jockeying for position. In an age where rank and precedence could enhance or reduce one's ability to translate a moral or intellectual stance into action, issues of political power and moral activism were inextricably intertwined.

Under the Carolina and its territorial elaboration, the *Württembergische Malefiz–Ordnung*, the final word in criminal proceedings was the duke's. The cases to be considered in this study occurred during the reign of Carl Eugen, Duke of Württemberg from 1744 to 1793. A man of conflicting impulses, the Roman Catholic ruler of a Lutheran territory, he was married to a niece of the Prussian king, Frederick II ('the Great'), at whose court he spent part of his teenage years. Goethe observed that

> Duke Carl [Eugen], to whom one must concede a certain grandeur of vision, worked nevertheless to gratify his momentary passions and to act out a series

> of everchanging fantasies... And even when his motives were less than noble, he could not help but further a higher cause.[26]

Goethe was referring to the cause of art, but his appraisal of the man's basic character applies to Carl Eugen's intellectual and moral stance as well.[27] Indeed, as Carl Eugen reached full intellectual maturity – he had taken up the reins of power at the age of only sixteen – the judicial climate in Württemberg underwent a dramatic change. In the early years of his rule, between 1757 and 1770, the privy council considered a total of twenty-five infanticide cases. Of these, eighteen ended with a sentence of death for premeditated infanticide (*infanticida dolosa*), while seven women were given workhouse sentences on lesser charges. By contrast, the next twenty-five cases, which came within a slightly shorter period (1771–81) resulted in only three death sentences. Sweat was replacing the sword, and frequently, it was problems with medical evidence that inhibited a judgment of *infanticida dolosa.*

But it is not numbers alone that carry significance. Just as important is the way that the relationship between medical evidence and judicial decision shifted. In the middle period of Carl Eugen's reign (1744–93), medical evidence was never truly at issue. In the cases where the women paid with their lives, apparent indications of violent death were accepted as obvious, and the medico-legal inspections by local physicians went unchallenged. One woman was subjected to judicial torture and condemned to death even though the infant's corpse had been defaced by birds.[28] Another case had a less tragic outcome. The cause of death was adjudged to be suffocation, but it was not medically certain that the child had been born alive.[29] Despite the accused's denial of intent and her testimony that she had fainted after the birth, the judicial faculty and high court decided that the half-proof criterion had been satisfied. But under judicial torture she exonerated herself of intent and was sentenced to two years in the workhouse.

Beginning in 1773, however, the role of medical evidence assumed a different character. The medico-legal report, written by the local health officers, was subjected to intensified scrutiny by the high court and, with increasing frequency, the medical faculty in Tübingen. At the same time, the faculty physician, in interpreting his autopsy results, became increasingly reluctant to insist on live-birth or unambiguous cause of death. The story begins not with intensified rigour of *corpus delicti* examination, but with a struggle over the question of judicial torture. As the tension between conservative and progressive legal philosophies escalated, medical evidence acquired enhanced priority.

Four landmark cases, 1773–4

In January, 1773, Margaretha Dorothea Dirolfin escaped the death penalty.[30] The medical inspection left no doubt that her child had been born alive. In the local inquisition, Dirolfin told several different versions of her story. But upon application of the 'Spanish Boot', she confessed to killing her child, and to having done so with intent. She said that she bore the child into a chamber pot, pulled it out by the feet and then dropped it in again, and, to make sure the child would die, tore the umbilical cord from its body. On the basis of this confession the law faculty and the high court demanded her execution. But a difference of opinion arose over the validity of a confession extracted under torture. The protocol attests to Dirolfin's being in 'a severe delirium' during the local inquisition. During the prescribed judicial torture process, after the required twenty-four hours waiting period, Dirolfin insisted that her child had *slipped* out of her hand and fallen back into the chamber pot. Under repeated questioning, she retracted that statement, and reverted to her original confession of intent. However, Dirolfin had introduced a shadow of doubt into a procedure that demanded proof 'clear as the light of day', and although they agreed that the full legal requirements for the death penalty had been met, the high court judges asked the duke to consider replacing the death penalty with lifelong workhouse incarceration. They were concerned that Dirolfin's erratic replies indicated a state of confusion induced by the torture process.[31] The privy council stood firm, arguing that even if the child had slipped back into the chamber pot, Dirolfin had committed an atrocious crime that should be punished by death. However, Carl Eugen disagreed and using his power of final decree, sentenced her to lifelong imprisonment in lieu of execution.

Six months later, in June 1773, the privy council struggled with the case of Catharine Barbara Wirthin.[32] The official documents portray Wirthin as what our grandmothers would have called 'a brazen hussy'. She threatened to countersue the townswomen who accused her of illegitimate pregnancy in the local court. She attempted to manipulate the physician who treated her for a strange white discharge – it turned red whenever she ate sauerkraut – into prescribing medication that might produce miscarriage. She lied to her mistress, who, believing her to be ill, attempted to make Wirthin comfortable during the early part of her labour, setting up a bed for her in the parlour. When the child was about to be born, Wirthin returned to her own bed to deliver, left the child in the cold room under the bedcovers and returned to the comfort of the parlour until morning.[33]

By her own admission the child was born alive, but she denied killing it or intending that it should die. Suspicious bruises on the child's head led the Stuttgart magistrates to suspect otherwise. However, the initial inspection report by the Stuttgart city physician (*Physicus*) L. H. Riecke, which noted the bruises, also insisted that the lungs of the child appeared undeveloped, which tended to support Wirthin's claim that the child had died of natural causes. In his medico-legal opinion for the high court, the Tübingen medical professor C. F. Jäger concluded that the evidence in Riecke's report was insufficient to establish that the child had been killed by a blow to the head.[34] Did the child die from exposure in the cold room, from bleeding through the cord, or possibly because the mother had prevented it from taking further breaths by holding her hand over its nose and mouth, or by pressing it between her thighs? The autopsy report could not answer these questions, at least not to a degree of certainty sufficient to warrant judicial torture on the basis of the material evidence. The firmest conclusion that Jäger could reach was just a possibility: that death could have resulted from a combination of the mother's deliberate attempt (which she had denied) to prevent the child from breathing and the way that she had wrapped the child's body after its birth. In light of Jäger's insistence on the inconclusive nature of the medical evidence, the high court was disinclined to allow the degree of judicial torture requested by the Stuttgart court, because it would signal reliance on 'a dangerous subsidiary mode of proof'. Several votes later, having considered the accumulation of conflicting evidence, the high court remained split. The majority recommended lifelong incarceration as a 'punishment close to the death penalty'. The minority felt that Wirthin's admission to having left the infant under the bedcovers for sixteen hours without seeking help was sufficient in itself to indicate intended murder. They wanted to allow the Stuttgart court to proceed with judicial torture in the hope of extracting a confession. Eventually, a compromise was reached, a recommendation for not lifelong, but an eight- to ten-year incarceration in the workhouse, without torture. The privy council, debating this 'troublesome' case, placed their trust in the *formale* part of the *corpus delicti*, that is to say, in the inference that her actions in themselves indicated intent to kill, and recommended a life sentence rather than the eight- to ten-year term. Significantly, the councillors made it clear in the final paragraph of the protocol that it was the *duke's* express intent to cease relying on judicial torture in such cases. The duke decided on a ten-year workhouse term.

Legally, what saved Wirthin from torture to induce a clear confession or denial of premeditated infanticide was the perceived unreliability of the material evidence in Riecke's initial medical-legal inspection and Jäger's reasoning in the medical faculty opinion. Jäger's autopsy was performed after twelve days had elapsed, and the external signs of possible violence had merged with those of natural deterioration (the child was born in

June). Also important was Jäger's unwillingness to draw firm conclusions from a medical report that did not meet the high standards required for legal evidence. But the duke, it should be noted, *could* have insisted on the death penalty for Wirthin; he did not have to accept the reduced sentence based on Jäger's reservations about the autopsy results.

Carl Eugen, like his father before him, had to strike power bargains with powerful Württemberg families, whose scions were heavily represented among his administrators.[35] His wish to join the ranks of 'progressive' thinkers who, like his model Frederick II of Prussia, were seeking to eliminate the use of judicial torture went against the intellectual grain of the more conservative members of his administration and the law faculty. The implications of the initial medico-legal report and opinion of the medical faculty quickly became apparent: without strong medical evidence for infanticide, judicial torture could be resisted. And without a confession of intent, and therefore without a *corpus delicti* to support intentional child murder, women could not be sentenced to death.

Two women had thus been spared from the executioner in the space of six months. In both cases, some jurists had voiced opposition to judicial torture. Dirolfin had cast doubt on her entire testimony by briefly negating a small detail, which happened to be a legally essential part of a capital confession. Wirthin was protected by the deteriorated condition of the corpse, which made the cause of the apparent bruises observed in the autopsy uncertain. As a result, neither the medico-legal inspection nor the faculty autopsy could provide definitive proof of a capital offence. In both cases, the judicial faculty and the privy council took a hard line, while the duke and the high court moved in the opposite direction, away from reliance on judicial torture and the extraction of a confession that would require the death penalty.

When confronted within a month by another possible controversy, the privy council went on the offensive, but was again effectively blocked by medical reservations about the physical evidence. Anna Catherina Härerin had her child outdoors under a hedge, and let it fall (accidentally, she insisted) twenty-six feet down into the snow, where it was found lying on its face. The baby clung to life for six days after its rescue, but then died. It seemed very clear to both the judicial faculty and the privy council that intent was involved, but once more, the medical report could not confirm that the fall and exposure were the absolutely certain causes of death. The material evidence was therefore insufficient and again judicial torture with a view to obtaining confession of intent was not legally permissible because the required half-proof did not exist. The privy council opted for a six-year workhouse sentence, noting pointedly that it was the smallest punishment that could possibly be levied. The duke concurred but made clear his displeasure with the longer-than-usual decision-making process.[36]

A case that threw the inconclusiveness of the material evidence into still sharper relief came the following summer, with a forester's discovery of not one but two tiny dead bodies in a basket. The widow Braitenmajerin, rumoured to be carrying on an illicit affair with a married man, was suspected of having borne them; indeed, the official midwife found milk in her breasts 'and other indications' that she had recently given birth. There was, however, a grave complication: the twins were a double conception. The smaller was judged by the local physician to have been only five or six months foetal age, having by all indications died *in utero* some weeks before birth. The larger twin was small for a full-term birth, had blood in its lungs, and had a fractured thigh bone.[37]

Braitenmajerin and her codefendant (her lover, a man named Schoch) insisted that the larger twin had been born alive but very weak, and had died within minutes. They claimed that they had not cut nor bound the umbilical cord because the infant died so quickly after birth. After considering the documents from the initial medical inspection and local inquisition, the Tübingen law faculty recommended judicial torture. Braitenmajerin had concealed her pregnancy and had given birth to a living child unattended by a midwife, both of which were formal grounds under Württemberg law for further inquisitorial proceedings – but only if the material basis (the medico-legal inspection of the corpse and the autopsy) showed sufficient evidence of mistreatment of the infant to constitute the required half-proof. But the high court refused to authorize judicial torture, because in the opinion of the medical faculty, the initial medico-legal report contained too many contradictions.[38] The most serious damage done to the child, the broken thigh bone, could be explained by the complications of birth caused by the dead foetus. If the leg of the child presented first, one of the most difficult positions for delivery, Braitenmajerin's lover would not have had the skill to extract the child and could inadvertently have caused the damage. Also, it was argued that the larger twin was contaminated *in utero* by the deteriorating foetus. That would explain its enfeebled condition, and suggest death from natural causes.

There were other medical ambiguities. According to contemporary medical opinion, blood in the lungs could have been caused, not only by wilful suffocation but as a consequence of the infant's first attempts to draw breath. Finally, the length of the child was more consistent with a seven- or eight- than with a nine-month pregnancy, which was also borne out by the widow's testimony as to the probable date of conception. An eight-month child was usually considered to have crossed the threshold of viability, but having to share the womb with another, damaged foetus would have lowered its chances of survival. The retarded development and attested weakness of the larger twin effectively negated a judgement of intentional infanticide; the charge was reduced to negligence, giving birth in circumstances that endangered life. Schoch was sentenced to only six months in the workhouse for adultery, and Braitenmajerin received two years, with the accompanying statement that hers was the greater crime.

What is remarkable in the Braitenmajerin case is the depth of argument about the medical evidence, which was far more extensive than that found in any previous infanticide protocol. In-depth medical investigation and rigorous scientific argumentation demonstrated the difficulty of assigning cause of death in any but the clearest case of intentional murder. The disruptive potential of medical testimony was rapidly becoming obvious: heightened demands for certainty applied to material evidence could effectively block the use of judicial torture.

Medical opinion and the torture question, 1774–93

In the final two decades of Carl Eugen's reign (he died in 1793), fifty-nine infanticide cases reached the high court. Although, with the exception of the duke, individual positions cannot be identified, the protocols made it clear that by 1774 a corner had been turned. The use of judicial torture in securing the *corpus delicti* was, with relatively few exceptions, an issue for extended and often acrimonious debate. In only three cases was there complete agreement among the various jurists and the duke, and in these the death penalty was levied.[39] Fifteen women were sentenced to long workhouse terms, 'the punishment closest to death'.[40] The ascertainable level of guilt for eleven women put them in confinement for four to six years.[41] Twelve received minimal punishments of one to three years.[42] In fourteen cases, the infants were too premature to be viable, and the mothers received workhouse sentences for fornication or abortion that ranged from three months to a year.[43] Four other cases were judged to fall outside the realm of infanticide delict.[44]

A chronological breakdown helps to make sense of these numbers in terms of the role of medical testimony in infanticide conviction. Between 1774 and 1780, seventeen cases of possible infanticide were referred to the high court by the localities. In six cases, the court refused to consider the charge of infanticide and imposed short workhouse sentences for abortion or fornication. Among the eleven cases where conviction for *infanticida dolosa* or *infanticida culposa* remained a possibility, judicial torture was authorized in only six cases; by virtue of that decision, the charge in the remaining five was reduced to one of *infanticida culposa*. Of the six cases actually tried on the more serious charge, four women were found guilty while the remaining two were finally exonerated of the capital crime and given lesser punishments.[45]

The duke in 1780, in retreat from his overt position of opposition to judicial torture, sought to avoid long delays caused by in-fighting and disputes over fine points of half-proof. These disputes more often than not involved points of medical evidence. His *Resolutione clementissima* demanded that the high court yield to him 'in special cases' the decision to recommend judicial torture.[46] And 'special cases' did abound. In only six trials during the next twelve years were the medical authorities agreed that a murder might have been committed. Between 1780 and 1793, as between 1773 and 1779, the outcome of the medico-legal inspection and autopsy was frequently indecisive: in eighteen cases out of thirty-seven the *materiale* of the *corpus delicti* was legally inadequate. Among these eighteen, the most common situation by far was indeterminate cause of death, with the law faculty, the majority and minority high court factions, the privy council and the duke expressing diverging opinions on the level of punishment justified.

After 1780, the high court was far more inclined to seek a medical faculty opinion (*Gutachten*) in addition to the medico-legal inspection of the local physician. Between 1757 and 1780, an opinion was requested in four of forty-eight cases tried: on average, one out of every twelve cases taken to the high court. In the thirty-seven cases tried from 1781 to the end of Carl Eugen's rule, the medico-legal inspection was supplemented by additional medical opinions in twelve cases, that is in practically every third trial, or four times more frequently than in the preceding period.[47] Significantly, in none of these cases was the undetermined cause of death resolved to legal satisfaction by the additional autopsy. Judicial torture was authorized just twice between 1780 and 1793. Medical authority was having the effect of displaying the uncertainty of the material evidence to the point where half-proof was becoming unachievable.

Further, the revealed instability of the *materiale* had the accompanying effect of shifting the burden of decision, especially concerning the harshness of punishment, onto the *formale*. In that regard, we see a notable evolution in the protocols: details of the woman's family relationships, her reputation for hard work or laziness, her moral comportment, her alleged physical and mental stability, appear with increasing frequency after 1780.[48] The protocol, of course, reflected the information the duke desired to have on hand when considering the recommendation of the combined judiciary. With his *Resolutione clementissima* of 1780, Carl Eugen introduced contingencies into sentencing that would make factionalism among jurists a feature of the last twelve years of his reign.

Thus increasing stringency within medicine had repercussions in law; it also nourished intra-professional tensions of long standing. In the eyes of the university and high-ranking government physicians, the medico-legal inspections done by local health officials were judged unsatisfactory. In six infanticide cases between 1780 and 1793 the carelessness or incompleteness of the initial autopsy raised the hackles of higher-ranking medical personnel.[49] The complaint was not new, but was becoming more frequent and more pointed. It resonated with an overall desire for reform of the medical administration and a new emphasis on the role of the official physician as medico-legal expert in criminal trials. Both gave impetus to simultaneous attempts to reform the medical curriculum of the territorial university in Tübingen.

The growth of forensic medicine instruction in Württemberg

As a problem in forensic medicine, infanticide presented a very special set of difficulties. The newborn child was an uncertain life at best: even when mothers were properly attended, infant mortality was high and not always explicable.[50] Second, in places where a woman was likely to bear a child unattended – in fields, in unheated servants' rooms, in barns – numerous natural hazards might affect the outcome. The child could be injured by the mother's attempts to help the delivery along, and could fall onto a floor if the mother gave birth unaided. The physician, then, had to distinguish between unintentional and intentional damage during and just after birth. Finally, if the child died, the desperate mother usually attempted to hide the body by burying it surreptitiously, throwing it into a well or dung heap or river. The dead body was therefore likely to undergo secondary damage that had to be distinguished from the actual cause of death.

Beginning with the 'landmark' infanticide cases of the mid-1770s discussed above, the two documents that comprised the *materiale* of the *corpus delicti* (the initial medico-legal inspection and the medical faculty opinion) came under heightened scrutiny in the judicial process. The inexactness of the initial inspection had been an ongoing problem: it was often carried out by a man with only the most basic knowledge of dissecting technique and little experience in the art of exact description. Most official physicians in the localities (*Physici*) were minimally qualified practitioners (*Licentiaten*) with two years' training at the University of Tübingen. There, students heard works by medical authorities read by faculty members, and observed anatomy demonstrations only when human cadavers were available.[51] At the end of the two years, the student defended a dissertation, usually one written by a faculty member. It was possible to supplement theoretical training by apprenticeships with experienced physicians and by private sessions with faculty members. Men who wished to compete for higher-ranking positions in the medical administration or in the faculty at Tübingen had to complete far more extensive studies for the *Doktorat*. These men commonly spent several years (*Lehrjahre*) travelling to faculties outside the duchy, and usually outside Germany – Leiden, Paris, Vienna.

But physicians of minimum and maximum qualification alike gained their positions via the time-honoured route of political patronage mediated through kinship networks. In most cases, one became an official physician (*Physicus*) in a provincial city by membership of or marriage into a family of local notables.[52] University chairs in medicine were the object of fierce competition and rarely moved outside the control of elite Tübingen families. Men in higher positions in the medical administration, for instance physicians to court personnel (*Hofmedicus*), most frequently had family ties with the court or the Stuttgart magistracy. To become a personal physician (*Leibmedicus*) to the duke it was necessary to possess prestige that would enhance the duke's glory, as well as the influence to press his health policies on recalcitrant local magistracies and, with no less a struggle, university physicians.

The initial medico-legal report and the faculty opinion, then, represented two extremes of medical sophistication and expertise. Frustration with inept initial reports, expressed in the protocols, was another manifestation of an ongoing struggle to upgrade medical education and wrest medical appointments from the control of local elites. Although legislation that would have instituted far-reaching reforms was blocked by political power networks in 1755, its intellectual spirit continued to prevail among progressive physicians in the upper ranks of government and university. They demanded higher standards of practice from local physicians and a higher level of scientific sophistication in the interpretation of autopsy results.

Improvements in the medical knowledge of local physicians responsible for initial medico-legal reports potentially offered something to both progressive and conservative interpreters of the law. A clear and unambiguous medical report might provide the evidence needed for conviction of deliberate infanticide. But as the four cases of 1773–4 demonstrated, the medico-legal inspection was also the element that was potentially most damaging to the case for intentional child killing. The move to upgrade forensic medicine pleased jurists in a non-political way as well, for whatever their stance on legal interpretation, they were dedicated professionals. And for high-ranking physicians, frequent denigration of the quality of medical reports by the jurists of the high court was a source of professional embarrassment. Thus no one involved had anything to lose from reform of the medical curriculum in a direction that would produce better-trained *Physici*, and potentially there was much to be gained. There was no opposition from the duke. His attention was now focused on his new military academy in

Stuttgart, the *Hohen Carlsschule*, where he was busy setting up a faculty whose appointments were an expression of his own wishes and not, as at Tübingen, a combination of patronage and kinship largely beyond his control.[53]

Forensic medicine was not new to the curriculum. Its origins at Tübingen reached back at least forty years before the heated debates of the 1770s. In 1736, Burkhard David Mauchart (1695–1751) was appointed Professor of Medicine at Tübingen and published the first of a series of medico-legal works to emanate from the faculty during the eighteenth century.[54] He was solidly behind the move to upgrade medical education and restructure medical legislation.[55] Under Mauchart's influence, legal medicine became a more-or-less regular feature of medical education at Tübingen. He lectured on the subject every third day during the winter semester of 1750.[56] His colleagues J. G. Gmelin and G. F. Sigwart included legal-medical topics in their lecture courses during the decade between 1750 and 1760, and by 1767 Sigwart (1711–95) was lecturing solely on forensic medicine.[57] Sigwart's early lectures were based on one of the standard texts of German legal medicine, Teichmeyer's *Institutiones medicinae legalis et forensis* (1723).[58]

A significant feature of Teichmeyer's treatise was his defence of the hydrostatic lung test. The so-called *Lungenprobe* had become standard practice in the states where the Carolina was the basis for criminal justice, because of the stipulation that infanticide could be committed only upon a living child, i.e. a child that had drawn breath. If the child had not breathed, conviction was sought on the lesser charges of fornication, concealed pregnancy, and/or attempted abortion. The difference was crucial because among these crimes only intentional infanticide was punishable by death.[59]

Christian Friedrich Jäger (1739–1808), who wrote the medical faculty opinion in the 1773 Wirthin case described above, lectured on medical theory and legal medicine as a member of the Tübingen medical faculty between 1767 and 1780.[60] He does not appear to have taught from Teichmeyer, however, perhaps because his training had led him to suspect that the experimental basis for Teichmeyer's defence of the lung test was faulty. Jäger studied the putrefaction of infants dead *in utero*, and found that the lungs of such infants, who had never drawn breath, would also float. He then used foetuses to test the hydrostatic lung test further. Teichmeyer's theory was based upon the lungs of calves that he anatomized, which were free from deterioration. Jäger, however, pointed out that physicians rarely tested the lungs of human infants for the courts under such ideal conditions. Autopsies for medical faculty opinions were often performed several days or even weeks after the infant's death, and under these circumstances gases from the decaying lung tissue could fill the lung cavities and could cause the lungs to float.[61]

Jäger rose rapidly through the ranks of official medicine in Württemberg, and in 1780 was appointed official physician to Duke Carl Eugen. This appointment followed the publication of his experiments on the lungs of newborn infants, which was dedicated to Carl Eugen. In this book, Jäger questioned three of the standard grounds for medico-legal decisions of live-birth and violent death: subcutaneous bleeding, the condition of the lungs, and the condition of the bladder. In all three cases, he argued, ambiguities and exceptions made the usual arguments invalid.

Jäger's career dovetails with that of the best-known practitioner of forensic medicine at Tübingen, Wilhelm Gottfried Ploucquet.[62] Unsuccessful at first in getting even an adjunct appointment to the medical faculty, which was experiencing a slump in student numbers, he caused an upset by publishing his first book, on nutrition, without ducal approval. He became an adjunct in 1770, but only one student matriculated with the medical faculty between 1770 and 1772. Ploucquet tutored privately to supplement his income and published two treatises on medico-legal topics.[63] In 1780 he succeeded to Jäger's chair in pathology and therapeutics, and in 1783 was appointed dean of the medical faculty. Interest in medico-legal issues was a constant theme in Ploucquet's career, which lasted four decades.

Ploucquet took up forensic-medical theorizing where Jäger had left it. In his studies on neonatal lungs, Jäger had discovered that there was a difference in the ratio between the weight of the lungs and the whole body weight between infants who had drawn breath after birth and those who had not.[64] Ploucquet developed a new lung test based on this finding after experimentally verifying Jäger's ratios and extrapolating the results for infants of low birth weight. His first publication as a faculty member was the treatise that proposed this substitute for the floating lung test; *De nova pulmonum Docimasia* (1781) hypothesized that changes in the distribution of the blood after initial respiration caused the specific weight of the lungs to increase. Ploucquet was the first Württemberg physician to publish for wider professional consideration a measurable rather than a phenomenological criterion for live-birth.[65] He thereby became a somewhat controversial figure, focusing the attention of German legal medicine on Tübingen.[66]

Ploucquet published anonymously, in 1783, on the Mannheim prize essay question, *Another Opinion on the Question: Which are the Best Workable Means to Stop Infanticide?*[67] His essay showed compassion for the predicament of the unwed mother, while revealing a predilection for rather repressive measures to prevent illegitimate pregnancy and secret birth. He argued that infanticide had its roots in social practice: the shame that the unwed mother experienced in the community, and her fear of punishment for concealing her pregnancy. He contended that statutes proscribing marriage between members of different social classes, prohibiting men in the army from marrying, and punishing the seduced woman far more severely than her seducer sealed the fate of unfortunate women; rather than facing ignominy, they killed their infants. Ploucquet proposed that public bathhouses be regulated and that women between the ages of fourteen and forty-eight be kept under close surveillance to prevent infractions of sexual morality. Finally, pregnant women were to wear special clothing that would make it impossible for them to conceal their condition.

Ploucquet's later *Treatise Concerning Death by Force, with an Appendix about Intentional Miscarriage* (1788) makes a crucial distinction between absolutely lethal acts and acts lethal under special conditions such as drunkenness, overeating, or poor health.[68] It contains echoes of Mauchart's 1736 treatise, but Ploucquet's treatise reflects clearly his long experience with the role of medical opinion in criminal prosecution.[69] Whereas according to earlier medico-legal theorists the physician would be called upon, in the report, to describe the wound itself as absolutely lethal or not, Ploucquet emphasized that the condition of the victim prior to the act made that judgement difficult. His categories reflect those of the *formale* of the *corpus delicti*: he distinguishes between murder with 'direct' intent and murder with 'indirect' intent, but emphasizes that the judge would make that decision, not the physician. It was the duty of the physician to produce an accurate report that would facilitate the legal process being carried out with maximum prudence. In his book on the education of the physician, he saw legal medicine as 'another type of application of medical knowledge, one that will assist medical policy': it had socio-political ramifications.[70] Ploucquet thereby highlighted the need for better training in legal medicine, not just for those who aspired to faculty or high administrative positions but also for the minimally trained practitioners in local posts.

The history of medical education in Württemberg during the second half of the eighteenth century is largely the history of the growth of training in legal medicine.[71] Yet Mauchart, Sigwart, Jäger, and Ploucquet struggled with inadequate facilities, the duke's fluctuating interest in the university, and not the least, with the moral dilemma of infanticide and justice. All of these men except Mauchart had studied theology, but even his thinking emphasized the ethical–moral aspect of legal medicine. The stand taken by Ploucquet pointed in the obvious direction of enhancing the facilities for hands-on experience in anatomizing, a solution that would begin to close the gap between the duty of the physician and his capacity to fulfil it.

Conclusion

The last two decades of Carl Eugen's reign saw a profound shift in the balance of forces affecting the outcome of infanticide investigations in Württemberg and the fate of the women accused. From the early 1770s, the quality of much of the material evidence in infanticide cases and the reliability of the methods used to obtain it were increasingly called into question by enlightened physicians and jurists, while growing scepticism about the reliability of confessions obtained under torture further inhibited its use. At the same time, intense public concern with infanticide as a social and moral problem, together with an increasingly widespread revulsion against the execution of women convicted of infanticide and the duke's own obvious reluctance to sanction the death penalty in such cases, made it almost impossible even for conservative councillors to enforce the full rigour of the law. The new enlightened criminal jurisprudence denied both the legitimacy and efficacy of torture in criminal cases, while Cameralist and Enlightenment political thought stressed the importance of preventing rather than punishing infanticide.

During this period, medicine's growing professional and scientific aspirations were reflected in demands for much higher standards in the conduct of medico-legal examinations and in the evaluation of causal explanations in the medical evidence. Conversely, the legal and political pressure placed on medical evidence by the infanticide question in the 1770s and 1780s clearly stimulated research and teaching on medico-legal aspects of infanticide in Württemberg at this time. The steady progress made by Jäger and Ploucquet in their academic and official careers in this period was doubtless bolstered by their substantial contributions to medico-legal knowledge bearing on infanticide.

The cumulative effect of these changes was to bring about a virtual cessation of the use of judicial torture in cases of suspected infanticide, and the *de facto* substitution of penal servitude in the workhouse for the death penalty. Indeed, following Carl Eugen's *Resolutione clementissima* of 1780, the whole focus of judicial inquiry in cases of infanticide gradually shifted away from the increasingly problematic search for material proof of the crime toward building an overall picture of the accused's past conduct and reputation as a means of determining the proper severity of her custodial sentence. The case of Anna Barbara Walterin (1792), decided during the last year of Carl Eugen's reign, exemplifies this alteration in focus. Walterin was charged with murdering her newborn by suffocating it with her hand and then throwing the body into an oven. The duke argued that the horror of her act itself proved her inability to make a rational decision, and thus to kill with wilful intent, because her actions were so 'contrary to the gentle nature of a mother'.[72] In this argument we see a complex blend of theological medical and socio-legal reasoning justifying a very different decision in 1793 than would have been possible in 1757. In Württemberg, as in many other parts of Europe, a combination of far-reaching changes in social attitudes, penal practice, and medical and legal reform were gradually to end the previously accepted penalty of death for women convicted of infanticide. The social, the political, the moral and the scienific were deeply intertwined in eighteenth-century Württemberg, and together they challenged the boundaries of legal decision, as they do in the present.

NOTES

1 Regina Schulte, for example, in *Das Dorf im Verhör* (Reinbeck bei Hamburg, 1989) treats the infanticide problem in later nineteenth-century Bavaria in the context of crimes in and against agricultural village communities, such as arson and poaching. Her 'Infanticide in rural Bavaria', in Hans Medick and David Warren Sabean, eds., *Interest and Emotion: Essays on the Study of Family and Kinship* (Cambridge, 1984), pp. 77–98, sketches most of her arguments.

2 For an interesting treatment of the implications of some recent discussions, see Barbara Duden, *Der Frauenleib als öffentlicher Ort: Vom Mißbrauch des Begriffs Leben* (Hamburg, 1991).

3 See Richard van Dülmen, *Frauen vor Gericht: Kindsmord in der Frühen Neuzeit* (Frankfurt am Main, 1991).

4 On punishment in early modern Europe, see Richard van Dülmen, *Theatre of Horror*, trans. Elisabeth Neu (Cambridge, MA, 1990), and van Dülmen, *Frauen vor Gericht*, pp. 39–57.

5 For an overview of the entries to the Mannheim prize essay competition and notions of judicial reform in the German Enlightenment, see Otto Ulbricht, *Kindsmord und Aufklärung in Deutschland* (Munich, 1990). Ulbricht's study is based on a thorough review of secondary literature as well as his own research in Schleswig-Holstein.

6 For a discussion of the Carolina in comparative historical context, see John H. Langbein, *Prosecuting Crime in the Renaissance* (Cambridge, MA, 1974), pp. 129–209.

7 The standard reference source for the law codes of the Duchy of Württemberg is August Ludwig Reyscher, *Vollständige, historisch, und kritisch bearbeitete Sammlung der württembergischen Gesetze*, 19 vols. (Stuttgart and Tübingen, 1826–51). While the Carolina is generally written in dispassionate language, the Württemberg code expresses the duke's concern for his duty as father to his people, i.e. guardian of the moral order, and justice as appeasement of God's anger over the destruction of innocents. It empowers and in fact obliges lords (i.e. nobles), masters (heads of households) and their wives to report suspicious women to the proper authorities: 'General-Reskript, das Verbrechen des Kinds-Mords betreffend. Vom 1. März 1658.', Reyscher, *Sammlung*, vol. 6, §152. Capital punishment for infanticide was reaffirmed in 'General-Reskript, die Bestrafung heimlicher Geburt und des Kinds-Mords betreffend. Vom 24. Mai

1715', ibid. §248, and the formal procedure for criminal trial clarified, 'Kriminal-Prozeß-Ordnung (Malefiz-Ordnung), Vom 4. April 1752', ibid. §299.

8 *Medizin vor Gericht: Gerichtsmedizin von der Renaissance bis zur Aufklärung* (Bern, 1983).

9 For an overview of medical education in eighteenth-century Germany, see Thomas Broman, 'University reform in medical thought at the end of the eighteenth century', *Osiris*, 5 (1989), 36–56.

10 See Mary Nagle Wessling, 'Official medicine and customary medicine in early modern Württemberg: the career of Christoph Friedrich Pichler', *Medizin, Gesellschaft und Geschichte*, 9 (1990), 21–44.

11 Fischer-Homberger, *Medizin vor Gericht*, pp. 85–9.

12 For the parallel phenomenon among British physicians, see Catherine Crawford, 'A scientific profession: forensic medicine and medical reform in British periodicals of the early nineteenth century', in Roger French and Andrew Wear, eds., *British Medicine in an Age of Reform* (London, 1991), pp. 203–30.

13 For the purposes of this paper, forensic medicine and legal medicine are interchangeable terms, following eighteenth-century usage.

14 'Commun-Ordnung vom 1. Juni 1758: Vierzehenden Abschnitt', Reyscher, *Sammlung*, vol. 13, pp. 584–5.

15 Opinions (*Gutachten, consilia*) were sought from the law and medical faculties of the University of Tübingen not just by localities of the duchy but also by independent polities such as imperial cities, and holdings of knights and nobles. Württemberg towns and cities sometimes sought opinions after the initial accusation, and, if the *corpus delicti* was deemed highly unreliable, declined to proceed further.

16 A spontaneous confession of guilt could be used to convict, or a combination of circumstantial evidence along with a confession obtained by means of judicial torture.

17 Both sets are extant in the archives of the University of Tübingen and contain supporting evidence. The legal opinions in particular often contain details of the local inquisition missing from the protocols.

18 Protocols for the infanticide cases are in the *Hauptstaatsarchiv Stuttgart* (hereafter cited as HSAS), divisional holding (*Bestand*) A202, which contains the working papers of the privy council. The records for years 1757 through 1793 are in bundle (*Büschel*) 1778. Each case cited will be identified by the date of ducal opinion, found on the first page of the protocol. Thus, Lenzin, sentenced 9 Dec. 1757; Maijerhöferin, 1 Mar. 1758, HSAS/A202/1778.

19 Wilhelm Wächtershäuser, *Das Verbrechen des Kindesmords im Zeitalter der Aufklärung* (Berlin, 1973). Wächtershäuser draws on a wealth of sources, including the writings of the Dutch physician Peter Camper and the compendia of case studies published by the Prussian jurists Georg J. F. Meister (1791) and Ernst Ferdinand Klein (1790–1801). However, this is a somewhat tendentious set of data: the cases were chosen by Meister and Klein for their jurisprudential interest, and do not constitute a representative spectrum of infanticide cases.

20 John H. Langbein, *Torture and the Law of Proof* (Chicago, 1977), p. 4. Langbein continues: 'In the two centuries preceding the abolition of torture, there occurred a revolution in the law of proof in Europe. The Roman-canon law

remained formally in force, but with its power eroded away.' The long workhouse term then became the punishment of choice for serious offences. My work in Württemberg indicates that the workhouse did provide an alternative to the death penalty, but that the process was much more complex than Langbein allows. In Württemberg, the workhouse was not much used as an institution where time was served as punishment for serious crime. See 'General-Reskript, die Benutzung des Ludwigsburgher Zucht- und Arbeits-Hauses, als Straf-Anstalt, betreffend. Vom 20 Mai, 1746', Reyscher, *Sammlung*, Vol. 6, §367.

21 See F.-C. Schroeder and P. Landau, *Strafrecht, Strafprozess und Rezeption* (Frankfurt, 1984), for a discussion of legal commentators.

22 See L. J. Jordanova, 'Natural facts: a historical perspective on science and sexuality', in Carol P. MacCormack and Marilyn Strathern, eds., *Nature, Culture and Gender* (Cambridge, 1980), pp. 42–69.

23 On the one hand, if the treatment of women is the 'moral barometer' of the society, then torturing women is the worst form of social barbarism. But if mothers are the moral guardians of society, then infanticide not torture is the worst social evil, and perhaps any effective means of stamping it out would be justifiable. I am grateful to Martin Pernick for this observation.

24 Albion Small, *The Cameralists* (Chicago, 1909). For the influence of Cameralism on Württemberg policy, see Heinz Schmucker, 'Das Polizeiwesen im Herzogtum Württemberg', Ph.D dissertation, Tübingen, 1958.

25 For example, the case of Arnoldin (1782).

26 Goethe to Duke Carl August of Saxe-Weimar, Tübingen, 12 September 1794, quoted in James Allen Vann, *The Making of a State* (Ithaca, 1984), p. 259.

27 On Carl Eugen, see *Herzog Carl Eugen v. Württemberg und seine Zeit*, Württembergischer Geschichts- und Altertums-Verein, 2 vols. (Esslingen, 1907–9); Vann, *Making of a State*; Erwin Hölzle, *Das alte Recht und die Revolution* (Munich, 1931).

28 Anna Maria Schmidin, sentenced 26 June 1770.

29 Catherina Steinhülberin, sentenced 5 March 1770.

30 Decision of 21 January 1773.

31 In the words of the protocol, 'wo die Confession durch die peinliche Frage extorquirt worden, einem Judici conscientioso immer einige formido oppositi übrig bleibe; nächst daß auch zur Zeit der ersten Verhör ein so starckes Delirium, daß sie auf zerschiedene Fragen verkehrt, theils gar nicht geantworttet, bey ihr verspührt worden wäre'.

32 The documents for the Wirthin case: protocol, HSAS/A202/1778 (7 June 1773); medical faculty opinion, signature 14/12, and judicial faculty opinion, signature 84/126, Universitätsarchiv Tübingen (hereafter cited as UAT).

33 The judicial faculty opinion, from which the details of Wirthin's behaviour are drawn, UAT 84/126.

34 Ludwig Heinrich Riecke was the son of Johann Viktor Heinrich Riecke, a high-ranking member of the medical bureaucracy and author of Württemberg's official manual for midwives. Riecke *père*'s office of *Stadtphysicus* was passed on to his son. See Walther Pfeilsticker, ed., *Neues Württembergisches Dienerbuch*, 3 vols. (Stuttgart, 1957), §2848. Jäger's *Gutachten*, comparing Riecke's inspection to an authority on head wounds, states, 'However, in the autopsy protocol, the words are not specified to be understood with the rigour and precision that legal

causation would demand' (Sind aber auch in dem Sections-Protocoll die angerführte Worte nicht in diesem rigore und so praecise, als man in sonsten in caussu legali forden kan, zu verstehen'), UAT 14/12, transcribed in Saskia Tilke Baur, 'Der gerichtsmediziner Christian Friedrich Jaeger (1739–1808)', MD dissertation, Tübingen, 1976, pp. 53–62.

35 Carl Eugen's struggle with the estates of the realm is presented in all its vicissitudes in Vann, *Making of a State*, the events of the 1770s on pp. 256–97, especially pp. 292ff.

36 See the duke's comments appended to the protocol, 24 July 1773.

37 The decision on Braitenmajerin and Schoch, 13 September 1774.

38 See protocol, 10 Sept. 1774.

39 In Schlitterin (1774), the signs of violence as recorded in the medico-legal inspection were not questioned. In Fehlin (1775), the infant 'before, during and after birth was lively and healthy' according to the opinion of medical professor Sigwart (UAT 14/12:33). The lung test was positive and uncomplicated; the pattern of blood accumulation clearly indicative of applied force rather than birth injury. Kozin (1778) confessed to bearing and letting die her own father's child; death was attributed to bleeding through the unbound cord. The protocol refers to a quarrel between medical authorities concerning the vitality of her seven-month infant, but the high court unanimously allowed judicial torture. Kozin was condemned to die despite the prematurity of her child, which could have undermined the *corpus delicti* for infanticide (all protocols, HSAS/A202/1778).

40 Protocols of Dirolfin (1773, reprieved 1785), Wilhelmin (1781), Klinckin (1788), lifelong incarceration; Wirthin (1773), Schneiderin (1776), Lutzin (1778), Schuppartin (1781), Ohnmeißin (1785), Walterin (1792), Baderin (1793), ten years; Ströhlin (1787), Beutelin (1787), Judain (1788), Bisreuterin (1788), Fischerin (1792), eight years.

41 Protocols of Tiroldin (1775), Unterbargerin (1776), Letschin (1776), Sattlerin (1781), Luzin (1782), Daubenschmidin (1783), Mäußlerin (1784), Locherin (1785), Höhingen (1786), Pfauin (1789), Epplin (1791).

42 Protocols of Barthin (1773), Härerin (1773), Braitenmajerin (1774), Schemppin (1775), Fischerin (1775), Kayserin (1777), Walckerin (1778), Abertinin (1784), Benzlerin (1785), Hauserin (1786), Lupferin (1791), Müllerin (1792).

43 Protocols of Hornungin (1771), Hirschmännin (1774), Hafnerin (1774), Groesin (1780), Haasin (1781), Fißlerin (1783), Baurin (1784), Vailin (1785), Ziglerin (1785), Lippin (1785), Adamin (1786), Schmidin (1790), Konzelmannin (1791), Loetterlin (1792).

44 Protocols of Leibrandin (1775), Schaafin (1781), Arnoldin (1782), Pfisterer (1791). In three cases, Tiroldin (1775), Unterbargerin (1776) and Müllerin (1792), the scribal protocols are missing, but information is provided by privy council communications to the high court, also in HSAS/A202/1778.

45 Schemppin, Fischerin (1775).

46 Information taken from the Maria Catharina Luzin protocol (1782).

47 Wirthin (1773), Tiroldin (1775), Lutzin (1778), all by Jäger, Härerin (1773) by Sigwart. After 1780: Sattlerin (1781), by Storr; Luzin (1782), Daubenschmidin (1783), by Jäger; Ohnmeißin (1784), Benzlerin (1785), Hauserin (1786), by Storr; Höhingen (1786), Ströhlin (1787), by Ploucquet; Ziglerin (1785), Pfauin (1789),

Lupferin (1791), author of opinion not identified; Baderin (1793), by Cannstadt *Stadtphysicus* Elwert. A 'medical faculty agreement' referred to in the protocol of the Epplin (1791) case may or may not mean that an opinion was formally requested; I have not included it in the figures.

48 For example, Schuppartin (1781), Ohnmeißin (1788), Klinckin (1788).

49 Sattlerin (1781), rebuke of *Physicus* Planer; Daubenschmidin (1783); Höhingen (1786), rebuke of local surgeons; Hauserin (1786), rebuke of *Physicus* Doerner; Judain (1788), corpse buried without dissection; Baderin (1793).

50 Two out of ten infants died before their first birthday. For infant mortality in eighteenth-century Württemberg, see James J. Sheehan, *German History* (Oxford, 1989), pp. 74–7.

51 In 1715, Duke Eberhard Ludwig decreed that bodies of executed criminals were to be taken to the university to be anatomized. In 1763 and 1765, Carl Eugen extended that to bodies of 'delinquents' who died in the winter months and indigent persons who died in hospitals. Reyscher, *Sammlung*, vol. 6, pp. 271, 582.

52 In 'Official medicine and customary medicine' (see note 10), I explore the network of power that kept local patronage practices intact. My 'Medicine and government in early modern Württemberg', unpublished Ph.D thesis, University of Michigan, 1988, examines university and court politics, pp. 27–76.

53 Kenneth Dewhurst and Nigel Reeves, *Friedrich Schiller: Medicine, Psychology, and Literature* (Berkeley, 1979), pp. 9–53, describes the regimen at the Carlsschule, and the *Cabale und Liebe* of the duke.

54 By all accounts aggressive, brilliant and controversial, he trained in Altdorf under the famed Lorenz Heister, in Tübingen, and in Paris under Woolhouse, an ophthalmic surgeon of international reputation. See Michael Reinhard, 'Burkhard David Mauchart (1695–1751)', MD dissertation, Tübingen, 1963.

55 See my 'Medicine and government', pp. 51–5.

56 UAT, 'Ordo studiorum Acad. Tubing, anno 1750. In Facultate Medica.'

57 A summary of the medico-legal topics taught to Tübingen medical students can be found in Bernhard Hubert Pfaff, 'Johann Geo. Gmelin, Philipp Fried. Gmelin, Geo. Fried. Sigwart, Karl Fried. Clossius und ihre Tätigkeit in Lehre und Forschung auf dem Gebiet der gerichtlichen Medizin in Tübingen', MD dissertation, Tübingen, 1976, pp. 128–34. Sigwart trained as a theologian before becoming a physician, and, as a student, heard lectures at Halle by Friedrich Hoffmann, the renowned medical theoretician and official physician to the Prussian king. Like Mauchart, he trained with well-known physicians outside the duchy and found ready entry into the medical officiate of Württemberg by marriage – to Mauchart's step-daughter (Pfaff, 'gerichtlichen Medizin', pp. 42–3). The list of thirty-one medico-legal books in his personal collection (ibid., pp. 54–7), reveals a man of broad medical erudition.

58 The seminar descriptions for Sigwart's teachings in 1766 and 1768 specifically single out Teichmeyer as the basis for the readings, according to Pfaff, 'gerichtlichen Medizin', p. 53. Of course we cannot know to what extent the numerous other authors in Sigwart's library may have featured in the discussions. The thesis was first published in Latin; the German translation, *Anweisung zur Gerichtlichen Arzneygelahrtheit* (Jena 1723, 1740, 1762, Florenz 1771; first published in German, Nürnberg, 1761) is generously abstracted ibid., pp. 58–63.

59 Baur, 'Jaeger', p. 121, traces the eighteenth-century use of the 'swimming lung test' in German medical jurisprudence; its theoretical origin is Galenic. Teichmeyer's teaching is abstracted in Pfaff, 'Gerichtliche Medizin', pp. 58–83. See also Robert P. Brittain, 'The hydrostatic and similar tests of live birth: a historical review,' *Medico-Legal Journal*, 31 (1963), 189–94.

60 Jäger had been promoted to the medical doctorate at Tübingen by Sigwart; like Sigwart, he studied theology before coming to medicine, and sharpened his medical skills by study outside the duchy, in Holland, in other German states and in Vienna. His marriage to the daughter of a Stuttgart magistrate positioned him well politically; he was appointed official physician to the city of Nürtingen in the year he received his doctorate, 1767 (Baur, 'Jaeger', pp. 3–5). Jäger published in 1767 'Observations de foetibus recens natis jam in utero mortuis et putridis, cum subjuncta epicrisi' ('Observations on newly born foetuses that died in the mother's womb, with a critical examination'), which contains important material relevant to the hydrostatic lung argument (see Baur, 'Jaeger', pp. 74–84).

61 'Disquisitio medico-forensis, qua casus et annotationes ad vitam foetus neogeni dijudicandam facientes proponuntur' ('A forensic medical investigation into the cases and observations that support the judgement of life of a newborn'), summarized in Baur, 'Jaeger', pp. 85–121.

62 Son of a pastor who was Professor of Logic and Metaphysics at the University of Tübingen, Ploucquet earned a master's degree in philosophy and started to study theology, but at the age of eighteen, changed direction once more and began to study medicine at Straßburg. After one semester there he returned to Tübingen, where, in August 1766, he was promoted to the doctorate in medicine. He spent a short time in Leiden and began private practice in Tübingen in 1767. See R. A. v. Duisburg, 'Der Gerichtsmediziner Wilhelm Gottfried Ploucquet (1744–1814)', MD dissertation, Tübingen 1974.

63 *Von den gewaltsamen Todesarten* (*On Death by Force*, 1777); *Über die physische Erfordnernisse zur Erbfähigkeit der Kinder* (*Concerning the Physical Requirements for Inheritance by Children*, Tübingen, 1779). On the intricacies of Württemberg's legal system as they are revealed in the everyday life of villagers, see David Sabean, *Property, Production, and Family in Neckarhausen, 1700–1870* (Cambridge, 1990).

64 See the 1780 Hennenhoffer dissertation in Baur, 'Jaeger', §XII, 'The scrutiny of a new method of testing the lungs', where Jäger discusses Ploucquet's test. This preceded Ploucquet's 1781 treatise; Jäger probably knew Ploucquet's work firsthand.

65 V. Duisburg, 'Ploucquet', includes a complete German translation of *De novo pulmonum Docimasia*, pp. 63–95.

66 See v. Duisburg, 'Ploucquet' p. 16. In §IX of *De novo*, Ploucquet credits Jäger for taking only two measurements of the proportional weights of foetal lungs. He describes his own procedure, in §X, the history of the discovery, §XI, and the dispute with the Leipzig professor Daniel over the issue of precedence, §XII (ibid., 75–84).

67 *Noch eine Meinung über die Frage: welches sind die besten ausführbaren Mittel, dem Kindermord Einhalt zu thun* (Tübingen, 1783).

68 *Abhandlung über die gewaltsame Todesarten, nebst einem Anhang von dem geflissentlichen Mißgebähren* (Tübingen, 1788).

69 In all, Ploucquet wrote seventeen opinions as a medico-legal expert. In the infanticide case of Rosina Küberlin (1795), where the initial medical report was careless and vague, he pleads for more precise medical evidence. Another of his medical opinions outlines hidden defects in prenatal development which would not have been detected in a medico-legal inspection but could have contributed to the infant's demise (Juliana Sperrin (1779), UAT 14/12, excerpted in v. Duisburg, 'Ploucquet', pp. 37–44). These opinions were not written during Carl Eugen's reign, but do reflect thinking that had matured in the 1780s when public interest in infanticide was at its peak.

70 *Der Arzt oder über die Ausbildung, die Studien, Pflichten, Sitten und die Klugheit des Arztes* (Tübingen, 1797), §95.

71 For lists of courses offered, see Wolfgang Albert Herzog, 'Carl Phillip Diez, Christian Friedrich Reuß, Georg Carl Ludwig Sigwart und ihre Tätigkeit in Lehre und Forschung auf dem Gebiet der gerichtlichen Medizin in Tübingen', MD. dissertation, Tübingen, 1974, pp. 17–31, 57–85; Walter Ulmer, 'Burkhard D. Mauchart, Christian L. Mögling, Ferdinand Chr. Oetinger und ihre Tätigkeit in Lehre und Forschung auf dem Gebiet der gerichtlichen Medizin in Tübingen', MD dissertation, Tübingen, 1980, pp. 32–4, 92–6, 125–31; Baur, 'Jaeger', 32–40; Pfaff, 'gerichtlichen Medizin', 128–34. If a professor did not teach a course as published, he was required by statute to submit his reasons in writing. See *Neglectus*, UAT 26/11, 27/2.

72 Walterin (1792):

> Especially when the reason can be understood, that, in the accomplishment of such a horrid assault against the fruit of her own body, [surely] inborn motherly tenderness would work against it; such a crime is only conceivable, which we have found it clearly and frequently to be the case, if, when the murderess is gripped by such a spiritual absence it makes her involuntarily capable of such an act.
>
> (Wann vorzüglich mit Grund angenommen werden kann, dass der Vollbringung eines solcher schweren Vergehens gegen eigene Leibesfrucht, schon die angebohrene mütterliche Zärtlichkeit entgegen strebt, mithin ein solches Verbrechen nur denkbar ist, wann wir zur Zeit der Entbindung so leicht und häufig der Fall eintritt, die Möderin von einer Geistes Abwesenheit befasst ist, die sie dazu allein, unwillkührlich, fähig machen kann.)

6

Training medical policemen: forensic medicine and public health in nineteenth-century Scotland

BRENDA WHITE

One of the many distinctive features of nineteenth-century Scottish medical education was the unique system of teaching forensic medicine and public health together under the heading of medical jurisprudence and medical police. Within the British Isles, Scotland was alone not only in teaching these subjects in tandem, but in doing so throughout the nineteenth century, and at some institutions well into the twentieth century. To the present-day observer, there would seem to be little in common between forensic medicine and public health, but throughout the nineteenth century these two subjects were intimately connected both at the level of academic teaching and in everyday practice. The link between them was their common concern with meeting certain requirements of the law. They did not train doctors to become more proficient in the healing arts, but equipped them to provide the courts and local magistrates with informed advice on the material facts of crime and squalor and the best means of dealing with them. This chapter focuses on two main aspects of this system. The first is the European origins of medical jurisprudence, sometimes referred to as *state medicine* or *medical police*, and the reasons why it was more attractive to Scotland than to England. It examines the circumstances surrounding the establishment of the first British chair of medical jurisprudence at Edinburgh in 1807, and the perceived radical implications of the subject. Secondly, the paper traces the progress of Scottish medical jurisprudence teaching, explaining why a formal system of medico-legal education was deemed necessary, who taught it and what its effects were.

Medical jurisprudence and medical police, considered as bodies of knowledge, were introduced into Britain from Europe via Scotland in the closing decades of the eighteenth century, when many facets of Scotland's cultural and educational life still bore the influences of its strong European links prior to the 1707 Act of Union. Scottish medical and legal ties with the Low Countries, Germany and France provided a fertile medium for the spread of Enlightenment thought, and its examination of man's relationship to society and to the state. In Germany, Johann Peter Frank, professor of medicine at Pavia and Vienna, formulated a system of state medicine congenial to autocratic rulers seeking to establish ordered healthy societies secure against invasion by either pestilence or foreign armies. Frank's encyclopedic work, *System einer vollständigen medicinischen Polizey*, published between 1778 and 1788 in Mannheim, and known in English as *A complete system of medical police* was a pioneering synthesis of many elements of what is now described as social medicine. George Rosen's seminal study of the history of social medicine compares Frank's work with other systems of 'state medicine' emanating from Italy and France in the eighteenth and nineteenth centuries. Rosen doubted that Frank's social philosophy could have been translated to Britain where 'administrative absolutism' had not been developed.[1] 'Administrative absolutism' was no more a feature of Scottish than English governmental tradition at this time. But in Scotland a unique combination of political and cultural circumstances enabled a modified form of medical police, shorn of its centralist trappings, to take root and flourish.

Politics and the regius chairs of medical jurisprudence

The conduit for Scottish acceptance of European models of legal medicine was Andrew Duncan, Sr (1744–1828). As founder-editor of the medical periodical *Medical and Philosophical Commentaries* in 1773, Duncan was in contact with a wide circle of influential European doctors.[2] Duncan was appointed Professor of the Institutes of Medicine at the University of Edinburgh in 1790. Shortly afterwards he introduced some of the principles of medical jurisprudence into his teaching from the chair, publishing his first *Heads of Lectures on Medical Jurisprudence* in 1792. By 1801, Duncan was conducting a winter series of extra-academical lectures on medical jurisprudence and a summer lecture series on medical police, held on Saturday mornings.[3] Duncan freely admitted that his lectures were inspired by Frank's writings. However, he inserted a strong measure of Scottish liberal thought into his teaching. Duncan's version of medical police replaced state intervention with a system based on private philanthropy, contributed to by doctors and laymen alike. In this system Duncan assigned a purely advisory role to doctors in their dealings with the magistracy on public health matters.

In 1798 Duncan presented a memorial to the university patrons on the value of medical jurisprudence teaching and requested the institution of a chair of medical jurisprudence similar to those recently introduced in France.[4] The subject, he claimed, was known in European countries as state medicine and consisted of both medical police to aid magistrates and the legislature in safeguarding the public health, and juridical medicine to assist the process of law in criminal, civil and consistorial courts. The university, however, rejected Duncan's arguments, saying that such a chair would add no credit or dignity to the university.[5]

Duncan's interest in the chair was to a certain extent motivated by family concerns. His eldest son, also named Andrew (1773–1832), had travelled extensively on the Continent during 1795–6 to widen his medical education.[6] There, using his father's earlier contacts, he met European medical jurists and studied clinical medicine under Frank before returning to Edinburgh in 1796. The younger Duncan held the position of Physician to the Queensferry fever hospital but had no other appointments.[7] Duncan's paternal anxieties may therefore have had some bearing on his advocacy of a chair to which his son would be eminently suited. However, discounting possible family ambitions, the point remains that in Scotland there was a sustained interest in the European development of medical jurisprudence and medical police. This interest sought to extend the medical care and attention normally given to human disorders to the treatment of social ones.

There are many reasons why Andrew Duncan's interest in medical jurisprudence and medical police found a favourable seeding ground in Scotland's capital. Although after 1707 Scotland's national identity was assured through the retention of its major institutions of Church, law and education, the Union of the Crowns in 1603 and the Union of Parliaments in 1707 had left Edinburgh as a capital without a royal court or the trappings of political power. However, by the late eighteenth century this vacuum was being filled by the rise of an influential professional class as Edinburgh society developed into a dense network of lesser nobility, lawyers, clergymen and doctors bound closely together by intricate familial relationships and political loyalties.

The establishment of the first British chair of medical jurisprudence at Edinburgh in 1807 drew on many of these factors, not least a fortuitous combination of inter-professional friendships and political loyalties. The latter point is particularly relevant. The regius chair of medical jurisprudence and medical police at Edinburgh owed its foundation to Andrew Duncan's lifelong friendship with Henry Erskine (1746–1817), a prominent Whig lawyer who became Lord Advocate when the Whigs enjoyed a brief spell of power in 1806–7 in what became known as 'The Ministry of All the Talents'.[8] The office of Lord Advocate, the chief legal officer, is a peculiarly Scottish political appointment: the incumbent is usually found a seat in Parliament. Until the re-establishment of a Secretary for Scotland in 1885, the Lord Advocate conducted virtually all Scottish business at Westminster.[9] Erskine, a radical Whig, readily saw the advantages of a medico-legal chair similar to those already founded in revolutionary France. In 1806 he successfully canvassed support for the chair in Parliament by submitting to the Crown a copy of Duncan's 1798 memorial to the patrons of Edinburgh University, together with a covering petition of his own dwelling on the usefulness of medical jurisprudence to the law in criminal and property-related cases.[10] It was thus Erskine, working within Parliament as Lord Advocate, who successfully obtained the creation of the first regius chair of medical jurisprudence and medical police in Britain in May 1807. The chair's first incumbent was Andrew Duncan the younger.

But the regius chair found no favour with the conservative medical faculty at Edinburgh, and it refused to house such a radical subject. For the first eighteen years of its existence the chair was therefore lodged within the faculty of law where, under the powerful protection of the Erskine family, it withstood repeated Tory attempts to suppress it. The earliest attempt came when the Tories returned to power in 1807, only months after the chair's foundation. In a much-quoted House of Commons debate on the excesses of the previous Whig administration, Canning is reported to have said of the chair of medical jurisprudence, 'He could alone account for such a nomination by supposing that after a long debate, in the swell of insolence, and to show how far they could go, they had said – We will show them what we can do – We will create a Professor of Medical Jurisprudence'.[11]

Regius chairs, created and funded by central government, are by definition political creations. The perceived radicalism of regius chairs of medical jurisprudence, and the continued reluctance of Scottish universities to accept them, is nicely illustrated by the controversy surrounding the establishment of the Glasgow regius chair in 1839. Although by 1839 medical jurisprudence and medical police were arguably less radical in their associations than in 1807, the circumstances surrounding the establishment of the Glasgow regius chair reveal a lingering political hostility to the subject. A Whig government was in power again when Robert Cowan (1796–1841), a staunch Whig supporter, was appointed first regius Professor of Medical Jurisprudence without consultation with the university's principal. Principal MacFarlan, a noted Peelite Tory, had previously ignored a recommendation in 1829, from the Royal Commissioners investigating university teaching, that a lectureship in medical jurisprudence should be established in the University of Glasgow. Queen Victoria's signature on Cowan's warrant for the regius chair surprised and angered Principal MacFarlan but, despite his strong opposition, the appointment stood. The last overtly political appointment to a Scottish regius chair of medical jurisprudence came in 1841 at Glasgow when Harry Rainy (1792–1876) succeeded Cowan after his untimely death. Just as the Whigs had done, the incoming Tory government chose Rainy because of his staunch party allegiance.[12]

When Andrew Duncan introduced the radical subjects of medical jurisprudence and police into his teaching from the chair of the institutes of medicine he was not whistling in the wind, but reflecting a fundamental concern about social order: a problem already recognized by some Scottish local government authorities. By the last decade of the eighteenth century, the onset of industrialism based on mining and textile manufacture had caused massive population shifts. Small villages and towns thrust into the vortex of social change emerged as large population centres with no adequate increase in living space or sanitary provision. New wealth juxtaposed with abject poverty made contemporary opinion more aware of crime, especially crimes against property. Under these stresses the old order of civic government gave way. Large Scottish burghs and towns, in common with large English towns such as Manchester, attempted to stabilize social order through local Police Acts. In the Scottish context, *police* does not just refer to constabulary, although that became part of it, but to the older, European meaning of civic government.[13] Scottish Police Acts covered the elementary civic amenities of cleansing, lighting and paving, and instituted uniformed police forces in Glasgow (1800) and Edinburgh (1806). The functions covered by the Acts were administered by police commissioners elected by local property owners and funded by local, property-based taxes. These commissioners were therefore not accountable to the established oligarchies in the unreformed town councils, but to a ratepaying electorate.[14]

Duncan and Erskine grasped the changing nature of society after the political revolutions in America and France and the onset of industrialization. They realized the ultimate value of inserting medical knowledge into the delicate balancing mechanism of the new social order. This explains their agitation for the formalized academic teaching of medical jurisprudence and police to combat the social evils of crime and squalor. The former offered medical expertise to protect the individual and his property, the latter offered medical aid to protect the health of the community.

In the introduction to his published *Heads of Lectures on Medical Police* (1801), Duncan stated clearly that he considered medical police to be of far greater importance than medical jurisprudence because it affected the health and well-being of the whole population, of society itself. Duncan saw medical jurisprudence as safeguarding the individual within society: not just in criminal cases, but in civil matters where personal liberty, property and marital arrangements were involved. In Duncan's time, civil cases involving property rights included testamentary disputes under the

Scottish law of death-bed; establishing the legitimacy or bastardy of offspring; and the confinement or release of lunatics. In such cases, the medical profession was especially visible, and consequently vulnerable. Duncan reminded doctors of the awful duty laid upon them in courts of law. Their medical evidence had to 'defend injured innocence against the shafts of groundless suspicion or malicious calumny, to detect atrocious guilt though concealed with the deepest art and to deal with the distribution of material justice where the person, property or life of an individual was at stake'.[15]

However, at a time when medical men sought greater public esteem and professional status, appearances in courts of law, whether criminal, civil or consistorial, meant that their own reputations, and that of the profession, were brought before the bar of the public. Whereas the fate of an accused person often depended, and still does, on answers given by doctors under oath to questions from advocates, the duty of defence counsel to their client is to expose medical error and magnify uncertainty. The teaching of medical jurisprudence was therefore necessary to impart a uniform body of knowledge to medical practitioners. Armed with this, they could enter any court of law with sufficient knowledge to rescue them from the snares of legal casuistry and to emerge with enough credit and dignity to impress the public.

Duncan's concern with sound medical jurisprudence teaching was therefore as much for the benefit of the profession as for the individual doctor, a concern which has been echoed throughout the teaching of forensic medicine from that time onwards.[16] In a sense forensic medicine taught the profession to police itself, and in part continues to do so through the teaching of medical ethics.

The teaching of medical jurisprudence and medical police

The elder Duncan's lectures on medical jurisprudence and medical police influenced many eminent doctors. John Gordon Smith (1773–1832), the first professor of forensic medicine in England, and George Edward Male (1779–1845), often referred to as the 'father' of English forensic medicine,[17] both attributed their interest in medical jurisprudence to his teaching. But Duncan's extra-academical lectures were not restricted to aspiring doctors and lawyers. They were popular lectures which the public were encouraged to attend. Thus Duncan conveyed to a wide audience his ideals of improving general health through the cooperation of doctors and laymen inspired solely by philanthropic motives.[18]

In its early years, the chair of medical jurisprudence became a steppingstone for young professors. Andrew Duncan the younger held the chair from its inception in 1807 to 1819, then succeeded his father in the chair of the institutes of medicine. There is little record of his teaching, and merely fleeting glimpses of his court appearances. In like manner, William Pulteney Alison (1790–1859) held the chair of medical jurisprudence for barely two years, from 1819 to 1821, then moved to the institutes of medicine, replacing Duncan. His detailed lectures on medical jurisprudence and police survive in the notes taken by his student James (later Sir James) Watson, who recorded or copied them verbatim.[19] Alison devoted practically the whole academic year to medical jurisprudence, which is scarcely to be wondered at while the chair still remained within the faculty of law. The few lectures on medical police reveal an Alison cast clearly in the mould of the elder Duncan, preferring persuasion to positive legal enactments on the grounds that unnecessary municipal health legislation infringed the 'private habits, liberty and comforts of individuals'.[20]

The chair gained in importance with the appointment of Robert (later Sir Robert) Christison (1797–1881). Christison held the chair from 1821 to 1832, then succeeded Duncan in the chair of materia medica where he remained until his retirement in 1877.[21] Christison revolutionized the teaching of forensic medicine and raised its reputation in courts of law. Through his constant prompting, medical jurisprudence finally found recognition in the Edinburgh faculty of medicine in 1825.[22] The subject joined a group of five optional subjects, from which students were obliged to choose two. But it was not until 1833 that medical jurisprudence became part of the Edinburgh medical curriculum because, as the *Edinburgh Medical and Surgical Journal* remarked with some acerbity, 'Medical jurisprudence has become so important a study and is required by so many inferior boards of education that its exclusion from a course of study, in a university where it is so well taught, would have been deplorable'.[23]

As a student in Paris, Christison had studied the effects of poisons under the French physiologist, François Magendie,[24] and as a teacher he made toxicology the touchstone of his long and brilliant career as a medical jurist. It was a timely choice. In 1819, a covert attempt to suppress the chair, made by the Scottish political manager, Henry Dundas, failed completely because Dundas was reliably informed that the teaching of medical jurisprudence was essential to the provision of expert testimony in cases of criminal poisoning in Scotland.[25] Christison's *Treatise on Poisons*, first published in 1829, became a standard text and went into four editions by 1845.[26] Students benefited from accounts of his court appearances and deductive reasoning, as shown in his detailed and frequently revised lecture notes.[27] But Christison was also interested in civil cases. He was the first chief medical officer of the Standard Life insurance company and one of his lectures reflected the actuarial nature of the doctor's role in medical examinations for life insurance policies.[28] However, Christison failed to deliver undergraduate lectures on medical police. The reason for this omission, made plain in the introduction to his lecture course, was the lack of time available to discuss its complexities.[29] But he was keenly interested in public health and related environmental problems, and wrote profusely on these subjects.[30]

When Christison moved to materia medica in 1832, the chair of medical jurisprudence fell to Thomas Traill (1781–1862), a 51-year-old chemistry lecturer and medical practitioner in Liverpool. Traill held the chair until his death in 1862. Although he made sporadic appearances in court, his interests lay more in scientific literature. His thirty year tenure covered years of great debate on British public health and the second edition of his published lecture outlines indicates a revival of the teaching of medical police, or public health, at Edinburgh.[31]

Although Edinburgh monopolized the university teaching of medical jurisprudence and medical police until the foundation of the Glasgow chair in 1839, medical jurisprudence was taught extra-murally in Glasgow from 1826 at the Portland Street Medical School.[32] James Armour (1792–1832) lectured on the subject in connection with midwifery, which perhaps reflected the legal disputes that could arise in connection with childbirth. On the one hand, doctors needed to be taught when to suspect, and how to detect, childmurder: on the other hand they could be faced with property-related disputed paternity cases in which the term of pregnancy was of paramount importance.[33]

The value of medical police teaching came into its own shortly before the first visitation of Asiatic cholera in 1832, when the visible progress of the disease across Europe demonstrated its life-threatening potential. Because of the poor state of medical tuition on community sanitary care, two extra-mural teachers of medical jurisprudence, James Armour and his successor John Pagan (1802–68), persuaded the Glasgow Faculty of Physicians and Surgeons to make courses in medical jurisprudence and police mandatory requisites for the faculty's Diploma in Surgery, which was essential for doctors practising in the west of Scotland.[34] To cater for this new requirement, the extra-mural Andersonian medical college introduced lectures on medical jurisprudence and police. Handbills printed during this period indicate that medical jurisprudence and police courses were accepted for the diplomas of the Royal Colleges of Surgeons of Edinburgh, London and Dublin, and for the Army and Navy Medical Boards.

Concern about the sanitary condition of Glasgow had favoured Robert Cowan's appointment at Glasgow in 1839, discussed above. The chair was essentially founded to promote the teaching of public health in the wake of Edwin Chadwick's enquiries into the health and living conditions of the

British labouring classes. Chadwick judged social conditions in Glasgow to be the worst he had encountered. Cowan wrote on health statistics and sanitary conditions, but his early death in 1841 brought a new professor and a change of direction. Harry Rainy's interests did not lie in public health. He styled himself professor of forensic medicine and made a significant contribution to the subject with his work on the cooling time of dead bodies.[35] He was considered a good teacher,[36] but his forbidding personal demeanour made defence and prosecution counsel alike reluctant to use him in court, and the chair lost active contact with current medico-legal casework.[37]

The University of Aberdeen appointed Francis Ogston to a new lectureship in medical jurisprudence in 1839, which was raised to an endowed chair of medical logic and medical jurisprudence in 1860, with Ogston as professor. Thus, by 1839 medical jurisprudence and police, examined in their own right, had gained recognition from three Scottish universities, two of the three Scottish medical licensing corporations and were also taught extra-murally. Moreover, in 1856 a course in medical jurisprudence became one of the prerequisites for admission to the Edinburgh Faculty of Advocates. Thereafter, no man was called to the Scottish Bar without first having been examined in forensic medicine, though not all lawyers agreed with this.[38]

The medical policing of crime and health

Overall, Duncan's broad vision of medical police was not sustained. Throughout the nineteenth century, private medical and lay philanthropy continued to address the problems of individual health by providing institutional care and treatment for diseased, aged and psychiatric patients. But, by the middle of the century, the health and sanitary condition of communities became the dominant strand of medical police. This had a paradoxical effect. While within Scotland, doctors seeking public health reforms by legal enactments remained inhibited by Duncan's philanthropic ideals, Scottish universities and medical licensing corporations exported socio-medical expertise to England in the boom years of Chadwickian health reforms. Scottish-trained doctors (especially those taught at Edinburgh) became an integral part of the developing public health movement in England.[39] Doctors with Scottish qualifications whose views supported Chadwick's philosophy included the medical sanitarians Thomas Southwood Smith and James Kay-Shuttleworth (Edinburgh) and Neill Arnott (Aberdeen). The list also includes Henry Duncan (1805–63), the first British medical officer of health, appointed by Liverpool under a private Improvement Act passed in 1847 to deal with the effects of immigrants fleeing the

Irish famine.[40] Duncan was the first of a long succession of Liverpool medical officers of health with Edinburgh medical degrees. Scottish-trained doctors were well represented in appointments made subsequent to the Public Health Act of 1848, covering England and Wales, which permitted local authorities to appoint medical officers of health and established the General Board of Health. The same holds true for members of the sanitary commission sent to enquire into army health during the Crimean campaign.[41]

However, in Scotland, where forensic medicine and public health were more thoroughly integrated, medical employment in public health was grafted on to the existing system of police surgeons. Discounting doctors employed by parochial boards, the first municipal medical officers of health in Scotland were appointed under general and local Police Acts passed in 1862.[42] They were not appointed under a Public Health Act. The first such Act for Scotland came five years later, in 1867. In Scotland, therefore, the police connection between crime and health was maintained, but requires further explanation.

Prior to 1820, there is no definite starting date for the first appointment of a police surgeon in Scotland.[43] The earliest appear to have been Alexander Black in Edinburgh and Francis Neilson in Glasgow, with James Corkindale acting as casualty surgeon and medico-legal examiner. Dundee appointed Alexander Webster in 1833 and Aberdeen appointed Francis Ogston in 1839.[44] Other large manufacturing towns followed suit. The duties of a police surgeon consisted mainly of examining the health of new police recruits, and attending sick constables and other members of the police establishment such as street cleaners, street lighters and firemen. They were also required to dress prisoners' wounds, attend at street accidents and generally act as casualty surgeons. All police surgeons appointments were part-time, and fees from post-mortem examinations and commissioned medical reports formed a valuable source of income. In large towns and cities, police surgeons gave evidence both in the summary courts and in serious criminal cases tried in the higher courts. Alexander Black was frequently employed as an expert on wounds, as was James Corkindale who also conducted chemical experiments to detect poison as a cause of death.

Until the 1830s it was not usual for police surgeons appearing in the higher courts to hold academic appointments, as medical evidence was not highly regarded. However, the position began to change, mainly through the efforts of Christison, Traill and James Syme (1799–1870), Professor of Clinical Surgery at the University of Edinburgh from 1833 to 1870.[45] Their joint publication in 1836 on how to conduct a post-mortem examination was directed towards lawyers and doctors.[46] Christison's writings on the detection of poison did much to enhance the standing of medical witnesses in court and heralded the rise of the medical expert.[47] This effectively encouraged lawyers to use informed medical testimony more often. Edinburgh High Court of Justiciary records reveal that, from the 1840s onwards, an increasing number of medical professors and lecturers appeared in court to lend the benefit of their experience, mainly to the Crown, but quite often on behalf of the defence.[48] Recognition of medical jurisprudence's utility to the legal system gradually altered the status of police surgeons in large cities on the high court of justiciary circuit. Ogston's appointment in 1839, noted above, was the first instance of a lecturer in the subject being appointed as police surgeon. Also in 1839, Glasgow appointed John Easton, lecturer on materia medica at the Andersonian medical college, as police surgeon.[49] Edinburgh made Henry Duncan Littlejohn police surgeon in 1854, shortly after his appointment as lecturer on medical jurisprudence and police at the Royal College of Surgeons, Edinburgh.

But in Scotland, in keeping with the close ties between medical jurisprudence and police, police surgeons also had health duties. In 1832, James Corkindale claimed to have had charge of all major epidemics in Glasgow from the time of his appointment.[50] There is no available evidence that Black had any epidemic disease duties for Edinburgh, but a successor, George Glover, kept the official cholera register in 1848.[51] At Aberdeen, Ogston supplied monthly health reports to the town council during the 1840s but it is not clear whether these related to the health of the police force or the health of the townspeople.[52]

This, then, was the role of police surgeons serving large Scottish towns and cities on the eve of long-awaited public health reforms in 1862. Amongst them was a proficient cadre of academic medical jurists, soon to undertake the duties of both of the subjects they professed, forensic medicine and public health.

The police surgeon as medical officer of health in Scotland 1862–1943

In the mid-nineteenth century, sanitary administration in urban Scotland was a recognized police function. This explains why the first wave of medical officers of health were appointed under general and local Police Acts. A medical input was necessary, but the administrative machinery still lay in the police committees of the large urban burghs. Street cleansing, nuisance removal and common lodging house inspection were functions of police establishments. Under various Scottish enactments police surgeons were empowered to enter common lodging houses to certify and remove occupants suffering from epidemic disease, to order the cleansing, fumigation and whitewashing of closes[53] and apartments during epidemics, and to certify nuisances dangerous to the public health. Police officers inspected common lodging houses, and general cleansing and fumigation duties were carried out by the cleansing departments of police establishments.

Scotland's separate legal system, and the different functions of its legal officers, made the general Sanitary Acts passed at Westminster unworkable in Scotland. The Nuisance Removal Act (Scotland) 1856, the first Act compatible with the Scottish system, permitted the appointment of sanitary inspectors. Almost without exception, urban burgh police chiefs and their lieutenants were appointed at executive level, with police constables used as proto-sanitary inspectors.[54] Therefore, it was quite natural for the new system of part-time medical officers of health introduced in 1862 to be grafted on to the existing, police-based, administrative structure. Police surgeons Littlejohn and Ogston were appointed as medical officers of health to Edinburgh and Aberdeen respectively. But in Glasgow, where high population density went hand in hand with high crime rates, the city had been divided into five separate police divisions, each with its own police surgeon. The five police surgeons were appointed as assistant medical officers of health to their respective divisions, acting under the supervision of the city's chief medical officer of health, William Tennant Gairdner, professor of medicine at the University of Glasgow.[55]

Departments created under this new system were *sanitary departments*: they were not termed *public health* departments until much later. Apart from medical officers of health, sanitary departments were staffed by sanitary inspectors drawn mainly from the police force, usually the detective branch.[56] The practice of using policemen as sanitary inspectors was not unique to Scotland. A study of the medico-legal aspects of British sanitary reform, published in 1867, included a table indicating that in most of the twenty-three towns surveyed – only four of which were Scottish – the sanitary inspectors were 'chosen from or assisted by the police', and in some cases the inspector of police was specified.[57]

Scottish police surgeons appointed as medical officers of health were, in the widest sense, true medical policemen, products of a medical education and a legal system peculiar to Scotland. While it is unrealistic to mention them all, the careers of Henry Duncan Littlejohn of Edinburgh, and Matthew Hay of Aberdeen, whose activities are particularly well documented, show the system at its apogee in the last quarter of the century.

Littlejohn served Edinburgh as police surgeon from 1854, and as medical officer of health from 1862. He lectured on medical jurisprudence and police at the Royal College of Surgeons, Edinburgh, from 1854 to 1897, when he succeeded Sir Douglas Maclagan as professor of medical jurisprudence at the University of Edinburgh. He retired from all these appointments in 1907. From 1873–1908 he was also the medical officer for Scotland's central public health authority.[58] As police surgeon, Littlejohn did not have an assistant until the latter years of his service and his day-to-day duties were quite demanding. In addition to caring for the health of the Edinburgh police force he was required to conduct post-mortem examinations in all cases of sudden or suspicious death, examine injured persons whose cases were under police investigation, examine all insane persons brought to the police office and, if necessary, to certify them. He was also required to visit the cells at least twice every twenty-four hours and, amongst many other duties, had to attend when the sentence of whipping was carried out on boys. He inspected food suspected of being unfit for human consumption and gave medical evidence when these cases were tried in the police court. More importantly, he was required to live within half a mile of the main police office and needed the permission of the Lord Provost or the Sheriff to name a deputy to cover any period of his absence. He was, however, allowed to practise independently of his duties as police surgeon, which was a part-time appointment.[59] This did not take into consideration his role as Crown medical examiner which, as his career developed, entailed Littlejohn appearing in virtually every notable murder case tried at the high court in Edinburgh, be it shooting, poison, child-murder, strangling or wounding.[60]

Littlejohn's public health duties, as medical officer of health for Edinburgh and for the Board of Supervision, engaged him in the struggle to raise the health, not only of his own city, but of all Scottish local authorities whose neglect of their duties was often so blatant as to incur the attention of the central authority. There were obvious difficulties for Littlejohn. When the Board of Supervision despatched him to a distant part of Scotland to deal with some public health problem, he had first to obtain permission from his civic employers to name a deputy as police surgeon. A striking instance of the dichotomy between the duties of policing crime and health came during Littlejohn's struggle to introduce into Scotland the compulsory notification of infectious diseases, finally incorporated into the Edinburgh Police Act of 1879. At the same time he was deeply involved in the sensational trial of Eugene Marie Chantrelle for the murder of his wife by arsenic.[61] In his lectures, Littlejohn brought to his students the accumulated experience of all these aspects of his work, and he encouraged them to attend in court when he was giving evidence.

Matthew Hay (1855–1932), professor of medical logic and jurisprudence at Aberdeen from 1883 to 1926, also lectured to undergraduates and postgraduates, and filled the offices of police surgeon and medical officer of health. His letter books from 1890 to 1905 provide a rare record of the day-to-day activities of a teaching medical policeman. His extensive forensic activities are interleaved with public health matters, students' references and private domestic worries.[62] Hay was an analyst of some note and, amongst other things, was often called upon to inspect the water supplied to whisky distilleries in northeast Scotland. His duties as police surgeon were similar to those of Littlejohn's, even down to the prescribed residential distance from the police station, but he was allowed to be absent from the city for twelve hours at a time. Hay gave evidence at the local police courts, and in cases tried at the Aberdeen sittings of the high court. His letter books for 1893 contain detailed correspondence on ballistics when, in the midst of his professorial and health duties, he was called to appear at the Edinburgh high court in the notable Ardlamont shooting case. Hay was called by the defence for Arthur Monson, accused of murdering Cecil Hambrough with a shotgun in the grounds of Ardlamont House. Henry Duncan Littlejohn appeared for the prosecution. The two professors of forensic medicine, Crown examiners, police surgeons and medical officers of health gave cogent, but contradictory, medical and ballistic evidence. The verdict was one of 'Not Proven', and both medico-legal experts returned to grapple with the health problems of their respective cities.[63]

The separation of forensic medicine and public health

The Scottish practice of teaching forensic medicine and public health in tandem at undergraduate level faltered at the end of the century with the rapid expansion of postgraduate public health teaching. Postgraduate qualifications had become essential for employment in large municipal and county public health departments.[64] Specialized public health courses, and the expansion in student numbers, made it impracticable to continue teaching it in conjunction with forensic medicine, which was itself experiencing the growth of certain sub-specialisms.

The University of Edinburgh severed the connection in 1897 when Littlejohn, now Sir Henry Littlejohn, took the Edinburgh chair of forensic medicine and a separate, endowed, chair of hygiene was founded. Similarly, Matthew Hay, who had resigned the post of police surgeon in 1909, relinquished his public health teaching when the University of Aberdeen instituted a separate lectureship in public health in 1914. When Hay retired in 1926, the University of Aberdeen took the opportunity to reduce the chair of forensic medicine to a lectureship.

The position was somewhat different at Glasgow. The university professor of medical jurisprudence and medical police, John Glaister (1856–1932), maintained the subjects' joint status until 1922 before accepting the inevitable. A separate chair of public health was then endowed at Glasgow by Glaister's friend, the industrialist Henry Mechan.[65] Despite, or perhaps because of, its acute problems with crime and health, Glasgow never conformed to the Scottish pattern of the police surgeon as medical officer of health. Glaister has found no place in this paper because, although he taught both subjects passionately, and would have considered himself a teaching medical policeman, he was never a medical officer of health.[66] Also, although an outstanding medical jurist, he was forced, by custom,[67] to relinquish his post of police surgeon when he took the Glasgow chair in 1898.

However, the traditional link between policing crime and health lingered on in some Scottish communities until the mid-twentieth century. In 1943, the deputy medical officer of health for the city of Inverness returned from active war service. Prior to leaving, he had also acted as the Inverness police surgeon. The town council, undecided on the value of continuing to combine the posts, approached fifteen burghs of similar size asking how they regulated these functions. Five of the fifteen burghs replied that they still combined the duties of medical officer of health with those of police surgeon.[68] Such was the strength of the nineteenth-century tradition of combining forensic medicine with public health. The Scottish medical policeman proved very hard to dislodge.

NOTES

Much of the material for this paper comes from research into the history of forensic medicine in Scotland funded by a generous grant from the Wellcome Trust.

1 George Rosen, 'The fate of the concept of medical police 1780–1890', in his *From Medical Police to Social Medicine* (New York: Science History Publications, 1974), pp. 142–56.

2 When it first appeared in 1773, *Medical Commentaries* was the only regularly published medical periodical in Great Britain. It contained news from British, European and American medical societies and was translated into German in 1775. See Lisa M. Rosner, *Andrew Duncan, MD, F.R.S.E. (1744–1828)*, *Scottish Men of Medicine* pamphlet series (Edinburgh: History of Medicine and Science Unit, University of Edinburgh, 1981). For full biographical details, see 'Andrew Duncan Senior, MD', in R. Chambers, ed., *Chambers' Biographical Dictionary of Eminent Scotsmen* (Edinburgh: Blackie & Son, 1854), pp. 498–9.

3 Andrew Duncan, *Heads of Lectures on Medical Police* (Edinburgh, 1801), introductory note.

4 'Memorial presented to the patrons of the University of Edinburgh, 1798', Edinburgh University Senate Minutes 1790–1811, vol. XI, pp. 146–7.

5 Ibid., p. 148.

6 A series of fascinating letters by Andrew Duncan Jr to his father, describing his medical education and adventures, especially those in Europe during the French revolutionary period, may be found in Edinburgh University Library, Special Collections, DC.1.90.

7 From 1796 to 1804, Andrew Duncan Jr co-edited, with his father, the periodical *Annals of Medicine*, which replaced the *Medical Commentaries*. In 1805 the *Annals* were in turn replaced by the *Edinburgh Medical and Surgical Journal*, with Andrew Duncan Jr as editor-in-chief.

8 Erskine's Whig principles were quite radical and he had some sympathy for the democratic ideals of the Scottish Friends of the People. See Alexander Ferguson, *Henry Erskine, his Kinsfolk and Times* (London and Edinburgh: William Blackwood & Sons, 1882).

9 For details of the Lord Advocate's role prior to 1885, see H. J. Hanham, 'The creation of the Scottish Office, 1881–1887', *Juridical Review*, (1965), 205–44, at pp. 238–42.

10 'Copy of Memorial presented by Dr Duncan to the Patrons of Edinburgh University, 1798, . . . recommended to the attention of His Majesty by the Right Hon. Henry Erskine when Lord Advocate for Scotland, 1806', Edinburgh University Library, Special Collections, Att.80 P.4/19. Also, in 1805, the younger Duncan reviewed and recommended to the profession François-Emmanuel Fodéré's *Les Lois éclairées par les sciences physiques, ou traité de médecine légale et d'hygiène publique*, and P. A. J. Mahon's *Médecine légale et police médicale* in the new *Edinburgh Medical and Surgical Journal*, 1 (1805), 330–42.

11 Quoted in Henry W. Rumsey, *Essays in State Medicine* (London: John Churchill, 1856), p. 67.

12 For further information on the Glasgow chair, see M. Anne Crowther and Brenda White, *On Soul and Conscience. The Medical Expert and Crime* (Aberdeen: Aberdeen University Press, 1988), pp. 5–25.

13 For a more detailed description of the early Scottish burgh Police Acts, see Brenda M. White, 'Medical police. Politics and police: the fate of John Roberton', *Medical History*, 27 (1983), 407–22.

14 The power struggles surrounding this new element in Scottish local government are discussed in Kit Carson and Hilary Idzikowska, 'The social production of Scottish policing 1795–1900', in D. Hay and F. Snyder, eds., *Policing and Prosecution in Britain 1750–1850* (Oxford: Oxford University Press, 1989), pp. 267–97.

15 Duncan, *Heads of Lectures on Medical Police*, introduction.

16 For the English case, see Catherine Crawford, 'A scientific profession: forensic medicine and professional reform in British periodicals of the early nineteenth century', in Roger French and Andrew Wear, eds., *British Medicine in an Age of Reform* (London and New York: Routledge, 1991), pp. 203–30.

17 Benjamin T. Davis, 'George Edward Male, MD, the father of English forensic medicine', *Proceedings of the Royal Society of Medicine*, 67 (1974), 117–20.

18 Duncan successfully instituted dispensaries for the sick poor and, from 1792, led the movement to build the Edinburgh lunatic asylum, which received a royal charter in 1807.

19 The lecture notes, in four volumes, are housed in the library of the Royal Society of Medicine, London, catalogue numbers MSS2–MSS5.

20 Ibid., vol. IV, pp. 2–3.

21 At this period, the younger Duncan, Alison and Christison appear to have played a confusing form of medical 'musical chairs'. Alison twice succeeded

Duncan, in the chairs of medical jurisprudence (1819) and institutes of medicine (1821). Christison succeeded Alison in the chair of medical jurisprudence (1821) and Duncan in that of materia medica (1832).

22 Robert Christison, *Memorial to the Principal and Professors of the University of Edinburgh, 24th June 1824*, Special Collections, Edinburgh University Library. For a discussion of the Edinburgh medical curriculum at this time and the place of medical jurisprudence within it, see Lisa Rosner, *Medical Education in the Age of Improvement* (Edinburgh: Edinburgh University Press, 1991), ch. 9.

23 *Edinburgh Medical and Surgical Journal*, 41 (1834), p. 254.

24 *The Life of Sir Robert Christison, Bart, Edited by his Sons*, 2 Vols. (Edinburgh: Blackwood, 1885), vol. I, pp. 224–48.

25 Letter from the Earl of Lauderdale to Henry Dundas, Lord Melville, Melville Castle Papers, Scottish Record Office GD51/5/699.

26 Robert Christison, *A Treatise on Poisons, in Relation to Medical Jurisprudence, Physiology and the Practice of Physic* (Edinburgh: Adam and Charles Black, 1829).

27 Christison's copious lecture notes are held in Edinburgh University Library, Special Collections, catalogue number DK.4.57.

28 For further details of medical insurance work, see M. Anne Crowther and Brenda M. White, 'Medicine, property and the law in Britain 1800–1914', *Historical Journal*, 31 (1988), 853–70.

29 'It has been my custom to confine myself to one department only of my professorial teaching, the branch of medical jurisprudence.' Christison, lecture notes, Edinburgh University Library, Special Collections, DK.4.57.

30 For a daunting list of publications covering all departments of Christison's long career, see *Life of Christison*, vol. I, pp. 471–9.

31 Thomas S. Traill, *Outlines of a Course of Lectures on Medical Jurisprudence*, 2nd edn (Edinburgh: Adam and Charles Black, 1840); 3rd edn (Edinburgh: Adam and Charles Black, 1857).

32 For a valuable table of university and extra-mural medical teaching at Glasgow, see John D. Comrie, *History of Scottish Medicine to 1860* (London: Baillière, Tindall & Cox for the Wellcome Historical Medical Museum, 1927), pp. 231–2.

33 Crowther and White, 'Medicine, property and the law', pp. 860–1.

34 Minutes of the Royal Faculty of Physicians and Surgeons, Glasgow, 4 April 1832, in the archives of the Royal College of Physicians and Surgeons of Glasgow (hereafter, RCPSG), 1/1/6.

35 Harry Rainy, 'On the cooling of dead bodies as indicating the length of time that has elapsed since death', *Glasgow Medical Journal*, 1, n.s. (May 1869), 323–30.

36 See notes taken by a student in 1866 on lectures on forensic medicine given by Professor Harry Rainy, in RCPSG 10/31.

37 For more on Rainy, see Crowther and White, *On Soul and Conscience*, pp. 16–20.

38 The compulsory requirement lasted until the end of the century, but courses in forensic medicine have remained popular with law students to the present day.

39 Jeanne L. Brand, *Doctors and the State: The British Medical Profession and Government Action in Public Health, 1870–1912* (Baltimore: Johns Hopkins University Press, 1965), p. 110.

40 At the time of his appointment, Duncan was lecturing on medical jurisprudence

at the Liverpool Royal Institution. See William M. Frazer, *Duncan of Liverpool, Being an Account of the Work of Dr. W. H. Duncan, Medical Officer of Health of Liverpool, 1847–63* (London: Hamish Hamilton Medical, 1947), p. 48.

41 Brenda M. White, 'Scottish doctors and the English public health', in Derek A. Dow, ed., *The Influence of Scottish Medicine: An Historical Assessment of its International Impact* (Carnforth, Lancs. and Park Ridge, NJ: Parthenon Publications, 1988), pp. 78–85.

42 Glasgow and Aberdeen each obtained private Police Acts authorizing, among other sanitary improvements, the appointment of medical officers of health. There was also a general Police Act enabling populous places to achieve police burgh status, which in turn enabled them to appoint medical officers of health.

43 For the early history of English police surgeons, see Ralph D. Summers, 'History of the police surgeon', *The Practitioner*, 221 (September 1978), 383–7.

44 Brenda M. White, 'The police surgeon as medical officer of health in Scotland 1862–1897', *The Police Surgeon*, no. 35 (1989), 29–37.

45 For details of Syme's career and his contributions to surgical knowledge, see his obituaries in *British Medical Journal*, 2 (1870), 21–6, and *Lancet*, 2 (1870), 31–2.

46 Thomas S. Traill, Robert Christison, and James Syme, *Suggestions for the Medico-Legal Examination of Dead Bodies*, pamphlet dated 30 January 1836, Scottish Record Office (hereafter SRO), AD/58/166. This pamphlet, published in Edinburgh in 1839 by the Crown Office, was intended to provide Scottish Procurators Fiscal (local public prosecutors) and their chosen medical examiners with a standard procedure for carrying out medico-legal autopsies. For the role of the Procurators Fiscal generally in Scottish criminal procedure and medico-legal investigations, see A. V. Sheehan, *Criminal Procedure in Scotland and France* (Edinburgh: HMSO, 1975), pp. 110–15, 128–30, 150–2, and Appendix 9, 'Sudden deaths'.

47 As well as his *Treatise on Poisons* (1829), Christison wrote many essays for readers of the *Edinburgh Medical and Surgical Journal* explaining in detail the methods that he used to detect poisons in his criminal cases. In this way, Christison reached many doctors who would otherwise have had no experience of suspecting, or detecting, poisoning.

48 Detailed records of criminal trials at the Edinburgh High Court of Justiciary are kept in the Scottish Record Office, JC 4 series. Papers relating to these trials are kept in the Small Papers series. Precognitions (written statements, etc. taken from witnesses), are filed under the name of the accused.

49 Minutes of the Statute Labour Committee, Strathclyde regional archives, E1–2–1.

50 'Testimonials in favour of Dr James Corkindale for the lectureship in medical jurisprudence', Glasgow University Library, catalogue number BG33–h.9.

51 George Glover was Henry Littlejohn's immediate predecessor. In 1854 Glover accompanied Hector Gavin, General Board of Health medical inspector, on a visit to Edinburgh when the town council proposed improvements to the affluent Water of Leith district. Glover provided Gavin with a damning report for the General Board of Health without informing his employers, the Edinburgh Police Board, and was dismissed for breach of professional etiquette. For

details, see Edinburgh Watching Committee minutes, vol. 4, 1844–53, Edinburgh city archives.

52 Aberdeen Police Committee minutes, vol. 9, p. 99, Aberdeen city archives.

53 In Scotland, the entrance and stairway of a tenement is referred to as a 'close'.

54 Glasgow, Paisley, Aberdeen and Dundee are prime examples of this system.

55 William T. Gairdner, newly appointed as professor of medicine at the University of Glasgow in 1862, was instrumental in changing the attitude of the Scottish medical profession towards employment in municipal sanitary administrations by delivering a series of lectures, later published as *Public Health in Relation to Air and Water* (Edinburgh: Edmiston & Douglas, 1862). See pp. 1–4 for his medical call-to-arms.

56 James Christie, *Medical Institutions of Glasgow* (Glasgow: Maclehose, 1888), pp. 146–55. For Edinburgh, see Haldane P. Tait, *A Doctor and Two Policemen: The History of Edinburgh Health Department* (Edinburgh: Mackenzie & Storrie, 1974).

57 Alexander Stewart and Edward Jenkins, *The Medical and Legal Aspects of Sanitary Reform*, 2nd edn (London: Hardwicke, 1867), reprinted with an introduction by Michael Flinn (Leicester: Leicester University Press, 1969), Table 11. Stewart was a doctor and Jenkins a barrister.

58 This function was vested in the Scottish Poor Law authority, the Board of Supervision for the Relief of the Poor, until its powers were transferred to the Local Government Board (Scotland) in 1894. See Ian Levitt, *Poverty and Welfare in Scotland, 1890–1948* (Edinburgh: Edinburgh University Press, 1988), pp. 22–43.

59 *Duties and Emoluments of Police Surgeon 1854*, miscellaneous pamphlets, YHV 8198, Edinburgh central public library.

60 Haldane P. Tait, 'Sir Henry Duncan Littlejohn: great Scottish sanitarian and medical jurist', *The Medical Officer* (21 September 1962), 183–90; William A. R. Thomson, 'An Edinburgh quintet', *Medicine, Science and the Law*, 22 (1982), 154–67, especially pp. 160–2.

61 For details of this trial, see SRO/JC 4 75, 7–10 May 1878, and related precognition files.

62 Matthew Hay, 'Medico-legal reports, December 1890–1905', Aberdeen University Library, Special Collections, MS. 2853. 1.

63 White, 'The police surgeon'; Thomson, 'An Edinburgh quintet', pp. 161–2. The verdict of 'Not Proven' was, and still is, a particularly Scottish verdict, which has no counterpart in English law.

64 For details, see Roy Acheson, 'The British Diploma in Public Health: birth and adolescence', in Roy M. Acheson and Elizabeth Fee, eds., *A History of Education in Public Health: Health that Mocks the Doctors' Rules* (Oxford: University Press, 1991), pp. 44–82.

65 Crowther and White, *On Soul and Conscience*, pp. 31–2.

66 In 1872, Glasgow revoked the 1862 appointments of all six part-time medical officers of health, including Gairdner, and appointed a single, full-time officer, James Burn Russell (1837–1904), the first such appointment in Scotland.

67 In the mid-nineteenth century, Sheriff Berry of Lanarkshire decided that his Crown examiners should not be drawn from the ranks of police surgeons.

68 Inverness town council minutes, 1943–5, Inverness city archives, 1B 1/1/76, p. 307; 1B 1/1/78, p. 57.

III

Special offenders

7

'I answer as a physician': opinion as fact in pre-McNaughtan insanity trials

JOEL PETER EIGEN

As the jury evolved from its original form – community members selected for their firsthand knowledge of the details of an offence – into a body of citizens chosen specifically for their *lack* of any such knowledge, witnesses played an increasingly important role in trials as suppliers of facts. Witnesses were, however, restricted to facts: the courtroom division of labour mandated that the jury alone drew inferences. A clear description of the separate roles of juryman and witness can already be found in the seventeenth century: 'a Witness swears but to what he hath heard or seen, generally or more largely, to what hath fallen under his senses. But a Juryman swears to what he can inferr and conclude from the Testimony.'[1]

Not all witnesses, however, were restricted to direct observation. There were numerous instances when special or 'skilled' witnesses were called to inform the court in areas of expertise supposedly beyond the ken of ordinary folk. Alone among witnesses, these men of skill – be they ship surveyors, insurance brokers, physicians, or grammarians – offered opinions on matters of fact relating to the offence in question. Was this a violation of the fundamental tenet that witnesses were not to offer inferences? To answer this objection, some jurists asserted that such opinion 'really has the flavor of a fact', that the testimony of skilled witnesses constituted a 'class of facts about which expert persons alone could have knowledge'.[2] But how was the jury to weigh such evidence? Did the expert's opinion constitute just another 'fact' for the layman to consider, or might the specialist's acknowledged expertise actually threaten the autonomy of jury decision-making? Were expert witnesses really witnesses at all, or were they in effect advisers to the juror whose testimony must necessarily sway the layman?

Although legal reasoning defending the use of expert opinion in court emphasized the 'witness' in expert witness, expert opinion in fact differed qualitatively from the layman's observations. An expert need not have had direct familiarity with the crime. His importance to the court lay in a different sort of experience, one which afforded a special acquaintance with a class of phenomena germane to a particular legal question. Expert witnesses gained this familiarity either in the practice of some skill or the pursuit of some livelihood, or by dint of systematic study of a particular body of knowledge. Either means of acquiring 'peculiar experience' was thought to be valuable to the court, and never more so than in the late 1700s. According to John Henry Wigmore, one finds in these years a growing recognition that there was a class of persons, skilled in matters of science, who while not personally knowledgeable about a particular offence, could nonetheless assist the jury's deliberations regarding what had transpired before and during the crime. In the end, it is experience which legitimates the testimony of both lay and expert witnesses: for the lay witness, the direct observation of the circumstances surrounding the crime; for the expert, special insight derived from sustained acquaintance with, and practice of, a particular activity.

Although these two kinds of experience are clearly different, the cognitive processes responsible for producing facts out of sensory experience, and opinion out of professional experience, resemble each other more than their separate designations imply. The associations an ordinary witness makes with visual or auditory stimuli are mediated through a history of past associations. From this experiential repertoire a judgement is formed, which is reported to the court as a 'fact'. Opinion is, by definition, a judgement, but just as the layman is likely to be influenced by past connections between sensations and ideas, so the expert's past experience of a particular occupation or professional training may substantially affect the formation of his opinions. In the eighty years which comprise the present study, there were several schools of medical psychology, each with its own proselytizers and fierce defenders. Medical opinions delivered in court were as likely to reveal their authors' philosophical affiliations as were medical opinions offered in any other context.[3] Given the element of a personal – even *professional* – investment in what one wants to believe as true, the difficulty of specifying the actual differences between fact and opinion has challenged historians to explain the privileged voice given to medical opinion in court.

Early medical precursors to forensic-psychiatric testimony

When medical men entered the courtroom to testify about the presence and effects of insanity, they were following in a longstanding tradition in which medical experience had translated into medico-legal expertise. As early as the fourteenth century one learns of a surgeon being summoned from London to render an opinion regarding the state of a wound.[4] Although we do not know how frequently surgeons, physicians, and apothecaries were called into court before 1800, case materials reveal that medical witnesses were examined by both the prosecution and the defence, and answered questions ranging from particular autopsy results to more general and even hypothetical questions. Did fever invariably accompany death due to wounds? Under what conditions could blood be absent from a victim's wounds? Why might a drowned man be found with no water in his lungs? The framing of hypothetical questions underscored the distinctive character of the medical expert witness. His testimony extended beyond the details of the case in question to consider contemporary medical opinion's general understanding of organic pathology.

Thomas Forbes assigns the role of what would now be called the first forensic psychiatrist to Edward Jorden, who appeared at a witchcraft trial in 1602.[5] Among the physicians who examined the alleged victim, medical opinion differed with regard to the nature of her distress: was she suffering from a physical ailment, or was her affliction due to 'some cause beyond the natural', i.e. witchcraft? Jorden argued that the unfortunate girl's distress was attributable to organic problems arising from 'the mother' (her uterus). Although Forbes underscores the historical importance of this case by noting that the experts disagreed fundamentally on a 'psychiatric' issue, his is a rather tendentious use of the term. Insanity as a medical condition with special clinical properties was not the focus of medical testimony in this trial.

In contrast, the particular symptoms of lunacy as a species of derangement were the focus of Dr John Monro's testimony during the celebrated trial of Earl Ferrers in 1760. Monro, who had not in fact examined the prisoner, averred that uncommon fury, jealousy, and groundless suspicions were signs of lunacy.[6] Ferrers endeavoured to fashion the medical man's images into a defence of 'occasional insanity' which would explain (and excuse) his intemperate fatal assault on a troublesome servant. 'Occasional insanity', however, met with stiff resistance from the Solicitor General. Echoing the sentiments of Sir Matthew Hale regarding the insufficiency of partial insanity to excuse 'the committing of any offence for its matter capital',[7] the Solicitor General reminded the House of Lords that an acquittal could follow only a total want of reason (permanent or temporary), but not a partial degree of insanity mixed with a partial degree of reason. According to the Solicitor General, if 'there be thought and design; a faculty to distinguish the nature of actions, to discern the differences between moral good and evil, then upon the fact of the offence proved, the judgment of the law must take place'.[8] The endurance of Hale's stricture regarding total insanity can be seen in a judge's instructions to a jury in 1786:

> it must be a total derangement of the mind – and it will be therefore for you to consider whether there is any evidence in this case that can go anywhere near that length – for unless it goes that length – it is my duty to tell you – however it may approach to that degree of disorder, it does not amount to justification.[9]

Although the attempt to reconstruct 'the law's' disposition relative to a specific area of jurisprudence at any one historical moment must be made with caution, the trial judges' instructions – infrequent though they may be – provide a valuable glimpse of the language and imagery that jury and court bystanders were asked to consider when derangement was raised as a possible exculpatory condition.

Source of data and overview of earlier findings

Judicial instructions are only one feature of an unusual publication which reports verbatim narratives of the eight (later increased to twelve) annual sittings of London's central criminal court, the Old Bailey. Appearing first as Elizabethan crime chap-books, these accounts offer graphic descriptions of criminal prosecutions, witness depositions, and eventual case outcomes printed by laymen for sale to the general public. Beginning in 1674, shorthand reporters employed by commercial printers recorded trial narratives to be sold on the street the following day. By 1775 the Common Council of the City of London had institutionalized the recording and printing of the proceedings, and the subsequent publication became known as the *Old Bailey Sessions Papers* (hereafter *OBSP*).[10] As these papers predate the advent of regular court reporting, they provide a rare opportunity to inspect the language employed by a variety of courtroom participants: witnesses, attorneys, judges, and prisoners.[11] Of particular interest for an investigation of the emerging role of the medical witness is the testimony and cross-examination of physicians, surgeons, and apothecaries who appeared in court to speak about mental derangement. Although prisoners in felony proceedings were not permitted full assistance of legal counsel until 1837, in reality this restriction only kept lawyers from addressing the jury directly or summarizing the prisoner's defence. The *OBSP* reveal that attorneys regularly appeared before 1837 to assist prisoners in questioning and cross-examining witnesses.

For the present study, the *OBSP* were surveyed to identify trials heard between the years 1760 and 1843 in which the mental state of the accused became a 'fact' for the jury to consider. This period spans John Monro's appearance in the Ferrers trial and the prosecution of Daniel McNaughtan which formalized the insanity plea by providing juries with a set of legal rules for assessing mental derangement. During this period, the possibility of mental derangement was raised in 331 trials. The question of mental impairment arose in a variety of ways. In some trials, family members, neighbours, or casual acquaintances testified to the aimless wanderings and flighty conversation of the prisoner. On other occasions, prisoners raised the issue themselves, characterizing their mental state as 'insensibility' or being 'out of my wits'. In still other hearings, a fully articulated insanity defence was introduced by an attorney, stating at the beginning of the trial his intention to 'prove the prisoner's insanity'. It should be stressed that during this period, the introduction of a formal insanity plea was by far the exception: most often it was a neighbour, co-worker, or the prisoner himself who mentioned derangement, incoherence, or madness in the course of other testimony regarding the circumstances surrounding the crime.

In the late eighteenth and early nineteenth centuries, medical men appeared at the Old Bailey with gradually increasing frequency. During this period, ninety-eight medical witnesses addressed the issue of mental derangement, most making only one court appearance, though several testified on a number of occasions. In the early years of this period, forensic witnesses did little more than legitimate previous testimony, declaring, for example: 'I have looked upon him as a man insane'.[12] If pressed for an explanation, the physician, surgeon, or apothecary might mention the prisoner's flighty and incoherent conversation or the want of connection between his ideas.[13] One searches in vain, however, for technical language or scientific explanations in the testimony of medical witnesses. The reason for the paucity of professional terms is not difficult to understand. Medicine had yet to formulate a distinctive – and exclusive – 'way of seeing' madness. Eighteenth-century terms such as lunacy, mania, and delirium were not unique to medical practitioners. Whereas their colleagues could speculate on the relative lethality of a wound, the presence of poison, or the probability that an apparently still-born child was in fact a victim of infanticide, eighteenth-century mad-doctors were testifying about a condition which was 'spectacularly on view'. As Roy Porter has written, doubts about 'nature's legibility' in cases of mental disorder troubled few observers in the eighteenth century.[14]

Given the legal insistence on total madness as the criterion for an acquittal, and the very obvious signs of raving mania which any neighbour or relative could report to the jury, it hardly seems surprising that medical witnesses played such a marginal role in the eighteenth-century insanity trial. Not only was their testimony practically indistinguishable from the layman's, they made relatively few court appearances as well. Only one trial in ten saw the appearance of a medical witness. This percentage remained fairly constant through the early decades of the nineteenth century, but grew dramatically after 1830. By the early years of the 1840s medical witnesses were appearing in over half of all trials at the Old Bailey in which derangement played a part in the defence. Such a dramatic increase in participation suggests that by the time of the McNaughtan trial, forensic psychiatric testimony had indeed 'arrived'.

But who were these witnesses? Was the nineteenth-century forensic-psychiatric witness merely a more frequent participant at the Old Bailey, resembling his earlier medical counterpart in all respects except for the frequency of his court appearances? An analysis of medical testimony offered from the years 1760 to 1843 reveals a fundamental shift in both the content of medical testimony and the occupational background of the forensic-psychiatric witness. One sees, for example, a decline in the use of the eighteenth-century symptoms of faulty association of ideas and incoherent conversation, and the introduction of a new set of 'understandings' which heralded a level of professional insight not shared by the lay observer. Further, forensic-psychiatric witnesses in the nineteenth century grounded their specialized knowledge in a new professional experience with the mad, which permitted them to rise above (misleading) sensory impressions. The content of their testimony, and the explicit references made both to sustained familiarity with the mad and to current medical literature about the causes and treatment of mental derangement, spoke directly to the common law's equation of 'peculiar experience' with expertise. The language used to assert expertise in court conveys not only a new 'way of seeing' (and hearing) but a contextual change of setting for this new perception. Asylums, madhouses, and gaols were fast providing the first clinical settings for the formation of a new field of expert opinion.[15]

The following five cases have been selected to illustrate various stages in the development of the medical claim to a privileged voice in criminal insanity. With the exception of the last case, these trials are noteworthy for their utter lack of celebrity. They concern ordinary prisoners on trial for ordinary crimes: stealing, forgery, assault. These trials feature an array of medical men whose testimony reveals first, the hazards encountered when conventional signs (facts?) of madness were cited by medical men, and second, the emergence of a specialized professional vocabulary and perceptual set regarding the acts of madmen. When their testimony is considered in relation to the differences between lay and expert witnesses, it soon becomes evident that expert opinion was more than just a claim to professional expertise; it was also a challenge to the layman's idea of a 'fact'.

How exactly does a madman jump about?

On 3 June 1789, John Glover entered a shop in Covent Garden and asked to see a ring. When he later refused to return the ring to the clerk –

maintaining that he had already replaced it – the Bow-Street Runners were sent for. During the search, Glover removed his shoes, stockings, breeches, coat, and waistcoat, although he kept his gloves on. Eventually he threw one of his gloves to the floor 'and it rung'. After hearing about the events in the shop, the jury then listened to three medical witnesses who offered a series of opinions regarding Glover's mental condition. Dr Joseph Hart Myers's acquaintance with the prisoner spanned two years, having attended Glover 'in the character of a physician'. Myers had originally been consulted because of the prisoner's 'great delirium' in which he evinced 'every symptom of insanity'. Although the prisoner's fever 'yielded to the treatment we administered, there was a degree of idiocy which remained, a perfect fatuity, absolute fatuity.'[16] The witness added that a 'want of recollection in his conduct' convinced him that Glover had not recovered.

Myers was followed by two medical men who attended the prisoner at the request of a Jewish society in London. Daniel Jacob De Castro found the prisoner 'in a state of melancholy', having just suffered the death of a son by fire. 'He had the appearance of a man whose mind was not right.' Dr Myers's diagnosis was next corroborated by the third medical witness, Benjamin De Castro. 'When that delirium went off, he was quite an idiot; it appeared quite a perfect idiotism.' Asked what conversation had passed between Glover and himself, the witness answered 'I asked him how he did, and he did not give me a proper answer, and I judged his mind was the same.' He was examined by the judge in the following manner.

COURT: How came you to judge it not a proper answer?

DE CASTRO: I knew he did not give me a proper answer.

COURT: Why not?

DE CASTRO: I remember it was not and I have seen him since that in the street.

COURT: Had you any conversation with him?

DE CASTRO: None at all, I judged of the state of his mind, by his raving about, jumping about the street; not walking in a manner that a man in his senses should do, he walked in a harum scarum manner.

COURT: Now describe a little?

DE CASTRO: Just as a madman does.

COURT: I really do not know how a madman walks till you tell me; I want to know?

DE CASTRO: By his raving and jumping about.

COURT: Did you see him jumping?

DE CASTRO: Yes, about the street.

COURT: In what manner, do describe a little?

DE CASTRO: Why, jumping from one place to another.

COURT: What to try how far he could leap?

DE CASTRO: I do not know ... I asked him how he did and I do not recollect what his answer was, but it was not a direct one.

COURT: Do you think that every man that does not give you a direct answer is mad?

DE CASTRO: No, certainly not; I think that the answer he gave me was not a direct one.

COURT: You cannot tell us anything like his answer?

DE CASTRO: No, I cannot.[17]

This exchange illustrates the hazards a medical witness faced when he invoked incoherent conversation or bizarre behaviour as signs of madness: his diagnostic inference could easily be challenged because he had no special criteria defining what constituted acceptable speech or conduct. What precisely made an answer 'improper'? How exactly does a madman 'jump about'? The cross-examination of this witness is noteworthy because De Castro's grounds for inferring insanity were well known to the court: laymen often invoked flighty conversation and burlesque antics as their basis for suspecting madness. When employed by medical witnesses, however, such grounds were no longer descriptions given by intimates, but were expected to constitute diagnostic bases for professional judgement. Medical witnesses who had nothing more to offer than flighty conversation or frantic behaviour to substantiate their inference of insanity were therefore likely to face tough questioning by the bench. Their 'facts' were only those of the layman. In the following four trials, we see how medical witnesses attempted to transcend conventional 'ways of seeing' madness by suggesting a level of insight which penetrated the mask of reason.

A mania for stealing spoons

A second trial for theft, heard in 1801, reveals a medical challenge to one aspect of the conventional lore surrounding derangement: the existence of lucid intervals. Because lunacy was by definition a variable condition, mad persons were often thought to alternate between bouts of derangement, and periods of sanity.[18] Even faced with evidence of marked derangement, a jury was likely to remain unconvinced of the prisoner's insanity if a witness could be found to relate occasions when the accused had appeared 'regular in his habits'.[19] Such testimony suggested that the criminal act might have been perpetrated during a 'lucid interval'. One certainly did not need a medical witness to describe the alternation of lunacy and lucidity that defined this species of madness. The innovation in nineteenth-century forensic-psychiatric testimony lay rather in the suggestion that the commission of a purposeful act did not necessarily indicate a 'return' to lucidity: mania could allow for surprisingly purposeful, yet deranged, behaviour.

Dr Luis Leo of Houndsditch was employed by the Society for Visiting the Sick and Charitable Deeds, an organization set up by the Sephardic

Jews of London. He first became acquainted with John Lawrence four or five months before the latter was arrested and charged with stealing three silver teaspoons and one silver salt spoon. Making his second appearance at the Old Bailey, Dr Leo was called 'For the Prisoner' and began by stating that he had first encountered Lawrence in a 'state of insanity', adding that 'it is often the case that persons in that situation have more scheme and artfulness than others'. Leo's comment was to become a recurring theme of medical testimony in the early nineteenth century as medical witnesses endeavoured to stress the coexistence of madness with heightened cunning. The witness was then asked a series of questions by the judge which were becoming standard by 1800. Was the prisoner *always* mad? Was he fit to have management of his own affairs? Did you advise his confinement? On occasion, the court might pointedly ask why the medical man had not *insisted* on confinement, given the graphic testimony of derangement he had just presented to the jury. In this trial, however, the examining attorney seemed most interested in establishing Dr Leo's credentials. Asked if he was 'particularly versed in the disorders of the mind', Dr Leo responded: 'I am':

COURT: Then you are what is called a mad doctor.

DR LEO: It is not my particular profession to attend persons under that complaint; I have attended them, we call it mania.

COURT: Did you recommend his relations to call in some persons whose particular profession it was?

DR LEO: I cannot say that I did; I recommended them to send him to St. Luke's, or some private place.[20]

Dr Leo was then cross-examined by Mr Knapp, one of a handful of attorneys who made frequent appearances at the Old Bailey, sometimes appearing for the prosecution, other times for the defence. In this trial, Knapp was clearly assisting the prosecution.

MR KNAPP: Though you do not profess this particular line, you have attended a great many under this complaint?

DR LEO: Yes.

MR KNAPP: It has occurred to you then to hear of a lucid interval, has it not?

DR LEO: Yes; several that I have attended have.

MR KNAPP: When they have these intervals, they have again the possession of their mind?

DR LEO: Yes.

MR KNAPP: Has it often happened to you to hear of a madman stealing spoons?

DR LEO: No.

MR KNAPP: Is it more likely for a man to do it in a lucid interval than in a moment of insanity?

DR LEO: He could do it in the paroxysm of mania.[21]

Dr Leo was the first medical witness at the Old Bailey to suggest that what might appear to the casual observer as a lucid interval might not be all that it seemed. With this response, he challenged the logic of Knapp's questioning: that the prisoner's act was consistent with a lucid interval, rather than a 'moment of insanity'. Instead, Dr Leo suggested an expanded meaning to the 'manic' phase of lunacy: a form of mania which evinced artful, rather than frantic behaviour. That Lawrence had sufficient possession of his wits to steal the spoons did not necessarily imply a temporary return to rationality, commonly referred to as a lucid interval. Rather, mania itself could encompass a state of mind which permitted the purposeful, if demented, pursuit of an objective. Hearing Dr Leo's response, the attorney abruptly changed the direction of his questioning and the following exchange ensued:

MR KNAPP: Have you ever given evidence here before?
DR LEO: I believe I have; is that any matter of consequence?
MR KNAPP: Have you not been here before as a witness and a Jew physician, to give an account of a prisoner as a madman, to get him off, upon the ground of insanity?
DR LEO: I attended here once, but for what defense I have forgot. I do not think I was here more than once.[22]

This trial in 1801 is noteworthy for Dr Leo's avoiding the pitfall of answering the 'either-or' question regarding criminal lunacy: either the prisoner was in a state of dementia – in which he barely retained sufficient thought process to carry out a plan – or he was experiencing a lucid interval in which he clearly knew what he was about. Instead, Leo sidestepped the forced choice and suggested that the prisoner could have stolen the spoons in a 'paroxysm of mania'. In such a state, a madman may give the appearance of having returned to rationality because of the artfulness with which he pursues his plan. But it is a *maniacal* plan, one which cannot be comprehended accurately in the conventional understanding of 'mania' or 'lucid interval'. One sees in Leo's testimony an early sign that at the turn of the century, some medical men were already chafing at the conceptual categories traditionally used to describe criminal lunacy. 'Paroxysm of mania' was just one of several new nineteenth-century forensic terms which would herald a level of insight claimed by a new generation of medical witnesses whose sustained experience with the mad would be invoked to claim an ability to 'pierce sanity's smokescreen'.

Delusion as a defence strategy

'Damn your eyes' cried Thomas Bowler as he fired his blunderbuss – loaded with gunpowder and 'divers leaden bullets' – at William Burrows, his longstanding friend and neighbour. The two men had recently quarrelled concerning Burrows's alleged lopping off of the tops of some trees on Bowler's estate. Bowler's subsequent trial for the attempted murder of his neighbour offers a glimpse of two important developments: the increasing role played by madhouse superintendents as expert witnesses, and a further challenge to the existence of lucid intervals by the introduction of an alternative construction of partial madness known as delusion.

Before the medical witnesses were called, the jurors learned that the prisoner's erratic behaviour dated from a fit of apoplexy suffered as the result of a riding accident in a hayfield. Bowler's son-in-law provided a vivid description of the prisoner's memory lapses, incoherent conversation, and unprovoked quarrelsomeness. When asked why he did not petition for a lunacy inquisition, he replied that it was 'from motives of delicacy; that the world might not say that we had locked up the man for the sake of taking his property'. The young man's anxiety was not groundless: the prisoner had recently become agitated about losing his estate because he was convinced that his 'land tax was purchased wrong. He was sure he should be exchequered.' Indeed, it may well have been this preoccupation with his property which magnified the dispute with his neighbour to homicidal intensity.

The first medical witness to appear was Mr Hyatt, a surgeon and apothecary who had originally attended the prisoner following the fit in the hayfield. When asked about the treatment he had prescribed, Hyatt answered:

> I bled him largely. In consequence of that bleeding he recovered, by degrees; in a few weeks he got tolerably well, so that he could walk about ... He complained of something in his head; from that time until this unfortunate business took place, he complained that he had an uneasiness in his head: but, he was so positive a man, I could not prevail upon him to take anything.[23]

Hyatt's answers to direct questions, however, revealed the prisoner to be only partially deranged, and the witness to be only partially helpful. When asked if Bowler's symptoms were of a continuing sort, Mr Hyatt replied, 'Either more or less.' When asked if he had the appearance of a man incapable of looking after his own affairs, he replied, 'He certainly has, latterly.' When asked if the prisoner 'was in a situation [that] he did not know what he did', Hyatt responded, 'I did not think he did at times.' Eventually, the judge interrupted the questioner and the following interchange ensued:

> COURT: My question is: during the whole of that time whether he was not in a state to exercise his mind, to know whether he was doing right or wrong.

MR HYATT: I do not think he was, perfectly. His recollection was much better at times than others.

COURT: Then you do not think, at any part of that time, he was a man that knew what he was about.

MR HYATT: Not entirely.

COURT: He might have a complaint in his head: do you mean to say that it was to that extent that he was incapable of acting as a rational being?

MR HYATT: I think he was, a greater part of the time.

COURT: Can you distinguish what part he was, and what part he was not?

MR HYATT: At times, as I observed before, he was better than at others, but never had his intellects perfectly clear.[24]

Surgeon-apothecary Hyatt epitomized the hapless medical witness whose acquaintance with derangement was merely that of a general practitioner, observing and considering the prisoner in much the same way as would any layman. That the insane could be 'better', that their intellects were clearer at some times than at others could easily be perceived by neighbours, lovers, friends, or relatives. Medical witnesses who lacked sustained experience with madness as a clinical entity had nothing to offer the court beyond their own, usually very slight acquaintance with the accused. Their language and imagery were familiar to the court; indeed, their discourse was anything but esoteric. When new medical terms and innovative conceptual categories entered the court early in the nineteenth century, it was not the general practitioner who employed them, but representatives of the new generation of madhouse keepers, superintendents, and practitioners who could claim extensive experience with the distracted.

Bowler's trial in 1812 in fact demonstrates the changing posture of the medical witness whose experiential credentials suggested a certain expertise. Following Mr Hyatt's rather lacklustre testimony, Dr Ainsley took the stand and was immediately asked, 'In the course of your practice you must have seen a great number of persons deranged', to which he answered, 'Certainly, a great number.' The attorney continued, 'From the experience that you have acquired, did it appear that his derangement might have been of a considerable standing?' Dr Ainsley replied, 'I have no doubt of it.' When asked whether the nature of Bowler's derangement was 'such as to act constantly, or subject to lucid intervals', Ainsley replied:

> Not to lucid intervals, but subject to various acts of violence, where there is a delusion on the subject; upon all other subjects the man can act as well as any person. Upon all subjects, except the subject of delusion they would think rationally and clearly. In the present state these parts of intellect are considerably weakened, and his memory imperfect, so that, perhaps, he has not a sound mind upon any subject, in any case where the derangement remains.[25]

MR GURNEY: The old delusion, acting on his mind, will lead him to do any act.

DR AINSLEY: Undoubtedly it will ...

COURT: Not conscious that he is doing wrong.

DR AINSLEY: Most likely.

Dr Ainsley's introduction of delusion as an alternative to the possibility that Bowler was 'acting constantly, or subject to lucid intervals' echoes Dr Leo's proffering 'paroxysm of mania' in the previous case. In both instances, the medical witness implicitly challenged the restrictive polarities of complete mania and lucid interval as suitable descriptions of the derangement suffered by these particular prisoners. What might appear to the layman to signify a return to purposeful conduct – hiding oneself by the road-side to wait for one's enemy – actually revealed a man tormented by a delusion which could 'lead him to any act'. Although the concept of delusion had been introduced into criminal jurisprudence twelve years earlier during the prosecution of James Hadfield for the attempted assassination of George III, Dr Ainsley's appearance in 1812 marks the first time that a medical witness at the Old Bailey used this term to call into question what appeared on the surface to be purposeful, intentional action.[26]

The two remaining witnesses in Bowler's trial also employed delusion in their explanation of the prisoner's conduct. Madhouse superintendent Thomas Warburton had visited the prisoner in confinement and began his testimony by declaring, when asked if he had the care of insane persons, 'I have seen many thousands in my time'.

MR GURNEY: Does his derangement consist in delusion of mind?

MR WARBURTON: Yes.

MR GURNEY: Is it common for deranged persons to conceive a dislike against some particular persons –

MR WARBURTON: It is a character of mental derangement, brought on by epilepsy. In that it is more characteristic than any other.

MR GURNEY: It is very common for them to conceive that enmity to the most dear friend –

MR WARBURTON: Frequently.

MR ADOLPHUS: You apprehend that he did labour under some particular delusion –

MR WARBURTON: I am satisfied it applied particularly to Mr Burrows. He imagined Burrows to be his secret enemy; he had instigated the whole country against him; that he could not pass from his own house to the next village without being insulted by the women and children, in order, as he imagined, so to deprive him of his property.

MR GURNEY: From the opportunity you have had many years of observing insane persons, have you any means of discerning whether they are deranged, or whether they are not –

MR WARBURTON: I have not the least doubt, in this instance, that he is insane. He is uniformly the same, since the commission of lunacy as before, from all my observations. I am quite satisfied that he has not imposed on me.

MR GURNEY: Is it not a common symptom of derangement of one man to suppose that another man means to deprive him of his estate, and, under that delusion of mind, they would proceed to vengeance.

MR WARBURTON: No doubt, they uniformly do, if not taken care to prevent it.[27]

After listening to the above examination, it would be difficult to say whose words the jury found most persuasive regarding the critical importance of delusion as a forensic-psychiatric term: the attorney's, or the medical superintendent's. The tone of Mr Gurney's questions unambiguously affirms delusion's existence, and the manner in which he invoked the medical witness's background clearly set the stage for the latter's unequivocal pronouncement of insanity. The attorney's effort to make the witness credible was not necessarily the extension of 'professional courtesy' to a recently arrived colleague: the testimony of medical witnesses was fundamental to the defence strategy. Just as one notices the active participation of contemporary American lawyers in the creation of various 'syndrome' defences (Child-Abuse Syndrome, Battered Woman Syndrome, Rape Trauma Syndrome, etc.), so one sees in the deftly phrased questions asked by early nineteenth-century barristers the implicit affirmation of morbid states of consciousness.

The language and images employed by Thomas Warburton and Dr Ainsley reveal the growing separation of lay from medical testimony in the early nineteenth century. Whereas neighbours and family friends continued to speak in terms of fits or head injuries following a riding accident, a noticeable current in medical testimony involved the questioning of conventional, popular notions of madness such as lucid intervals. Indeed, the entire notion of a *return* to sanity was under scrutiny. The possibility that derangement was limited to a particular subject rendered potentially meaningless the layman's testimony regarding the apparently sane behaviour that immediately preceded the crime. Even the act itself, seemingly *reasonable* to the untrained eye, might reveal to the experienced eye the maniacal pursuit of an objective. The layman's error was his inference that the cessation of maniacal fury betokened a return to composure and lucidity.

An unconscious forgery

The connection between delusion and mental states in which the accused was 'unconscious that he was doing wrong' was further explored in a case two decades after the Bowler trial. In 1833, Elizabeth Wratten was indicted for forging a cheque for four pounds and nine shillings. The prisoner stood mute throughout the trial, and drew the following comment from the recorder of the *OBSP*:

> The prisoner being repeatedly desired by the Court and by her Counsel to enter upon her defence; made no reply for some time; but at last said, 'The four corners of the earth and the strength of the hills is his also.' 'I said, they were all going down to the Red Sea.' During the whole trial she kept distorting her feautures [*sic*], working her fingers about, and conducting herself in an incoherent manner.[28]

After several witnesses recounted their dealings with the eccentric Mrs Wratten, Dr David Uwins, author of several tracts on phrenology, took the stand. He first informed the court of his considerable experience in cases of insanity, having been connected with a lunatic asylum for five or six years. At the request of her relatives, Uwins had visited Wratten in gaol. Although he first suspected that she was acting, he now considered her to be irresponsible. When asked about the possibility of cases in which the mind had become deranged all at once, but partly recovered 'and very high duties have been performed' the witness agreed that such had been known to happen. The judge then posed the following question:

> COURT: That being the case, would you not judge of the state of mind, by the degree of contrivance exhibited at the time of the transaction; should you deem a person insane who appeared aware of what he was about, and contrived and took measures for his own benefit?
>
> DR UWINS: I cannot say that an act itself sane, might not be coupled with insanity.
>
> COURT: You have heard of the prisoner obtaining a writing, and presenting one resembling it, and obtaining through that, a sum for her own benefit?
>
> DR UWINS: I have heard of aberration of mind, being manifested before that took place – I can conceive a great deal of contrivance in the process of effecting a design.[29]

The witness was then asked pointedly by the judge: 'Would such a degree of contrivance be consistent with imbecility or idiocy: would it be consistent with the absence of reason?' Uwins answered the hypothetical question by invoking his professional experience: 'Among my patients at the Institution, they have gone through the process of reasoning for the object they have in desire, as a sane person would.' The act itself did not reveal sanity or insanity: 'there may be considerable imbecility of mind, and yet the process of reasoning exist'. However, such 'reasoning' did not necessarily convey an understanding of the responsibility which flowed from one's actions: 'I conceive it possible for an individual to act as the prisoner did with respect to this cheque, without knowing the degree of responsibility under which she herself must stand in reference to it.'[30]

It is important to note here that Uwins was introducing a novel way of looking at consciousness, and by implication, intention. The law's concern with culpability speaks to the individual's capacity to understand the circumstances surrounding his or her actions. In this trial, Uwins suggested that one could perform purposeful actions, yet fail to recognize the criminality of one's conduct. He was not suggesting a form of *partial* insanity; in fact, when asked by the court whether many persons partially insane are perfectly capable of knowing they are doing a wrong act, he averred, 'That more refers to cases of monomania.'[31] Mrs Wratten had not been *propelled* into forgery against her will – conscious that she was doing wrong but unable to help herself (monomania). Rather, Uwins argued that she knew what she was doing, but 'without a consciousness that there was anything wrong in it'. How was it possible for him to know this, when the lay observer would naturally infer that forgery presupposes a criminal intent? Uwins asserted that it was possible to act without consciousness because he had seen it happen before. Among my patients, he informed the jury, I have 'seen several instances where the object has been of less importance'.

In the evolving tradition of 'Counsel for the defence' (as he was referred to in the *OBSP*) leading the emerging forensic psychiatric witness by posing carefully worded questions, Uwins was then asked, 'Have you known persons labouring under insanity pursue an object with a cunning you would only expect from very clever persons?' He replied 'Certainly: in the only instance of suicide which has occurred since I have been physician of the Asylum at Peckham, the cunning evinced for months and weeks to accomplish the purpose would surprise every body.'

Beyond his identification of single-minded pursuit and 'contrivance' with types of behaviour fully 'consistent with insanity', Uwins's courtroom appearance was also important for what he did not say. He neither declared the prisoner sane nor insane. Indeed, his familiarity with the prisoner was slight, and he does not claim on such short acquaintance to be able to fit a diagnosis to her particular case. Instead, he appeared neutral and professional. His role was to inform the court participants (and the many readers of the *OBSP*) about medical insight into the mind of the mad gained through professional experience. Indeed, he underscored his impartiality by declaring, 'I do not come here as an advocate, nor do I positively say she was not conscious of the delinquency of the act.' He was in court to advise the jury about how insane people may act – of the fact that their deluded thought and subsequent behaviour may quite remarkably mimic the actions of rational beings.

Uwins was followed in the witness box by an apothecary called by one of the prosecuting attorneys. Thomas Halifax attended the prisoner's family and testified that he had always considered her 'perfectly sound in mind'. Apothecary Halifax contradicted Uwins by saying that the act itself was really all one need go on: 'I consider a person sane at the time, whose conduct is sane, and whose view of things is the same as persons in their ordinary senses.' He acknowledged, however, that he could not recall how many insane persons he had treated over the past ten years, adding 'I believe Dr Uwins has an experience of 200 a week.'

The final medical witness was Gilbert McMurdo, who made no fewer than seventeen appearances at the Old Bailey during the years that spanned 1830 to 1843. As surgeon of Newgate Gaol, McMurdo found himself in an advantageous position to observe prisoners' behaviour, notice any changes over the course of confinement, and to detect any proclivity towards 'counterfeited madness'. Though one might imagine that he was therefore ideally suited to become an authoritative voice in forensic-psychiatric testimony, he actually exemplified the general practitioner of the mid-eighteenth century more than the nineteenth-century asylum keeper and medical attendant. His testimony rarely rose above his professed skill at detecting shammed madness. Although he did not always contradict prior medical testimony asserting a prisoner's insanity, in Wratten's case he certainly did.

> I have observed her manner at the bar, she can conduct herself different at times in the gaol; and when I was sitting in the box just now, the moment I spoke to her to try the effect of my observation, she instantly began to assume the position of the eye, which has been observed; she was perfectly right before, and she began moving her mouth as she does now.[32]

Elizabeth Wratten's trial in 1833 affords an interesting opportunity to compare the three professional roles which typified the early nineteenth-century medical community's encounters with the mad: the general practitioner who treated the deranged 'in the character of a physician' (usually for a fever, a fit, or a head injury of some sort); the gaol surgeon sent by the court to observe the prisoner, and the asylum superintendent or medical attendant. Not until a generation of specialist asylum doctors came of age did the general practitioner's degree of familiarity with insanity come to be thought insufficient. By the second third of the nineteenth century, the general physician, surgeon, or apothecary was making fewer and fewer appearances at the Old Bailey. The gaol surgeon was everywhere in evidence, but his capacity (or willingness) to comment upon the protean nature of madness was subsumed under a more pressing concern: unmasking fakery. One suspects that this was a primary reason for his employment in visiting prisoners thought to be contemplating an insanity defence. In another trial in the same year as the Wratten case, McMurdo accounted for his appearance in court as follows:

> I go to the Compter daily to see the prisoners ... [T]he Clerk of arraigns told me it was very likely I should be wanted, and I had better be in attendance; on one occasion the Lord Mayor met me and said, 'Mind you see that prisoner, for it is very likely we shall want your evidence.'[33]

The third and most recent type of medical witness was the asylum superintendent, typified by Uwins in the present case, and by Warburton in Bowler's trial. They were the new specialists whose reference to professional experience and elaborate exposition of the varieties of madness clearly set them apart from the first two types of witnesses. Even though they were questioned closely, their cross-examination did not fundamentally challenge their claims to expertise.[34] Though the moment when experience becomes expertise is obviously difficult to specify, it is doubtless true that successful claims to cognitive territory generally follow years of professing unique insight and skill in as public a forum as possible. The voice of the forensic witness was neither strident nor self-aggrandizing, but nor was it diffident. By the second third of the century, the employment of ideas such as 'delusion' and maniacal 'contrivance', as well as a willingness to address medical testimony to legal questions was well underway. As physician to Peckham Asylum, David Uwins stated simply in court, 'I don't think she was in a state to distinguish right from wrong at the time of this affair.'

A lesion of the will

The last in this series of five cases differs from the previous ones by virtue of its notoriety, although in the area of landmark insanity cases the trial of Edward Oxford in 1840 ranks considerably behind the prosecutions of Daniel McNaughtan and James Hadfield. Had Oxford injured the Queen, his trial would certainly be among the most famous; indeed, had proof existed that his pistols were in fact loaded, the case would very likely have received more attention.[35] Yet from the standpoint of the history of forensic psychiatry, Oxford's trial is significant because it marks the formal introduction of the conception of moral insanity – which originated in the French school of *médecine mentale* – and the first claims by a forensic witness that insanity was indeed a medical matter about which medical practitioners were uniquely qualified to speak with authority. The Oxford case also provides further examples of how assertions of professional expertise surfaced in response to particular questions asked in cross-examination.

Following the reading of Oxford's indictment, a host of witnesses appeared to report the facts of the shooting. They were followed by a number of Oxford's acquaintances who informed the court of an episode in which the prisoner had been 'raving mad . . . [we were] obliged to put cords on him'. Eventually he was admitted to Greenwich hospital, behaving 'like anybody *quite gone*' [emphasis in the original].[36] The prisoner's mother next testified, graphically recounting her son's periods of causeless violence, gloomy fits followed by hysterical laughing, and a particular fondness for firearms and gunpowder: 'he would amuse himself with letting off cannons'.[37] Altogether, the witnesses gave an account of a decidedly eccentric, even violent man, who might go berserk for no apparent reason – a characterization of madness with which the Old Bailey was only too familiar.

Dr John Birt Davies, sometime physician to the Oxford family, Warwickshire magistrate and, since 1839, coroner for the city of Birmingham, was the first medical witness to appear. His acquaintance with the prisoner was limited to an encounter sixteen years before, of such short duration that he had insufficient 'opportunity of judging as to the state of his mind'. He reported hearing of Oxford's odd conduct, and stated that he had been present in the court during the trial, but he had not visited the prisoner in confinement. Given this decidedly superficial acquaintance, it seems curious that Davies was even called as a witness. Even more curious was the direction his testimony took, embarking on a hitherto unknown characterization of criminal insanity when he was asked the following:

> Supposing a person in the middle of the day, without any suggested motive, [were] to fire a loaded pistol at Her Majesty . . ., to remain on the spot, to declare he was the person who did it – to take pains to have that known, and afterwards to enter freely into discussion, and answer any questions put to him on the subject, would you refer such conduct to a sound or unsound state of mind?[38]

When Davies declined to answer with a simple yes or no but instead replied, 'if to that hypothesis were added what I deem a proof of hallucination –', the judge interrupted and asked, 'You mean to state, upon your oath, that if you heard these facts stated, you should conclude that the party must be mad?' Acknowledging that he would make this determination without undertaking any further inquiry, the witness explained the grounds for his inference: 'the absence of motive, the absence of precaution, the deliberate owning, and the free discussion afterwards, of his own conduct, criminating himself in that way immediately afterwards, with the danger staring him in the face'. When a prosecuting attorney asked whether the existence of papers written before the transaction clearly announcing his violent intent would strengthen or weaken 'the inference that you have already told us you draw', the witness answered: 'It would greatly strengthen the inference.' Dr Davies's testimony ended with the following cross-examination, put to him by Sir Frederick Pollack:

SIR FREDERICK: You have answered some hypothetical questions put by my learned friend opposite, I beg to ask you whether you give that answer from your knowledge, as a physician, or from your experience as a Coroner, or as a Magistrate, or merely as a member of society?

DR DAVIS [*sic*]: I answer as a physician – I think the circumstances which have been supposed, have, medically speaking, a tendency to prove insanity.

COURT: We do not exactly understand what you mean when you say medically?

DR DAVIS: If as a physician, I was employed to ascertain whether an individual was sane or insane, in whom I found those facts, I should undoubtedly give my opinion that he was insane.

COURT: As a physician, you think every crime that is plainly committed to be committed by a mad man?

DR DAVIS: Nothing of the kind; but a crime committed under all the circumstances of the hypothesis.

COURT: What are the circumstances in the crime itself, which you think show madness?

DR DAVIS: The crime is committed in open day, it being obviously of great magnitude and danger; of great atrocity; it is committed without any precaution, without any looking for the means of escape; it is afterwards spoken of openly, so far from concealing the criminating facts; facts which might afford a chance of escape; the existence of the balls is acknowledged, the free discussion of the circumstances, the absence of motive – by the free discussion, I mean a free respondence to the questions put to him immediately afterwards in the cell – the questions which Lord Uxbridge stated yesterday he did put – he said, on Lord Uxbridge entering the door, 'I did it'.[39]

Although Davies did not label it as such, the derangement he described to the court was by the 1830s widely referred to as moral insanity. Its origin can be traced to Philippe Pinel's *manie sans délire*, a form of distraction in which the afflicted was under the most abstract fury, yet experienced no defect in reasoning. For Pinel, and others of the French school of *médecine mentale*, reason was no longer the sole wellspring of human activity; reason could in fact remain intact while the individual was swept into fury by a morbid state of the passions – or by the force of an autonomous and deluded imagination. As insanity thus became 'de-intellectualized', reason increasingly became separated from the will, and the emotions from reason.[40] Speculation on the relationship between the emotions and insanity preoccupied other members of the French circle such as Jean-Etienne-Dominique Esquirol and Etienne-Jean Georget, who coined the new categories of *monomanie instinctive* and *monomanie homicide* respectively. Their approach was further elaborated by James Cowles Prichard, and by writers in the Scottish Common Sense tradition of philosophy. Prichard's formulation of moral insanity fits all the particulars of the Oxford case. Eschewing the notion that the mind was overcome by confusion or preoccupied by delusion, Prichard averred that 'some ruling passion seems to have entire possession of the mind'. The impulsive nature of the will impelled the person into motiveless criminal activity. Indeed, the very want of any logical reason for the act suggested a blind force which 'neither reason nor sentiment determine' and which the will no longer has the power to control.[41]

It is difficult to gauge how widespread was acceptance of this 'volitional insanity'. Certainly, popular beliefs encompassed a view of the passions as capable of carrying one away in their thrall. Given psychiatry's proclivity to be shaped 'from below'[42] it comes as little surprise that romanticism should find expression in nineteenth-century psychiatric conceptions of the passions as no longer subjugated by the intellect. For Davies, the very want of a motive signified the insanity of Oxford's act: the effect of unrestrained passions in which intellect played no part. Delusion was not an integral part of this line of reasoning; indeed Prichard had lamented the courts' reliance on delusion as the necessary element of madness. What was crucial in Prichard's view was an appreciation of the independent role of the passions and the emotions.

When Davies stated that Oxford's lack of any delusion and his awareness of the nature of his act were themselves proof of insanity, his opinion was given so matter-of-factly that it is hard not to infer that all evidence of bravado and recklessness were regarded as clear proof of madness. In the tradition of previous medical witnesses, Davies was reminding the court that things are seldom what they seem; *folie* masquerades as *crime*. Madness could lie behind the most seemingly purposeful acts, but like so many medical phenomena, could not be detected by the naked, or rather, the untrained eye. As the next medical witness was to explain, an informed opinion regarding the soundness of a man's mind required the 'careful comparison of particular cases'; by implication, precisely the sort of professional experience which medical men alone were gaining through their asylum work.

'I have been a physician about fourteen years – I have been lecturer on morbid anatomy, and have written some works: lectures on pathological anatomy, and lectures on the promotion of health.' With these words, Thomas Hodgkin began his testimony, agreeing with Davies that lack of motive, readiness to deliver oneself to the law, and appearing 'reckless of the consequences', were indeed 'circumstances of strong suspicion' of insanity. Departing from Prichard's ideas, Hodgkin added that evidence of a previous delusion would certainly strengthen the inference, as would evidence of hereditary insanity. He was then asked: 'Are there instances on record of persons becoming suddenly insane, whose conduct has been previously only eccentric?' Hodgkin replied that there certainly were, and that such a form of insanity 'exists and is recognised'. When asked for the name by which he called such insanity, Hodgkin replied:

> *Lesion* of the will, it has been called by Le Marc, insanity connected with the development of the will – I should not consider a headstrong person to be under such an influence – I mention *lesion* of the will, as a term which a highly reputed writer on insanity has chosen to designate a form of insanity ... [I]t means more than a loss of control over the conduct – it means morbid propensity – moral irregularity is the result of the disease ... [I] have had cases under my observation, in which this form of insanity existed, one case in particular, that person was in perfect health – I do not think I ever met with a case where the only apparent symptom was moral irregularity, where I had no medical indication of physical disease – I think that, committing a crime without any apparent motive, is an indication of insanity – doing anything of any sort, without motive, is not an indication of unsoundness of mind in every instance.[43]

At this point the judge interrupted:

> COURT: Do you conceive that this is really a medical question at all which has been put to you?
> DR HODGKIN: I do – I think medical men have more means of forming an opinion on that subject than other persons – I am supported in that opinion by writers on the subject, by Loura [Leuret], and by Le Mark [Marc], who I have alluded to, who is a particularly eminent writer – my reasons for thinking so is, because it is so stated by those writers.
> COURT: Why could not any person form an opinion whether a person was sane or insane from the circumstances which have been referred to?
> DR HODGKIN: Because it seems to require a careful comparison of particular cases, more likely to be looked to by medical men, who are especially experienced in cases of unsoundness of mind.
> COURT: What is the limit of responsibility a medical man would draw?
> DR HODGKIN: That is a very difficult point – it is scarcely a medical question – I should not be able to draw the line where soundness ends and unsoundness begins – it is very difficult to draw the line between eccentricity and insanity.[44]

By its very name, 'lesion of the will' endowed moral insanity with materialist overtones while nevertheless giving full expression to more traditional ideas of the will as an autonomous force in human functioning. An organic basis for insanity was hardly new to the court: brain fever, epilepsy, head injury, and fetid breath were commonly mentioned in the medical literature and sometimes in court to account for aetiological and/or somatic correlates of madness. What was novel in Hodgkin's testimony was the casting of the legal community's essential element of culpability, a wicked will (Bracton's will to harm) as the agent *responsible* for producing in the afflicted person's mind a 'morbid propensity' quite beyond a mere loss of control. The pathological turn of the will was not the secondary *result* of mental derangement; the will *itself* was diseased. Some morbid growth, some *lesion* had distorted its nature.

Lesion of the will was first articulated by Georget in 1825 in his initial separation of monomania into affective and ideational components.[45] The particular construction, lesion of the will, was further described by Marc and Leuret in a number of publications beginning with the 1829 inaugural issue of the *Annales d'hygiène publique et de médecine légale*. Hodgkin's assertion that it was only the careful comparison of particular cases which afforded insight into the contours of mental (and moral) pathology resonates with these French works published ten years earlier. In the *Annales* and in other publications, Marc and Leuret defended the concept of instinctive monomania against medical critics who insisted that intellectual delirium must attend any disturbance of the will. Such ill-informed detractors, they argued, lacked the sustained professional experience necessary to compare and observe the variation of disturbance among the mentally ill.[46] Marc, in particular, took issue with those who doubted the existence of non-delirious insanity when he referred to his monitoring of asylum inhabitants over a sixteen-year period. His examination of 200 persons suffering from this particular malady had left him with no doubt of the reality of lesions of the will.[47] Quoting a patient of Leuret's, Marc provided what is doubtless the most familiar expression attributed to these patients: 'I can't help myself, it is stronger than me!'[48]

Although a 'lesion of the will' might appear to challenge fundamentally the legal element of intent and 'wicked will', it is well worth noting that Hodgkin claimed to respect the courtroom division of labour. His role, he maintained, was to inform the court of the *fact* of this condition, ' a form of insanity which exists and is recognized'. Responsibility, however, 'is scarcely a medical question', and he carefully avoided appearing to encroach upon the jury's prerogative. As he averred, the line separating eccentricity and insanity was difficult to draw; perhaps at no time more so than after his testimony.

John Conolly, physician to Hanwell Lunatic Asylum, Middlesex, made his first appearance at the Old Bailey during the trial of Edward Oxford. Announcing that he had 890 patients under his care and 'some experience in the treatment of disorders of the mind', he informed the jury that his conversations with Oxford led him to conclude that he was indeed of unsound mind. When he asked the prisoner 'if he was conscious that he had committed a great offense in shooting at such a young and interesting person as the Queen', Oxford said, 'Oh, I might as well shoot at her as anybody else.' Conolly then proceeded to read to the court the notes he had made following his meeting with Oxford:

> A deficient understanding; shape of the anterior part of the head, that which is generally seen when there has been some disease of the brain in the early period of life – an occasional appearance of acuteness, but a total inability to reason – a singular insensibility as regards the affections – an apparent incapacity to comprehend moral obligations, to distinguish right from wrong – an absolute insensibility to the heinousness of his offence, and to the peril of his situation – a total indifference to the issue of the trial; acquittal will give him no particular pleasure, and he seems unable to comprehend the alternative of his condemnation and execution; his offence, like that of other imbeciles who set fire to buildings, &c., without motive, except a vague pleasure in mischief – appears unable to conceive any thing of future responsibility.[49]

Conolly's notes constitute a kind of check-list of late eighteenth- and early nineteenth-century medical conceptions of madness: deficient reasoning capacity, insensibility to affections, inability to comprehend moral obligation (to distinguish right from wrong), and in an echo of the law's concern with intent, an implicit failure to understand the consequences of one's actions. There may even be a trace of phrenology: 'shape of the anterior part of the head' which would indicate imperfect development. Although Conolly mentions a part, not an 'organ' of the brain, his remarks clearly resonate with the ideas of early nineteenth-century phrenologists, who contended that irregular cranial shape revealed the dominance of a particular faculty due to overdevelopment of its associated organ.[50] Conolly does not elaborate on brain 'parts' or any other grounds for inferring insanity. Still, he provides the historian with a list of nineteenth-century correlates of madness, and the first evidence of 'case notes' entering directly into expert testimony.

Dr Chowne, a physician to Charing Cross Hospital, returned to the question of lesion of the will. Identifying himself as a lecturer on medical jurisprudence, he answered a question about the mental state of a person who committed a motiveless crime, regardless of consequences, without 'anything like consciousness of responsibility for the act' in the following way: 'a propensity to commit acts without an apparent or adequate motive under such circumstances is recognized as a particular species of insanity, called in medical jurisprudence, *lesion* of the will – I do not know a better term – it is an old term – it has been called moral insanity'.[51] He next recounted examples of patients being 'impelled with a strong disposition to suicide, of the madness of which there can be no doubt', yet totally lacking any other symptoms of mental disease. They report nothing to complain of, no 'unhappy news', no disappointment. 'My husband is kind to me', one patient had told him, 'nothing at all to impel me to the act but a strange impulse'. When asked by an attorney whether this sort of 'mental disease is consistent with a person performing all other functions and duties of life with accuracy', the witness replied, 'There is no doubt of it.' Dr Chowne concluded his testimony with a report of his conversation with Oxford, which had taken place in the company of three other medical men. He had informed the prisoner that he was quite wrong if he believed that no proof existed that there were indeed balls in his pistols, 'that his responsibility was a terrible one', and in all likelihood decapitation would be his punishment. To this, Oxford replied that 'he had been decapitated in fact a week before, for he had a cast taken of his head'.[52]

The final medical witness called was a family physician who had interviewed the prisoner together with Drs Conolly and Chowne. James Fernandez Clarke, surgeon to the Dorcas Charity and honorary secretary to the Westminster Medical Society, recalled a particular episode when he had visited the Oxford home. The prisoner ignored the visitor's presence, and eventually responded furiously to his mother's entreaties that he be civil to the surgeon, swearing that he would 'stick her'. At Oxford's trial, Clarke was asked whether in cases of hereditary insanity there was a particular period of life during which 'medical writers consider it likely to break out, to appear', and Clarke replied:

> In the kind of insanity, particularly, which is connected with acts of violence, Escoreaux [Esquirol] says, in several cases which bear great analogy to the one which we might suppose to exist at present – in six of these cases I think that three of them took place at the age of puberty, between the ages perhaps of fourteen and twenty.[53]

Although Mr Clarke's testimony contains no innovative terms nor an expressed basis of familiarity with madness, his testimony affirms the existence of at least one authority, Esquirol, and the 'great analogy' of Oxford's case to others already in print. Together with Hodgkin's reference to Marc's lesion of the will, and Chowne's affirmation that this condition was recognized as a particular species of insanity, it could hardly have been lost on the jury that there existed a body of opinion which supported medical claims to special insight into the mind of the mad. Lecturers on morbid anatomy and medical jurisprudence claimed it, and superintendents of asylums who recounted their experience in the treatment of disorders of the mind explicitly referred to it. Even Mr Clarke, a general practitioner with neither special training nor experience in the detection of mental disorders, could cite a written source to support his opinion about Oxford's manifest insanity.

Medical opinion and 'the fair range of dispute'

One sees in this fifth and final case the dynamics of an evolving forensic psychiatry: professional experience in treatment, claims to expertise thus acquired, and an attempt to move the grounds of professional inference beyond surface impressions to the correlation of physical with mental pathology. Although the case of Daniel McNaughtan has certainly received more attention in the history of law and insanity, there can be little doubt that the trial of Edward Oxford provides the historian of medicine with compelling evidence of the extension of claims to professional expertise from medical text to medical testimony. A familiar theme in nineteenth-century medical texts had been the layman's errors of perception regarding insanity, most specifically his reliance on histrionic exhibitions, and 'caricatures of disease which the stage represents, or romances propagate'.[54] In a similar vein, medical witnesses stressed the naïvety of the layman's acceptance of surface calm as proof of a return to rationality. One can well appreciate the physicians' lamenting a 'state of affairs whereby laymen comment on insanity ... [and] medical knowledge is thought to come by intuition'.[55] When Hodgkin asserted that 'medical men have more means of forming an opinion on that subject than other persons', his was not a novel claim. It was, however, the first time that such distinctions were clearly made in court.

The demarcation drawn by Hodgkin helps to add historical and contextual framing to Judge Learned Hand's delineation of various types of courtroom evidence. 'Fact and opinion are actually distinguished by merely a practical consideration, i.e. whether the inference is one which is within the fair range of dispute, or whether, given the impression of sense, the inference from them is so self-evident as to make any attempt to question it frivolous.'[56] Nothing could have been more 'frivolous' in the eighteenth century than questioning a deranged prisoner's Lear-like rantings, or the single-minded pursuit of his criminal ends. Would anyone even have suggested that something *beyond* plain observation was needed? By the mid-nineteenth century, however, what was plainly seen or heard by laymen was no longer self-evident, and any inference drawn from such superficial impressions was itself likely to be called into question. Leo's 'paroxysm of mania', Uwins's idiosyncratic employment of 'contrivance' without accompanying moral consciousness, and Hodgkin's 'lesion of the will' each placed a seemingly straightforward action under the rubric of mental derangement. In terms of Learned Hand's separation of fact from opinion, there simply were no *self*-evident facts when the acts of madmen were reported by nineteenth-century laymen. Whatever impressions they may have made on the organs of sense, no report or interpretation of these 'facts' could be accepted without careful consideration of like cases, informed by extensive experience in the day-to-day observation of the afflicted. Medical opinion became expert opinion once it had succeeded in moving mere observation into 'the fair range of dispute'.

The further distinctive element of medical opinion was the notion of hidden, treacherous forces which undermined the prisoner's capacity to control his conduct. The early nineteenth-century juror listened to novel conceptions of the mind – paroxysm of mania, contrivance unattended by consciousness, delusion – which suggested the prisoner's inability to resist or control a morbid criminal impulse. If the forger, assaulter, or thief could not recognize a delusion for what it was, how could one say that the prisoner acted deliberately? And consciousness was not the only conceptual entity to appear fragmented: the independence of the will – and the implications this carried for the question of self-control – also figured prominently in the growing professional literature on medical witnessing. In medical texts, witnesses were advised to say whether in their opinion, the alleged lunatic had 'at the time he committed the offense, sufficient control over his actions'.[57] In fact, *self-control* was considered by medical authors to be the proper subject of medical testimony, not the prisoner's ability to tell right from wrong, or the 'fit' of the prisoner's delirium with an inclusive definition of insanity. 'Nothing is so easily seized upon than a definition', cautioned one textbook author.[58] Witnesses were further advised to prepare thoroughly for their time in court, to 'give sufficient reason for the foundations of opinion' and to be wary of the 'subtle underminings of cross examination'.[59] Although the fraught nature of medico-legal dialogue gave rise to some unease, medical witnesses did not avoid the courtroom nor fail to assert their importance in print. As Forbes Winslow claimed in 1832: 'Medical evidence materially influences the jury; if of no value, why are so many witnesses examined?'[60]

Although there is no way to subject Winslow's assertion to empirical scrutiny, there is little doubt that by the 1840s, the forensic-psychiatric witness had indeed 'arrived'. But one suspects that the acceptance of forensic testimony bearing on insanity attests to more than medicine's success in claiming superior insight into madness. Medical evidence was not simply offered; it was actively sought and subpoenaed. Although it is certainly true that the courtroom provided medical specialists with a most visible (and audible!) forum in which to assert their professional expertise, an analysis of trial narratives suggests that medical men succeeded in no small part because their evidence was fast becoming an important element for the 'Counsel for the Defence'. Even though the time period surveyed predates the formal granting of full legal representation, one cannot miss the strategic way in which questions were formed to elicit the most legally salient elements of medical testimony. The Lord Mayor *employed* gaol-surgeon McMurdo to detect counterfeited madness; counsel for the defence used asylum superintendents and lecturers on medical jurisprudence to expose the inadequacies of the layman's self-evident 'facts'. The historian of forensic psychiatry must be therefore ever mindful of parallel developments in advocacy representation and the likely reciprocal relations that obtained between professionally-conscious medical witnesses and ambitious barristers.

In the end, forensic-psychiatric witnesses succeeded in establishing a role in the courtroom because they skilfully employed medical ideas to address basic elements of intention: consciousness, control, contrivance. They did not ride into court on the back of their professional reputation nor did they automatically benefit from pre-existing deference to men of science. Rather, their testimony reveals a gradual but persistent effort to question the perceptual sets of laymen who lacked the experience to distinguish, for example, Elizabeth Wratten's maniacal *contrivance* from consciousness, Edward Oxford's 'lesion of the will' from intentional assault, John Lawrence's 'paroxysm of mania' from purposeful theft. Trial narratives of the testimony and cross-examination of medical witnesses reveal not only an evolving professional consciousness but a growing self-confidence in medicine's claims to a privileged role in the detection of criminal lunacy. Given the choice of placing his testimony under the professional sign of the magistracy or of the coroner's office, Dr John Birt Davies, witness in the trial of Edward Oxford, stated simply: 'I answer as a physician.'

NOTES

1 Bushell's case (1671). Quoted in Learned Hand, 'Historical and practical considerations regarding expert testimony', *Harvard Law Review*, 15 (1901), 40–58. For a discussion of the historical development of the jury trial, see James Bradley Thayer, *A Preliminary Treatise on Evidence at the Common Law*, (Boston: Little, Brown & Company, 1898), pp. 47–182.

2 John Henry Wigmore, *Evidence in Trials at Common Law*, 4th edn (Boston: Little, Brown & Company, 1985), vol. VII, p. 4.

3 Andrew Scull, 'Mad-doctors and magistrates: English psychiatry's struggle for professional autonomy in the nineteenth century', *Archives Européennes de Sociologie*, 17 (1975), 279–305; Scull, 'From madness to mental illness: medical men as moral entrepreneurs', *Archives Européennes de Sociologie*, 16 (1975), 218–59.

4 Hand, 'Historical and practical considerations', pp. 42–3. For a discussion of the evolution of the role of medical evidence in coroners' inquests, see Thomas

Rogers Forbes, 'Crowner's quest' (an account of London coroner's inquests, 1788–1829), *Transactions of the American Philosophical Society*, 68, part 1 (1978), 5–50.

5 Thomas Rogers Forbes, *Surgeons at the Bailey: English Forensic Medicine to 1878*, (New Haven and London: Yale University Press, 1985), pp. 168–9.

6 For a discussion of Monro's testimony and his examination by Ferrers, see Nigel Walker, *Crime and Insanity in England, Vol. I: The Historical Perspective* (Edinburgh: Edinburgh University Press, 1968), pp. 58–63.

7 According to Hale, the legal criterion to be met was total, or *perfect*, insanity. Only total insanity would convincingly preclude the 'will to harm', the essential element which rendered an action morally and legally culpable. By partial insanity, Hale referred either to those people who normally enjoyed the use of their reason except in relation to some particular subject, or to those unfortunates whose partial derangement was a matter of 'degrees'. In this latter category, the author named melancholics whose condition consisted in 'excessive fears and griefs'. A full statement of the separation of total from partial insanity may be found in Sir Matthew Hale, *The History of the Pleas of the Crown*, (London, E & R Nutt, 1736), pp. 30–7.

8 The principle of *Voluntas nocendi*, a will to harm, was first articulated by Henri de Bracton in the thirteenth century. For a discussion of the evolution of legal thinking relative to insanity from Bracton to Hale, see Anthony Platt and Bernard Diamond, 'Origins and development of the "wild beast concept" of mental illness and its relationship to theories of criminal responsibility', *Journal of the History of the Behavioral Sciences*, 1 (1965), 355–67, and Robert Dreher, 'Origin, development and present status of insanity as a defense to criminal responsibility in the common law', *Journal of the History of the Behavioral Sciences*, 3 (1967), 47–57.

9 *Old Bailey Sessions Papers* (hereafter, *OBSP*), 1786, Sixth Session, Case 591, p. 875.

10 Forbes, *Surgeons at the Bailey*, p. 18.

11 The *OBSP* have been checked for historical credibility by comparing them with shorthand trial notes taken down by Judge Dudley Ryder during the decade of the 1760s. When the judge's notes have been set alongside the corresponding trial narratives in the *OBSP*, the latter have been deemed to be a reliable account. See John H. Langbein, 'Shaping the eighteenth-century criminal trial: a view from the Ryder sources', *The University of Chicago Law Review*, 50 (1983), 1–36.

12 For a discussion of the early years of forensic testimony bearing on madness, see Joel P. Eigen, 'Intentionality and insanity: what the eighteenth-century juror heard', in W. F. Bynum, Roy Porter, and Michael Shepherd, eds., *The Anatomy of Madness, Vol. II: Institutions and Society* (London: Tavistock, 1985), pp. 34–51.

13 The imagery found in eighteenth-century medical testimony resonates with the fundamental tenets of associationism, the dominant school of psychology in the mid-to-late 1700s. Based on the Lockean belief that all knowledge originated in sensory experience and the subsequent patterns of thought built up from one's impressions of the external world, associationists maintained that the repetition of certain sensations and the consequent revival of their associated ideas gave rise to 'trains of thought'. See Robert Hoeldtke, 'The history of

associationism and British medical psychology', *Medical History*, 11 (1967), 45–65. A discussion of the decline of associationist imagery and the rise of terms connected with early nineteenth-century medical psychology can be found in Joel P. Eigen, 'Delusion in the courtroom: the role of partial insanity in early forensic testimony', *Medical History*, 35 (1991), 25–49.

14 Roy Porter, *Mind-Forg'd Manacles: A History of Madness from the Restoration to the Regency* (Cambridge, MA: Harvard University Press, 1988), p. 35.

15 For discussion of the world of the asylums, see William L. Parry-Jones, *The Trade in Lunacy: A Study of Private Madhouses in England in the Eighteenth and Nineteenth Centuries* (London: Routledge & Kegan Paul, 1972), and Andrew Scull, *Museums of Madness; The Social Organization of Insanity in Nineteenth Century England* (New York: St Martin's Press, 1979). For a specific account of the evolving role of asylum management in the rise of psychiatry, see Porter, *Mind-Forg'd Manacles*, especially pp. 169–76, and J. Doe, *Reports of Cases Argued and Determined in the Supreme Judicial Court of New Hampshire*, 50 (1870), 409–44.

16 *OBSP*, 1789, Fourth Session, Case 494, p. 605.

17 Ibid., p. 60. While the *OBSP* prints the name of the witness each time he responds, questioners are named only at the beginning of their examination of a series of witnesses. For the testimony extracts which appear in this paper, questions are attributed to the last recorded examiner. Most often this was an attorney, but often it was the judge, referred to as 'Court' in the *OBSP*.

18 Hale, for example, equated lucid intervals with partial insanity: 'But such persons as have their lucid intervals, (which ordinarily happens between the full and change of the moon) in such intervals have usually at least a competent use of reason, and crimes committed by them in these intervals are of the same nature, and subject to such punishment, as if they had not such deficiency' (*History of Pleas*, p. 31).

19 In the trial of James Bellingham for the murder of Spencer Perceval, Mr Justice Mansfield went out of his way to emphasize the 'rational' actions of the prisoner on the day of the killing. *OBSP*, 1812, Fifth Session, Case 433, pp. 272–4.

20 *OBSP*, 1801, Fifth Session, Case 446, p. 319.

21 Ibid., p. 320.

22 Ibid. Cf. Joseph Mason Cox: 'it often proves a perplexing as well as painful duty to the physician to decide on the Innocence or Guilt of the person accused, especially where any doubts exist whether these acts were perpetrated during a maniacal paroxysm or in a lucid interval'. *Practical Observations on Insanity* (London: C&R Baldwin, 1806), p. 203.

23 *OBSP*, 1812, Sixth Session, Case 527, pp. 331–2.

24 Ibid., pp. 332–3.

25 Ibid., p. 333.

26 Thomas Erskine, who introduced the term 'delusion' into courtroom testimony during the Hadfield trial, later elaborated on the fit of the concept to criminal responsibility by stipulating that the exculpatory potential of delusion was restricted to an act which was the direct, positive result of the derangement. It is therefore significant that in questioning Dr Ainsley, the attorney did not attempt to link the prisoner's action to his particular delusion, but instead asked whether

'the old delusion, acting on his mind, will lead him to do any act', to which Ainsley replied, 'undoubtedly it will'. Ainsley's implication was that a 'logical' connection between the subject of the delusion and the act did not have to exist: the delusion was sufficient evidence of derangement. For the Hadfield trial, see Walker, *Crime and Insanity*, pp. 74–83; Jacques M. Quen, 'James Hadfield and medical jurisprudence of insanity', *New York State Journal of Medicine*, 69 (1969), 1221–6; and Richard Moran, 'The origin of insanity as a special verdict: the trial for treason of James Hadfield (1800)', *Law and Society Review*, 19 (1985), 487–519.

27 *OBSP*, 1812, Sixth Session, Case 527, p. 339.

28 *OBSP*, 1833, Seventh Session, Case 1304, p. 729.

29 Ibid., p. 733.

30 Ibid.

31 For discussion of the origin of monomania and the controversy surrounding its use in court, see Raymond de Saussure, 'The influence of the concept of monomania on French medico-legal psychiatry (from 1825 to 1840)', *Journal of the History of Medicine*, 1 (1946), 365–97, and Jan Goldstein, *Console and Classify: The French Psychiatric Profession in the Nineteenth Century* (Cambridge: Cambridge University Press, 1987), pp. 162–96.

32 *OBSP*, 1833, Seventh Session, Case 1304, p. 736.

33 *OBSP*, 1833, Fourth Session, Case 815, p. 402.

34 Although the *OBSP* have passed scrutiny as a credible source of trial narratives, they nevertheless suffer from considerable condensation, apparently at the whim of the editor. While the reader can trust the narrative which survives, there is no way of knowing what might have transpired in the trial, but was deleted in the actual publication. Because of this, one cannot say with assurance that the testimony of a particular medical witness went unchallenged, simply because the *OBSP* record no follow-up questions. Still, the content of medical testimony is reported in such elaborate detail, and the cross-examination that does appear in the *Papers* is given so much space, that it seems very unlikely that spirited legal-medical exchanges would have escaped the attention of the shorthand writers or the interest of the editor.

35 As the prosecution was unable to prove that the firearms Oxford discharged actually contained any bullets, his crime of firing pistols at the Queen's carriage should only have constituted a misdemeanor. Instead, the prisoner was found not guilty by reason of insanity to the charge of high treason, which put him securely into confinement under the Safe Custody Act, rushed through Parliament during the trial of James Hadfield in 1800. For a discussion of the Crown's conduct in this case, see Richard Moran, 'The punitive uses of the insanity defence: the trial for treason of Edward Oxford (1840)', *International Journal of Law and Psychiatry*, 9 (1986), 171–90.

36 *OBSP*, 1840, Ninth Session, Case 1877, p. 482.

37 Ibid., p. 490.

38 Ibid., p. 494.

39 Ibid., p. 495.

40 For discussion of the conceptualization of emotional, in contrast to intellectual, insanity, see J. G. Spurzheim, *Observations of the Deranged Manifestations of*

the Mind, or Insanity (London: Baldwin, Cradock, and Joy, 1817), and Henry Werlinder, *Psychopathy: A History of the Concepts. Analysis of the Origin and Development of a Family of Concepts in Psychopathology* (Philadelphia: Coronet Books for Uppsala University Press, 1978).

41 Prichard has left a rich corpus of works in which he explained his notion of moral insanity. See for example *A Review of the Doctrine of a Vital Principle* (London: Sherwood, Gilbert and Piper, 1829); *A Treatise on Insanity and Other Disorders Affecting the Mind* (London: Sherwood, Gilbert and Piper, 1835); *On the Different Forms of Insanity in Relation to Jurisprudence, Designed for the Use of Persons Concerned in Legal Questions Regarding Unsoundness of Mind* (London: Hippolyte Baillière, 1847).

42 Porter, *Mind-Forg'd Manacles*, p. 31.

43 *OBSP*, Ninth Session, 1840, Case 1877, pp. 504–5. Emphasis in original.

44 Ibid., p. 505.

45 Etienne-Jean Georget, *Examen médical des procès criminels des nommés Léger, Feldtmann, Lecouffe, Jean-Pierre et Papavoine, dans lesquels l'aliénation mentale a été alléguée comme moyen de defénse, suivi de quelques considérations médico-légales sur la liberté morale* (Paris: Migneret, 1825), pp. 68–70.

46 François Leuret, review of Elias Regnault, in *Annales d'hygiène publique et de médecine légale*, 1 (1829), 289.

47 Charles-Chrétien-Henri Marc, 'Considérations médico-légales sur la monomanie et particulièrement sur la monomanie incendiaire', *Annales d'hygiène publique et de médecine légale*, 10 (1833), 357–474.

48 Charles-Chrétien-Henri Marc, *De la folie, considérée dans ses rapports avec les questions médico-judiciares*, part 1 (Paris: J. B. Baillière, 1840), p. 88.

49 *OBSP*, 1840, Ninth Session, Case 1877, p. 506.

50 For a discussion of phrenology's claims regarding the relationship between the size of an organ and the dominance of its associated faculty, see Robert M. Young, *Mind, Brain and Adaptation in the Nineteenth Century: Cerebral Localisation and its Biological Context from Gall to Ferrier* (Oxford: Clarendon Press, 1970), pp. 54–79, and Roger Cooter, *The Cultural Meaning of Popular Science: Phrenology and the Organization of Consent in Nineteenth-century Britain* (Cambridge: Cambridge University Press, 1985).

51 *OBSP*, 1840, Ninth Session, Case 1877, p. 507.

52 Ibid., p. 508.

53 Ibid., p. 509–10.

54 J. A. Paris and J. S. M. Fonblanque, *Medical Jurisprudence* (London: W. Phillips, 1823), p. 316, and John Haslam, *Medical Jurisprudence as it Relates to Insanity According to the Law of England* (London: C. Hunter, 1817), pp. 7–10.

55 Forbes Winslow, *The Plea of Insanity* (London: Royal College of Physicians, 1840), p. vii.

56 Hand, 'Historical and practical considerations', p. 50.

57 Winslow, *The Plea of Insanity*, p. 75.

58 Ibid.

59 John Haslam, *Medical Jurisprudence*. For a list of questions often asked of medical witnesses in cases of insanity, and advice concerning possible answers, see George Edward Male, *Elements of Juridical or Forensic Medicine: For the Use of Medical Men, Coroners, and Barristers* (London: E. Cox & Son, 1818).

60 Forbes Winslow, *The Principles of Phrenology as Applied to the Elucidation and Cure of Insanity: an essay read at the Westminster Medical School, January 4th, 1832* (London: Sherwood & Piper, 1832), p. 26n.

8

Understanding the terrorist: anarchism, medicine and politics in *fin-de-siècle* France

RUTH HARRIS

Between 1892 and 1894, dozens of self-professed anarchists were tried in the French courts following a series of murderous assaults. Although there were just a handful of notorious cases, the outrageousness of crimes such as the bombing of restaurants and the assassination of the President meant the incidents were immediately seized upon to exemplify the perniciousness of all anarchist ideas.[1] The defendants combined violence, political idealism and extreme individualism, and the mixture stimulated a wide-ranging commentary among all strands of the national political community. The press, particularly the illustrated weeklies, feasted on a sumptuous diet of horror, graphically portraying the destruction caused and the expressions of terror on the victims' faces. Although some anarchists used the old-fashioned assassin's dagger, the most feared were those who resorted to explosives, new weapons which lent a lethal unpredictability to the terrorists' acts. A lurid picture was painted of a handful of fanatics gathering to read subversive tracts and share the simple chemical knowledge needed to fabricate bombs. The bombings themselves were seen as indicating a special kind of criminal mentality, a cold and calculated willingness to hurt unknown people against whom the offender had only an abstract political, rather than personal, grudge.[2]

While the technical paraphernalia of anarchism – chemicals, sieves, measuring-spoons, nails, fuses etc. – excited morbid interest when displayed in court, the people who used them to terrorize Paris and other cities fascinated both the lay public and officials. Every detail of their lives and characters was examined – their love letters perused, antecedents investigated, *mémoires* recorded. The anarchists themselves generally responded with alacrity to such attention, the more articulate using their notoriety as a means of advancing their cause still further. Their trials, often precipitately brought to court, were major news events, complete with massive security procedures, armed guards, and jurors visibly worried that a verdict of guilty would trigger attempts at revenge.

The intense interest in these men becomes more comprehensible if one examines their deeds. The incomparable Francis-Auguste Koenigstein, alias Ravachol, claimed not only to have set off two deadly explosions on the Boulevard St-Germain and later at the Lobau barracks, but also to have robbed graves and murdered an old defenceless hermit for money. In 1893, Léon-Jules Léauthier used a shoemaker's knife to murder the foreign minister of Serbia in a restaurant on the Avenue de l'Opéra. In the same year, Auguste Vaillant threw a makeshift bomb into the Chambre des Deputés, injuring forty-seven people, including himself, in an attempt to strike a death blow to the government's nerve-centre. Emile Henry, the 'St Just' of anarchism, bombed the crowded Café Terminus at the Gare St Lazare, and went on to assert that such actions 'awake the masses, jolt them with a violent blow of the whip, and show them the vulnerable side of the bourgeoisie, still all atremble at the moment that the revolutionary walks to the scaffold'.[3] Finally, the Italian anarchist Santo Caserio journeyed to Lyons where Sadi Carnot was making a public appearance and managed to stab the President of the Republic to death. It was during and after this final outrage that the so-called '*lois scélérates*' were introduced to curb freedom of political association and allow the police new powers to hunt down all manner of political dissidents.

It was clearly not enough merely to catch the perpetrators of such crimes, just as the anarchists themselves were not content simply to blow up a building and then keep quiet. The attacks were only the starting point of a lengthy political, moral and social debate between accused and accusers which used the courtroom as a forum. The defendants exploited their notoriety to further their cause and spread their doctrines through the press, while the representatives of authority and ranks of professional experts – jurists, doctors, alienists, politicians – joined battle to undermine the anarchists' ideas and to condemn them for their acts. The straightforward political debate was inflected by considerations of masculinity and family, philosophical ethics and the pervasive criminological discourse of the era. Ultimate blame for the bombings was variously ascribed to materialism (especially Darwinism and evolutionism), to Roman Catholicism, the republican political system, deficient heredity, insufficient or excessive education for the masses, and, finally, to the influential legacy of the Great Revolution and the Terror on contemporary politics, a diversity of ascriptions which itself suggests the variety of political interests and passions involved. As I will show, all these positions are important not only for understanding how contemporaries sought to 'know' the anarchist, but also how they tried to exploit his violence to further other political positions in the partisan struggle.

Anarchism and the 'man of honour': politics and passion in a corrupt world

Throughout the interrogations and trials, the defendants succeeded in putting the authorities on the defensive. In the judicial culture of *fin-de-siècle* France, the long process of pre-trial interrogation conducted by the investigating magistrate was inquisitorial in nature. During the months of examination and confrontation, defendants generally sought to represent themselves in the most flattering light possible, to bring the magistrate round to an interpretation which either attenuated or excused their crimes. It was a demanding exercise for both sides, but in general the magistrates, having authority behind them, were in command. However, the anarchists seemed to escape the psychological rigours of this process and often seemed more in control than those who were interrogating them. Nonchalant in their attitude to authority, they expected and even demanded the highest penalties, and were therefore only concerned to use their trials as a way of propagating their ideas. The men who tried and examined the anarchists were, in effect, challenged to justify a legal and moral system which the defendants rejected on first principles.

However, there was one area where even the anarchists were susceptible to the moral criticisms of their era. They claimed to be 'men of honour', a simple assertion which was as hotly disputed as any of their more self-consciously 'political' statements about class exploitation and the need to destroy the state. Throughout their trials, they used the positive stereotypes of the period to create an image of honourable working men betrayed by a corrupt society. This self-presentation was not so easily countered, despite the terror and anger caused by their acts, and the debate over their responsibility for their deeds was heavily conditioned by an analysis of masculine identity and honourable values on which the anarchists themselves insisted.

The image they developed of themselves was one which contrasted their implacable pursuit of the bourgeoisie with altruism towards the dispossessed of their own class. Often portrayed as ingrates, and as '*fainéants*' (layabouts) who did not wish to work like honest men, the defendants sometimes successfully countered this accusation by portraying themselves as sons, fathers, and husbands willing to take on the burdens of adult manhood, but thwarted by an emasculating bourgeois society. Finally, even the most rudely educated among them vaunted learning as the key to the development of their political consciousness. Fiercely proud of their various intellectual attainments and convinced of the power of learning, the anarchists were none the less most forcefully criticized for misusing their education, with the harshest mockery coming from those who belittled their intellectual pretensions.

All the men accused of great anarchist crimes, except for Emile Henry, came from the working classes. Henry himself was a very special case, a candidate for the Ecole Polytechnique, a young man of considerable talents who, in the view of his judges, had thrown away an 'honourable' bourgeois career for the adventurism and rebelliousness of the anarchist cause. He represented a particularly brilliant ne'er-do-well, the symbol of a youthful generation led astray.

If Henry represented the danger from within bourgeois society, then the other clearly symbolized the threat from the masses outside. They sought to show what they regarded as true loyalty to the dispossessed by avenging the penalties meted out to their comrades. Ravachol began the cycle by bombing a building on the Boulevard St-Germain, targeting the judge who had directed the trial of anarchist demonstrators the year before at Clichy, and followed up this assault with another on the Lobau barracks. Vaillant later sought to avenge Ravachol, and Léauthier both of them; finally, Emile Henry threw his bomb into the Café Terminus to avenge them all. Throughout the investigations and trials, each scrupulously avoided implicating any comrades, insisting, often against the evidence, that he had acted alone.

The assertion that each had been engaged in a solitary struggle was not only crucial in avoiding the accusation that they were a band of conspirators – an important element in the criminological account – but also as a means of magnifying the heroic individualism of their deeds. Far from subsuming his identity in the socialist parties which he despised, or in a front, faction or liberation army like later generations of revolutionaries, the anarchist found legitimacy in eschewing all such connections.

On top of their willingness to protect their comrades, the anarchists also stressed their physical courage. This stylized manliness reached a peak at the moment of execution when the condemned man embellished a rich tradition in criminal folklore by acting out the role of insouciant hero until the very end; only the Italian assassin Santo Caserio was seen to tremble before the scaffold. The inimitable Ravachol set the pace, and his performance was never surpassed. He joked with the executioner, enjoining him to do it gently, and even sympathized with him for his 'very dirty job'! He contemptuously dismissed the chaplain: 'I don't give a damn for your Christ ... I spit on all of that.'[4] This was an important gesture of obstinacy, as Ravachol had been raised a Catholic, but had rejected the Church in favour of anarchism.

Perhaps his most remarkable performance was to sing a blasphemous and witty song as he was led among the crowd to the scaffold:

> Pour être heureux, nom de Dieu
> Il faut tuer les propriétaires,

Pour être heureux, nom de Dieu
Il faut couper les curés en deux,
Pour être heureux, nom de Dieu
Il faut mettre l'bon Dieu dans la m[erde].[5]

Even at the last moment, he tried to deliver a speech but was prevented from doing so, only managing to cry 'Vive la Ré...' before, in the words of one observer, 'the blade fell, cutting the word with his throat'.[6]

Those who followed Ravachol to the scaffold sought to imitate his style. Léauthier was spared the death penalty and died in captivity, but Vaillant was executed in the Place de La Roquette, and in a voice which was purportedly clear and level cried out: 'Death to bourgeois society ... and long live anarchy.' Clemenceau attended the execution of Emile Henry and likened him to 'a vision of ... Christ, with his mad air, his frightening pale face seeded with sparse red ... hair. Despite everything, his expression is still implacable'.[7] Like the others, Henry also proclaimed: 'Long live anarchism.' For those who admired the anarchists' courage – and there were a considerable number who espoused the same cause, even if they did not themselves believe in 'propaganda by deed' – the executions were examples of masculine heroism, strength and fortitude. However, as we shall see, for some criminologists this 'courage' was a part of the pathology of anarchism; the emotional coldness and 'intentional suicide' or martyrdom were sorry signs of the political fanaticism which characterized the modern age.

Anarchists often described their political development in the context of deprived childhoods and exploited working lives. Vaillant, who threw the bomb into the Chamber of Deputies, was illegitimate, abandoned by his parents and forced to live off his wits, often barely having enough to eat. He spent two years in Argentina where he hoped to make a success of a land grant. Abandoned by his business partner, seeing his *compagne* and daughter on the brink of starvation, he returned to France to take revenge against a cruel society which made it impossible for an honest man to feed his family.[8]

Léauthier, at nineteen, was also poor, although it was clear from the judicial interrogation and the anti-anarchist press that his condition was not considered any worse than that of most other workers, especially since he had a small inheritance of 1,000 francs. However, while a hardworking and well-qualified shoemaker, he had the very low wage of five-and-a-half francs a day and was fired because he was once late with a delivery. By the time of his arrest, Léauthier had eaten only one substantial meal a day for several months, and had been going to bed perpetually hungry.[9]

Of all the anarchists, the one who gave the most details of his past was Ravachol. During his stay in the Conciergerie, there was enormous public interest in his character and motivations, so much so that his guards began in the spring of 1892 to record his account of his life, love, crimes and politics. The director of the Conciergerie was also fascinated by him, questioning him on his family, education, religion, and so on 'to distract him' from the isolation of his cell. The prison director sincerely wished to catechize the anarchist, insisting that Ravachol's atheism was misguided, hoping that, by flattering his intelligence, the prisoner might be persuaded of the 'immortality of the soul' and the existence of God. Like so many others, he wanted to show the anarchist the error of his ways and to bring about his spiritual redemption. It seemed that punishment was not enough; a public repudiation of anarchism was also earnestly sought by the authorities, even though they never obtained it.

If the document produced bears any resemblance to his actual statements, it seems likely that Ravachol enjoyed dictating his 'portrait of a revolutionary'.[10] Born in the Loire in the small commune of St Chambond, Ravachol was the son of a Dutch father and a French mother. He said his father beat his mother and that he was confided to a nurse and then to an institution when his father left. His early childhood was presented as a life of solitary misery: hired out as a shepherd at the age of seven, forced to winter in the mountains without proper shoes, to live among strangers, separated from his beloved mother, and to survive the several different masters who commanded him. He insisted that he was a 'good' child, going to church and believing its teachings.

But finding work on the peasant farms in the area too hard – and annoyed especially by one farmer who always hurried his labourers at mealtimes to limit the amount they ate – Ravachol tried to change to industrial and urban labour, beginning, like so many of similar origins, in a coal mine and continuing as an unskilled metallurgical worker, where the noise began to make him go deaf. He then became an apprentice in a silk-dyeing workshop but had no chance of learning the trade well, as the trade secrets were too closely guarded by the owners and master artisans. Only when the foreman ate could the apprentices sneak into the workroom and experiment on their own.

From the age of sixteen, when he was fired from the dye-shop, Ravachol's life was one long struggle to feed his family. He worked in Lyons and St Etienne, sometimes finding work, sometimes not. He played the accordion at Sunday dances, and began to steal chickens from peasants when his sister gave birth to a child. He describes a slow but seemingly inexorable descent into part-time criminality, first in contraband alcohol, then counterfeiting, burglary, tomb-robbing and finally murder.

This was also the period when, as he sought to explain his own penurious state, he first came into contact with anarchism, took part in the first strikes in Lyons, and began to question his religion. He listened to the great figures of the anarchist movement, and was shaken by an anti-clerical speech delivered by the famous revolutionary woman, Paule Minck. He read books on anarchism and became obsessed by the massacre of the Communards. He went to nightschool and even attempted to enrol in day classes when unemployed but was turned away because of his age. The transition from struggling worker to revolutionary anarchist seems, from the way he explains it, a logical, indeed inevitable, outcome of a life in which he was obliged to support a family but could not do so by honest means.

Ravachol and other anarchist defendants often dwelt on their sense of responsibility to mothers, children, and sometimes mistresses. Society might feel no concern for 'defenceless' women and children, but they, in contrast, took their duties very seriously. This constant reference to their keen masculine desire to protect their weaker dependants was used as a way of showing an honest, manly sensibility. Ravachol adored his mistress and acknowledged his love for her in a tearful confrontation in court;[11] Vaillant claimed that it was the callous attitude of his employer to his duties as a breadwinner and father that finally persuaded him to bomb the Chamber of Deputies.[12]

Emile Henry was in a slightly different category, maintaining a resolutely cold attitude, almost daring those who defended him to find some extenuating circumstances for what, by his own admission, was a horrible crime. Although only twenty-one, he could express himself with wit. Asked for his address, he replied drily that he had recently been living at the Conciergerie; described by the court president as an assassin covered with blood, he snapped back: 'My hands are not more covered with blood than your red robe, M. le Président.'[13] But even he could not hide certain feelings of warmth and affection, and he protested strongly when his mother was called to the stand: 'I declare that I condemn her presence. I do not want the spectacle of my mother suffering before the jury.'[14] Once again, by breaking down at this moment, he presented himself as a man with 'natural' sentiments of love for a female member of his family.

In almost all the trials, the anarchists disdained the flights of oratory which their lawyers wanted to deploy in their defence. Instead they read out their own statements, except for Ravachol, who reckoned that he was not a good talker. However, his memoir showed that he had painfully acquired a certain culture, largely from books like Eugène Sue's *Le Juif Errant* and the popular anarchist journals of his day. Vaillant's closely-written declaration railed against the judges and the bourgeois society that they represented. Above all, he was careful to refer to authors who, in his view, prophesied the end of the class society:

> [J]ust as in the last century no authority was able to prevent people like Diderot and Voltaire from sowing emancipatory ideas among the people, so now not all the governmental powers will prevent the Reclus, the Darwins, the Spencers, the Ibsens, the Mirbeaus from sowing ideas of justice and liberty which will annihilate the prejudices which hold the masses in ignorance.[15]

He ended his statement by declaring that his judges would live in infamy, a tactic which did not exactly endear him to the authorities, who were in turn irritated at being scolded and instructed by a mere '*employé de commerce*'.

Henry could not be so easily dismissed. In a simple and extremely eloquent statement, he explained his transition from personal disillusionment to active anarchism. He maintained that, like most of his generation, he was 'accustomed to respect and even to love the principles of fatherland, family, authority and property'. However, with time he realized that social and political institutions ostensibly based on 'justice and equality'[16] merely gave the capitalist licence to exploit his workforce, the politician to steal from the electorate, and the military to shoot strikers down in the streets. First attracted to socialism, he soon became disenchanted with a doctrine which had so little 'respect for individual initiative'[17] and instead turned to anarchism.

The miner's strike at Carmaux in 1892 strengthened his revolutionary zeal and led him to his first bomb attempt against the Carmaux Mining Company. Later, while in Paris during the furore over Vaillant's bomb attack, he witnessed the authorities' campaign of persecution against anyone even mildly associated with anarchism: 'the anarchist wasn't a person anymore, he was a wild beast stalked everywhere, with the bourgeois press – vile slave of authority – demanding [his] extermination'.[18] In revenge, he decided to bomb the Café Terminus, aiming to annihilate as many bourgeois as possible. As he explained in a remark that was to become famous: 'Why? It's simple enough. The bourgeoisie treats the anarchists *en bloc* ... so we strike [at them] *en bloc*.'[19]

Henry's account plainly indicates the way the anarchists sought to alter the terms in which moral and social responsibility were discussed by suggesting that essentially corrupt and unjust social relations, not they themselves, were ultimately to blame for anarchist violence. This claim, while not accepted, none the less touched a nerve. The early Third Republic had done nothing, it seemed, either to stem the tide of revolutionary ardour or to guarantee the social welfare of its poorest citizens. And, as will be seen, in structure the anarchists' analysis did not differ significantly from that being put forward by the most advanced experts in the new science of criminology.

The judicial representation of the anarchist

While the anarchist presented himself as a loyal and courageous man of honour defending family and comrades, prosecuting lawyers and bourgeois commentators took a very different view. For them, anarchist 'altruism' was a mask for greed, selfishness and anger at not having succeeded in a world which rejected the anarchists' deranged ambitions. The anarchists represented a special kind of monstrosity, a criminality which required the support of amoral intellectuals who took no responsibility for the impact of their ideas on a strangely violent and directionless youth. The influence was ubiquitous; it corrupted the minds of workers like Ravachol and the cream of French bourgeois youth like Henry. Throughout the trials, judges and journalists were determined that these young men should not succeed in presenting themselves as heroes.

One way of undermining this self-presentation was through a description of the anarchists' physiognomies. As much as any criminal anthropologist, the public and journalists were concerned to discover the defendant's 'true' nature from his physical appearance. Albert Bataille, a leading observer of crime who wrote a yearly round-up of the major criminal trials in France, attempted to cut through Ravachol's superficial charm by detailing his animality: 'The eye is hard, the jaw bestial, the hue leaden.'[20] Vaillant revealed a shifty, puny, slightly megalomaniacal appearance: 'The face is bony; the eye, small and blinking, is hard and pitiless. Nothing generous, nothing open in this ungrateful face that at moments is contracted by forced mockery.'[21] Léauthier was characterized as a sybarite despite his emaciated and impoverished appearance, 'a skinny boy ... with a goat's face ... thick rabelaisian lips'.[22] Henry had a peculiarly tight and sullen countenance: 'thin, pursed ... lips'.[23] Finally, Caserio was a pale, meagre fanatic, a man whose true personality was difficult to grasp: 'with jug ears, shaved head, a [face] like a mask of a faun-like Pierrot'.[24]

The easiest way to attack the anarchists was to portray them as nothing more than common criminals. Ravachol was, in fact, the only one of the major defendants who could be described thus, as none of the others had any significant criminal record. A series of unsolved murders was laid at his feet, and he was accused of murdering a couple and another man in two robberies. Ravachol denied these accusations, and indeed no proof was ever provided to link him with these crimes, although he willingly admitted murdering an old man for money.

> I did indeed enrich myself! I hadn't another penny (laughter). But I didn't want to kill the hermit; I wanted only to take away his money, which he didn't need, being old and a bachelor.[25]

He even expressed regret over the murder, although he recognized that nothing would undo his deed. And once again, he resolutely maintained that he had the right to do anything to guarantee his own subsistence.

The murder was in fact brutal, and it was difficult for anyone to see much idealism in the killing of a helpless old man. On the contrary, the fact that Ravachol then went off and spent some of the money on an enormous meal – six eggs, fish, and a steak downed with punch – suggested strongly that greed, not politics, was the prime motive for the assault. Equally, for all his identification with the underprivileged, everyone was struck by Ravachol's bourgeois demeanour and appearance:

> Ravachol walks in first, moustache in the air, self-satisfied, very bourgeois, with his immaculate collar and his proprietor's frock coat ... the fop of anarchism.[26]

A similar view was taken of Léauthier's near-fatal attack on the Serbian minister. What bothered the court was Léauthier's seeming desire to copy the 'sublime Ravachol', 'to consume according to his needs' in a good restaurant. His needs, it was noticed, were fairly considerable, as part of the stalking of his prey involved him in eating a meal of game accompanied by champagne and good burgundy, all of which he refused to pay for.

> You had yourself served a roasted quail, champagne, and, since dinner was no doubt good, you lingered over it for so long that when you had finished there was no longer a single bourgeois left [in the restaurant] ... in the end, when M. Marguery came to ask you to settle your bill, you replied that you didn't have any money.
> M. Marguery observed that in that case, one shouldn't drink champagne.
> 'The bourgeois drink it!' you replied.
> 'But they pay for it', riposted M. Marguery.
> 'With our money', you said.
> M. Marguery, who had had enough, took you by the arm and threw you out.[27]

According to the judge, this restaurant had not suited Léauthier's purpose, so he went to another on the Avenue de L'Opéra and there stabbed the minister.

Thus, in contrast to the anarchists' image of themselves as honourable and idealistic, the judicial critique portrayed them as greedy, violent criminals. While the anarchists claimed to be courageous, the jurists accused them of cowardice. To stab complete strangers, to throw bombs without warning or regard for the victims, even though they might be women and children, were seen as particularly despicable acts. Moreover, sometimes they took flight and sought to evade capture. There was considerable debate over this last point. Léauthier, for example, initially ran away only to give himself up eventually. It was not clear whether he surrendered because he had left his hat in the restaurant and hence could be traced or whether, like other anarchist terrorists, he sought capture to prove his deed was political rather than criminal.

Giving oneself up was important for the authorities in assessing motives for crimes, and hence the perpetrator's degree of culpability. Crimes of passion, for example, normally ended with a voluntary submission, and the apparent willingness to accept the consequences was interpreted as showing the lack of a 'criminal personality'. There was nothing to be gained from locking such people up, as they were unlikely to repeat the crime, and the result was normally either a light sentence or complete acquittal.[28]

Although the anarchist was in a very different category to the *criminel passionnel*, they shared similar styles as defendants. The anarchists' long disquisitions on personal and political philosophy and the reiteration of their honourable intentions were clearly reminiscent of the *crime passionnel*. Equally, both insisted on the right of individuals to take matters into their own hands, disregarding legal processes. While a betrayed husband might maintain that the stain on his honour as a man prompted him to stab or shoot his wife, Ravachol invoked bad working conditions, insults, physical abuse and exploitation as violations of his masculinity and citizenship and as justifications for his act. Occasionally, defence lawyers would explicitly compare the two types of offenders. The attorney Hornbostel argued, for example, that Henry was nothing more than a misguided *criminel passionnel* who was led astray by the strength of his romantic illusions,[29] while Vaillant's attorney Labori contended that the defendant's deed was a *crime d'exception*, a product of human misery, not a revolutionary act.[30] Such a line of defence sought to distinguish the anarchist from the common murderer or 'criminal personality' by stressing that he was moved by lofty idealism and poverty rather than by avarice, vengeance or ambition.

Such arguments did not greatly impress the courts. It was accepted in a 'true' crime of passion that a man could lose his mind when a wife or mistress betrayed him and when his honour was besmirched. Hotblooded emotion animated the *criminel passionnel*, while the anarchist chose his target coldly and abstractly. The former was pushed by impulses which could be easily comprehended, while the latter acted out of political motivations, which were deemed pathologically destructive. Léauthier, for example, only regretted not having pulled off a spectacular bombing rather than a mere stabbing, while Vaillant would have preferred to have 'hit all the deputies rather than wounding only one of them'.[31]

While seeking to redefine the anarchists' 'courage' as brutality, commentators also attempted to undermine the quality of their convictions as well, drawing parallels between the anarchists and the fanaticism of religious martyrs in the past, an important tactic to be discussed below. Even more dismissive was the verdict that they were nothing more than 'egotistical suicides' who had turned to anarchism to escape from personal difficulties. This charge was above all levelled against the penniless Léauthier and Emile Henry who, some suggested, had turned to murder after a hopeless affair with a married woman.[32]

Of all the defendants, Henry produced the most ambivalent reactions. He appeared threatening precisely because of his superior social and educational background, a young man who exemplified the disenchantment of a whole generation. How, it was asked, could such intelligence become so perverted? The discussion concentrated on the crisis of values *within* middle-class society, the lack of moral principles which led young men to analyse social situations without the requisite moral understanding. He was a 'victim of books', perverted by contemporary literature – Stendhal's *Le Rouge et le noir*, Zola's *Germinal*, and Barrès's *Culte du moi.*[33] The selection of titles was important: Stendhal's Lucien had delusions of grandeur; Zola's Etienne had a misguided revolutionary ardour which brought disaster; while Barrès's early work epitomized the decadent self-obsession of the younger generation. The result was a harmful moral relativism. In short, Emile Henry was dangerous because he could have been *any* gifted middle-class youth; intellectually adept, but overly impressionable, he had become morally unsound. He was the nightmare of every respectable family.[34]

Medicine, criminology and the revolutionary

One of the most interesting groups to react to these crimes were the so-called *criminalistes* whose speciality was virtually created in the period between 1870 and the First World War. The new discipline comprised professionals from many fields: medico-legists and forensic psychiatrists involved in aiding magisterial investigations within the inquisitorial system of continental justice; progressive jurists and magistrates who sought changes or re-adjustments in penal law, especially the criminal code; and, finally, penal administrators, moralists, and clergy active in criminal rehabilitation. Their interests were wide-ranging, their opinions diverse. As a field of endeavour, criminology may be said to have had orientations and directions, rather than unanimously endorsed aims.[35]

In France, the growth of the field was conditioned by its development in contradistinction to the views of the founder of the Italian school of criminal anthropology, Cesare Lombroso.[36] Lombroso's assertion that criminals were born and not made was swiftly recognized as a revolutionary challenge to the European criminal justice system. In effect, his school argued that punishing offenders either for purposes of deterrence or retribution was philosophically misguided and practically useless. A better response, in his view, was a dispassionate system of penal management which would identify those likely to become criminal by hereditary disposition and remove them from circulation.

Where Lombroso emphasized heredity and the 'born criminal', the French school stressed the interaction between individual and environment, or 'milieu', as a cause of crime. However, for all their greater subtlety, the various French *criminalistes* also emphasized the deterministic aspects of criminal behaviour, the abnormal functioning of 'criminal psychology' and criminal societies. Their shared reliance on deterministic explanations led both Italian and French schools to diminish the field in which moral agency could operate and to promote a view of criminality as a social disease which required expert strategies of intervention and prevention.

For all the *élan* associated with the new field of criminology, the anarchists posed a particular challenge to the experts. They claimed to be able to identify and even predict the onset of criminal behaviour, but found themselves peculiarly deprived of means when dealing with a group of offenders who, except in rare instances, had no criminal histories. Like everyone else, they were obliged to find the unifying features of the anarchists' psychological dispositions and sociological characteristics after the event. Their reflections focused primarily on two key areas. The first was the nature of individual anarchists, their psycho-biological characteristics and the social influences which had most deeply affected them. The second was the wider social and cultural dimension of the anarchist phenomenon as *both* an atavistic regression and a symptom of the evils of modern civilization.

By virtue of Article 64 of the Penal Code of 1810, which stated that insane individuals were not to be punished for their crimes, magistrates were obliged to call in medical experts or risk accusations that they were wrongfully condemning a morally innocent madman. Since the 1820s, alienists had given expert testimony in the courts in an attempt to spare heinous offenders from the guillotine by arguing that the murderers had acted upon an 'irresistible impulse'.[37] Using the new medical diagnosis of 'monomania', the physicians had maintained that individuals might intellectually comprehend the difference between right and wrong but be unable to control emotional and instinctive urges to commit crimes. Alienists' early, and often sensational, intervention in legal proceedings helped them carve out a role within the judicial setting, but at the same time contributed to the growth of a deep-seated antagonism between medical and judicial appraisals of human behaviour and responsibility. The alienists favoured deterministic explanations of disease to account for crime, while jurists invoked free will and moralistic interpretations of wrongdoing to condemn and punish offenders. At times, it seemed as if the two professions were to be locked in an interminable struggle.

However, the apparent irreconcilability of the two approaches hid other, less divergent tendencies in the professional relations between jurists and psychiatrists. The French criminal justice system was based on a paradox which partially undermined the jurists' position. On the one hand, the criminal code of 1810 envisaged a perfect and invariable fit between crimes and penalties. Indeed, so strong was the calculus which bound particular misdeeds to particular punishments that it was only in 1832 that any formal provision was made for extenuating circumstances. In sum, the criminal code made no provision for flexibility in sentencing, tailoring its punishments to fit the crime rather than the criminal.

On the other hand, the inquisitorial French system seemed to encourage another, virtually opposing trend. French justice relied upon the investigating magistrate who, during months of pre-trial examination, conducted elaborate inquiries, requesting expert opinions and interrogating at length not only the defendant, but also his or her accomplices, family members, and associates. The procedure obviously favoured the development of criminal biography and even criminal self-dramatization as integral parts of the judicial process. Records of the investigatory procedure show the frequency with which magistrates requested memoirs from defendants, who, in turn, eagerly provided self-justificatory accounts of their crimes. Often, in fact, after months of repeated interrogations and confrontation with witnesses, the defendant and magistrate seemed almost to have reached agreement on the underlying motivation for the crime.

Alienists' reports constituted one of the principal channels whereby the personality and biography of defendants came into play in this larger process. Although their accounts retained a deterministic language of disease, their own interpretation of the genesis and development of mental pathology was itself profoundly moralistic. It was not that judicial and psychiatric accounts were identical – far from it – but rather that a shared preoccupation with 'knowing' the individual on trial and condemning his anti-social propensities helped to shape an emerging criminological approach. In their obsessive preoccupation with 'moral' pathology and physical abnormalities, the reports of alienists were often as sensational as anything that the popular press had to offer, and journalists, in turn, eagerly plundered medical concepts and terminology to add an esoteric, sometimes even morbid, element to their portraits of great criminals.

By the end of the nineteenth century, alienists' attitude to the criminally insane had also shifted profoundly since the days of the monomania controversies. These early struggles with the judiciary had been inspired by an evangelical ardour, an optimistic assessment of the possibility of cure and rehabilitation for the insane. In succeeding decades, alienists increasingly hardened their position when faced by the masses of incurable patients, often considered 'degenerate', whom they guarded in large and underfunded public facilities. Moreover, they were reluctant to become the custodians of those who seemed wedded to criminal activity, whether they were merely the 'detritus' of urban living – vagrants and beggars – or 'professional' criminals who robbed, cheated and killed. By the 1880s, most of the idealism associated with the early enterprise of legal psychiatry had dissipated, despite the continued presence in the courts of alienists as expert witnesses. Legal psychiatry in the old-fashioned sense was increasingly giving way to criminology and the 'science of social defence'.

Nowhere were these changed attitudes more evident than in the anarchist trials. Alienists were wary of overt intervention during the actual trials. While eager to provide social-scientific explanations of anarchism and accounts of the perverted psychology of the defendants, they wanted to avoid any imputation that psychiatrists were condoning terrorist violence. Equally, the anarchists refused to defend themselves by turning to the psychiatrists, and rejected any attempt to 'de-moralize' or depoliticize their deeds. Indeed, escaping a medical diagnosis of diminished responsibility was an essential condition for entering the pantheon of anarchist heroes.

Some anarchists did become the object of psychiatric investigation, and were thereby dismissed as pathological aberrations. For example, a little-known anarchist, Gaston Richard, decided to murder a boss [*patron*], much being subsequently made of his political sympathies and the anarchist papers he read. He chose his victim apparently at random, but at his trial affirmed that he had been 'pushed by a force' stronger than himself. This assertion raised the possibility that an irresistible impulse, rather than political conviction, was the cause of his crime. Once Richard himself had made this remark, physicians were no longer faced with the possibility that their diagnosis might serve to extenuate or excuse the defendant's political ideas. On the contrary, by raising the possibility of an '*idée fixe*', Richard opened the way towards his own pathologization and that of his anarchist ideas. For Henri Vallon, an expert witness, Richard was nothing more than a 'degenerate', one of the vast number of unstable, potentially pernicious, but not necessarily irresponsible individuals whom physicians regularly identified in their medico-legal work.[38]

Henry, however, strenuously resisted the medicalization of his acts. A physician and family friend, Dr Goupil, began to sketch Henry's childhood medical history in such a way as to suggest that typhoid fever might have made him susceptible to disturbed ideas, or that his father's cerebral congestion might have been passed on to him. Henry seemed well aware that this tactic was a means of saving him from the guillotine, but none the less tried to head the doctor off:

> Doctor ..., I thank you. But I assume responsibility for my acts. My head does not need to be saved. I am not mad. I am perfectly conscious ... I claim absolute responsibility for what I did.[39]

On the whole, the criminological community seemed content to agree with Henry, although this did not stop more rarefied debates taking place outside the courtroom. Lombroso, for example, examined a large number of anarchists for mental and physical abnormalities. For him, Caserio's background as a Lombard peasant and the pellagra which demonstrated the malnutrition and misery of his upbringing were chiefly responsible for his criminal urges.[40]

More systematic approaches, such as that of the Lyonnais physician and criminologist, Emmanuel Régis, incorporated 'a clinical description' of Caserio into a broader analysis of regicide as a phenomenon caused by mental instability.[41] Régis's work unified and pathologized any number of historical actors through retrospective diagnoses. Rather than assassins operating in different eras having different political aims, he united a mass of individuals into a new 'clinical type', with monks like Jean Châtel, the murderer of Henri III in 1589, differing little from Charles Guiteau, the assassin of President Garfield in 1881. All had tendencies towards mysticism and political fanaticism. Suicide, epilepsy and eccentricity loomed large; they were marked by a 'defect of equilibrium', and a 'morbid instability'.[42]

While Régis sought to universalize the 'regicide' as an aberrant category in human history, other criminologists were less willing to take this potentially indulgent approach. For them, anarchists were neither martyrs nor apostles fighting for oppressed humanity, but rather savages, a social excrement of which society needed to be rid. For the jurist and mainstream republican Alexandre Bérard, the anarchists epitomized 'the struggle for life of the savage, the primitive, who has no concern for the rights of others. It is the principle set out for all criminals, the brutal and savage principle of absolute, triumphant force, of the negation of law and liberty.'[43]

Bérard considered the anarchists to be particularly dangerous because their attacks from the left also made the Republic vulnerable to assault from conservatives. He believed that the anarchists, rather than denouncing the regime, should have appreciated the advances it had made. Most importantly, anarchist violence seemed to compromise the political mission of the republican mainstream, whose defenders had always sought to venerate the early, 'moderate' stages of the Great Revolution and to discard the legacy of the Terror. But for conservatives like the jurist and *criminaliste* Louis Proal, the anarchists represented a latter-day reincarnation of the blackest, most irredeemable phase of the Terror in 1793:

> The Terrorists, like the anarchists today, gloried in their crimes; they boasted about having drowned priests and gunned down aristocrats. Saint-Just, Robespierre, Couthon, Collot-d'Herbois, Billaud-Varennes experienced no remorse. They believed the drownings, the shootings and the massacres were legitimate because of the ends they had in sight. They thought that the blood-lettings purified the social body. The anarchists who throw bombs to terrorize society also excuse their abominable crimes on the basis of the ends they are after. They do not blush at their attacks because they want to achieve universal happiness through dynamite, in the same way that the Jacobins wanted to achieve it through the scaffold.[44]

Bérard saw himself as sandwiched between two enemies and he endeavoured to fight them off with tried and tested republican weapons. As an anti-cleric, he saw the mystical fanaticism of anarchism as yet another perversion of Catholicism, a dangerous attack on rational values and civic morality. Anarchism was 'the old and antique tendency of the inquisitors of the middle ages which the anarchists, these primates, apply to the nineteenth century'.[45] While acknowledging that Henry was not the direct product of a religious education, Bérard pointed to testimony given by Henry's mother as evidence of a fanatical predisposition: she had claimed that her son had been inspired by a portrait of St Louis that he carried in his pocket.

Nor was Henry the only one 'afflicted' by religion. Caserio was, in Bérard's view, a mystic, a former altar boy who was always chosen by the priests to appear in religious processions. He also cited Sébastien Faure, one of the great anarchist theorists, who was the son of royalist parents and himself a defrocked Jesuit novice. Bérard's argument was important to the development of psychological theorizing on the nature of revolutionary action, and was shared by many others in the criminological debate. When the Catholic right accused the republicans of creating a secular, amoral society which bred criminal misfits concerned only with material gain, the republicans responded by pointing to the dangerously 'mystical' tendencies which stemmed from Catholicism and clerical systems of education.

Such a desire to make anarchism appear derivative of the creed of one's opponents, rather than accepting it as a political theory in its own right, shows the strength of the political passions and interests involved. No one among the criminological community seemed more affected by anarchist violence than the progressive physician and eminent medical jurist

Alexandre Lacassagne of Lyons, whose whole professional life had been dedicated to establishing an understanding of crime which linked it to biological and social conditions, rather than to notions of sin and retribution. But, although theoretically against the death penalty, he was willing to make an exception for Sadi Carnot's assassin, Caserio.[46] Like Bérard, he saw anarchist deeds in quasi-religious terms, 'like demonic agitation, possession, sorcery that occupied all of the middle ages'.[47] But he did not think Caserio was mad, nor would he class him as one of Régis's *régicides*. Rather, he insisted that the man was a common criminal and was reassured by the way he apparently trembled with fear on the scaffold. Lacassagne maintained that a clinical regicide would have met death with the radiance of a martyr and he concluded: 'when his head fell, there were "bravos" and applause. The great voice of the people is sometimes unjust, but it can also be the spontaneous cry of justice, of truth. Never perhaps has the death penalty won so much approval.'[48]

If some expert commentators sought to comprehend anarchism and its deeds by harking back to medieval mysticism, others believed that such deeds represented a revived form of primitive tribalism. For example, Gabriel Tarde, one of the leading social theorists of the day, believed that anarchist crimes represented 'a new criminality ... which, without any sure signs of atavism, seems to take us back to the heyday of primitive vendettas ... It is the vendetta raised to the highest power yet seen.' Anarchist atrocities were, in his view, animated by 'this very old dogma of collective sin, mutually transmissible from man to man', in which the target was an entire class rather than a responsible few. Tarde summed up this line of analysis when he remarked that anarchist crimes exemplified 'collective hatred, above all, the anonymous and impersonal hatred of the masses, the hatred of innumerable strangers, [all the] more vilified because they are unknown.'[49]

Associating the anarchists with the vendetta in turn evoked a host of secondary associations. Seen in this light, the anarchists were like rural brigands or bandits, men who devoted themselves to a bloody cause in order to save their own honour or that of their families. They showed contempt for authority, and sometimes even successfully competed with it.[50] They flourished above all in rural areas, especially Corsica, Sicily and Creole societies, and, like the anarchists, evoked contrasting reactions. Were these men true heroes protecting their honour, or were they merely cowardly lawbreakers? Were their grievances, and unwillingness to go through proper channels, symbols of excessive vanity or a justified response to an unjust society? However, whether they abhorred or admired them, all commentators agreed that the vendetta was a form of crime associated with 'backward' societies which had not attained a sophisticated division of labour or governmental structures based on the consent and respect of the population.[51]

But while it was thus possible to dismiss the vendetta as a sorry residue of a primitive past, the anarchists – despite such analogies – could not be so easily explained away. Tarde himself acknowledged this when considering the danger that such groups posed. In analyses which condemned their instinctual primitivism, he also noted the anarchists' 'modern' and unprecedented characteristics. Tarde believed that in a society with widespread literacy, a popular press and universal suffrage, every kind of mental 'contamination' was possible. The outrages of anarchism were just one example of the dangers of mass society and mass politics.

Tarde's ideas were part of a broader debate over crowd psychology and mass communication which preoccupied many criminologists.[52] They were concerned to uncover the unconscious wellsprings of group behaviour, often arguing that 'degenerate' and psychically undeveloped individuals were susceptible to the urgings of harmful suggestions, especially in the area of revolutionary politics. While Tarde's discussion was of a higher calibre than most, his ideas did little but give scholarly credence to the conventional arguments about the role of suggestion and mental contagion in the spread of anarchist ideas. Men like the physician and *criminaliste* Paul Aubry, looking at terrorist phenomena and the wealth of anarchist newspapers and pamphlets, concluded that revolutionary ideas were like dangerous microbes, infecting an already debilitated social organism. He and many others painted a baleful portrait of the anarchist menace, arguing that these young men were hypnotized by the atmosphere of conspiracy and peril, and by the promised joys of self-advertisement. Such views led him to argue that the only solution was widespread censorship, a policy designed to keep anarchist ideas under wraps. Liberal society had to defend itself, he argued, against the attacks of misguided, half-educated individuals.[53]

Criminologists like Aubry returned again and again to the conclusions of crowd theory to justify their repressive political inclinations in the wake of anarchist violence. Yet they were also vaguely aware that such arguments were not entirely sufficient to explain anarchism as a social phenomenon. Rarely, it seemed, were anarchists criminally motivated, and only a very few chose violence as an option. One investigator from Lyons, Augustin Hamon, who sympathized with the anarchist cause, went so far as to conduct a survey to define the anarchist personality and was struck by the strong strain of altruism which marked anarchist discourse.[54] Much more than other people, it seemed, the anarchist cared for his fellow human beings: the most persistent theme was his desire to help the poor and underprivileged. The problem was how such concern for others came to be linked with the diabolical practice of 'propaganda by deed'. This question struck at the heart of the debate but was not seriously addressed. If there were links between the violence of the terrorists and the humanitarianism of the rank-and-file, investigators seemed wary of exposing them. At least, there seemed to be no cogent political or psychological theories which enabled them to address the issue.

The anarchist offenders deftly employed the language of honourable masculinity to further their political views and gain support for their cause. They and their opponents sought to conquer the moral high-ground, to contrast heroism and cowardice, altruism and aggression, self-sacrifice and selfishness in a debate about the revolutionary tradition, the Republic and social and economic justice. The criminological debate added another dimension, the esoteric analyses of psychological and physical types merging into a broader sociological discussion of anarchist deeds. The stress on primitivism both alarmed and reassured: the threat of a dangerous political throwback was mixed with the belief that such anachronisms would pass away in time. Less complacent comment focused on the 'modern' aspects of anarchism, the way it used modern technology and the media to spread its 'disease' in an unprecedented and dangerous fashion.

Both anarchists and *criminalistes* were keenly concerned with issues of individual action and responsibility. The anarchists wanted to present themselves as figures apart, untrammelled by organization and bureaucracy, unlike the socialist reformers whom they so despised. For the bourgeois public, however, the anarchists were necessarily conspirators, the mere tip of an iceberg of subversion and decadence. When the issue of responsibility was raised, both sides adjusted their positions. Those who demanded harsh punishment saw the anarchists as fully conscious of, and hence fully responsible for, their crimes. The anarchists, like the criminologists, availed themselves of the socializing discourse of the era, blaming society and its crimes for their own attacks, while accepting their 'martyrdom' as a small price to pay in the struggle for liberation.

These many paradoxes and shifts in position were based on one underlying contradiction which ran throughout the trials. The Third Republic was hardly the first French regime to be threatened by political violence and assassination. Napoleon and Louis Napoleon were the objects of such assaults, as was Louis Philippe in his turn. But in each of these instances, the attack was directed against the current embodiment of imperial or monarchical power and prestige, the very person who symbolized the unjust political regime which the assassin sought to bring down. In contrast, the Third Republic was ostensibly based on the sovereignty of the people. In attacking its high-ranking officers, its parliament and its 'innocent' citizens, the anarchists asserted that the principle of popular sovereignty was a sham. Ungrateful, embittered and armed with powerful weapons, the anarchist terrorists were unimpressed by the Republic's achievements and were proud of any deed which eroded its legitimacy. It is perhaps because of this challenge – this underlying assault on everything which the Republic stood for – that the trials were as much an exercise in discrediting, redeeming or pathologizing the anarchist as they were the means of convicting and beheading them.

NOTES

1 For the classic account of these cases see Jean Maitron, *Histoire du mouvement anarchiste en France, 1880–1914* (Paris: Société universitaire d'éditions et de librairies, 1951), pp. 195–230.
2 For the world of the anarchists see André Nataf, *La Vie quotidienne des anarchistes en France, 1880–1910* (Paris: Hachette 1986), particularly pp. 121–35.
3 Maitron, *Histoire du mouvement anarchiste*, p. 221.
4 Henri Varennes, *De Ravachol à Caserio (Notes d'audience)* (Paris: Garnier Frères, 1895), p. 47.
5 Ibid.

> To be happy, in the name of God
> We must kill the property-owners
> To be happy, in the name of God
> We must cut the priests in two,
> To be happy, in the name of God
> We must put the good Lord in the s[hit].

6 Ibid., p. 48.
7 Maitron, *Histoire du mouvement anarchiste*, p. 226.
8 Varennes, *De Ravachol à Caserio*, pp. 109–11.
9 Ibid., pp. 167–9.
10 For his memoir see the dossier in the Préfecture de la Police, Paris, BA/1132.
11 Varennes, *De Ravachol à Caserio*, pp. 45–6.
12 Ibid., p. 117.
13 Ibid., p. 223.
14 Ibid., p. 233.
15 Ibid., p. 119.
16 Jean Maitron, *Ravachol et les anarchistes* (Paris: Collection Archives/Julliard, 1964), p. 103.
17 Ibid., p. 104.
18 Ibid., p. 108.
19 Ibid., pp. 109–10.
20 Albert Bataille, *Causes criminelles et mondaines de 1892* (Paris: Dentu, 1893), p. 6.
21 A. Bataille, *Causes criminelles et mondaines de 1894* (Paris: Dentu, 1895), p. 2.
22 Ibid., p. 26.

23 Ibid., p. 50.
24 Ibid., p. 111.
25 Varennes, *De Ravachol à Caserio*, p. 36.
26 Bataille, *Causes criminelles et mondaines de 1892*, pp. 5–6.
27 Varennes, *De Ravachol à Caserio*, p. 170.
28 For the way *criminels passionnels* were represented and perceived by contemporaries see my *Murders and Madness: Medicine, Law and Society in the Fin de Siècle* (Oxford: Oxford University Press, 1989), chs. 6 and 8.
29 Varennes, *De Ravachol à Caserio*, p. 242.
30 *Gazette des tribunaux*, 11 January 1894.
31 Varennes, *De Ravachol à Caserio*, p. 113.
32 Maitron, *Mouvement anarchiste en France*, pp. 221–2. It seems that Henry was passionately in love with a Madame Gauthey, the wife of one of his brother's friends. The publication of his love letters at the time of the proceedings helped to launch this hypothesis.
33 Reg Carr, *Anarchism in France: The Case of Octave Mirbeau* (Manchester: Manchester University Press, 1977), pp. 65–6.
34 For more on the problem of 'educated' youth and their attraction to 'decadent' social values and crime see Harris, *Murders and Madness*, pp. 312–20.
35 Martine Kaluszynski, 'La criminologie en mouvement. Naissance et développement d'une science sociale en France à la fin du 19ème siècle', Thèse de 3ème cycle, 2 vols., Université Paris–VII, 1988.
36 For the history of this school and the French response to it, see Robert Nye, 'Heredity or milieu: the foundations of European criminological theory', *Isis*, 67 (1976), 335–55 and his *Crime, Madness and Politics: The Medical Concept of National Decline* (Princeton: Princeton University Press, 1984). For an illuminating perspective on Lombroso, see Daniel Pick, 'The faces of anarchy: Lombroso and the politics of criminal science in post-unification Italy', *History Workshop Journal*, 21 (1986), 60–86. See also my remarks in *Murders and Madness*, pp. 80–98 and Gordon Wright, *The Guillotine and Liberty: Two Centuries of The Crime Problem in France* (New York: Oxford University Press, 1983).
37 For the most illuminating discussion of the development of psychiatric intervention in the French courts see the chapter on monomania in Jan Ellen Goldstein, *Console and Classify: The French Psychiatric Profession in the Nineteenth Century* (New York: Cambridge University Press, 1987). See also Robert Castel, *The Regulation of Madness: The Origins of Incarceration in France*, trans. W. D. Halls (Berkeley: University of California Press, 1988), pp. 142–9.
38 *Gazette des tribunaux*, 15 June 1894.
39 Varennes, *De Ravachol à Caserio*, p. 233.
40 Cesare Lombroso, *Les Anarchistes*, trans. M. Hamel and A. Marie from the second Italian edition (Paris: Flammarion, 1897), preface.
41 Emmanuel Régis, *Les Régicides dans l'histoire et dans le présent* (Lyons: Storck, 1890).
42 Indeed, Régis even went so far as to plead for Caserio's life, a move which caused some friction within the close-knit criminological community in Lyons where the trial took place. See his 'Le Régicide Caserio, Lettre à M. le Dr. A. Lacassagne', *Archives d'anthropologie criminelle*, 10 (1895), 59–71.

43 A. Bérard, 'Les Hommes et les théories de l'anarchie', *Archives d'anthropologie criminelle*, 6 (1891), 609–36, at p. 611.

44 Louis Proal, *La Criminalité politique* (Paris: Alcan, 1895), pp. 41–2.

45 A. Bérard, *Documents d'études sociales: sur l'anarchie* (Lyons: Storck, 1897), p. 20.

46 The circumstances of his conclusions were unique – the death of the President of the Republic took place in his native city and Lacassagne was responsible for examining both the President and the defendant. His emotion is clearly displayed in his writings on the subject. For the abolitionist tradition which sought to exempt political offenders from the death penalty see Nye, *Crime, Madness and Politics*, pp. 178–9.

47 A. Lacassagne, 'L'assassinat du Président Carnot', *Archives d'anthropologie criminelle*, 9 (1894), 513–43, at p. 517.

48 Ibid., p. 543.

49 G. Tarde, 'Les Crimes de haine', *Archives d'anthropologie criminelle*, 9 (1894), 241–54, at p. 241.

50 For the classic introduction to the problem see E. J. Hobsbawm, *Bandits* (London: Weidenfeld & Nicolson, 1969).

51 See Armand Corre, *Le Crime en pays créoles: esquisse d'ethnographie* (Lyons: Storck, 1889), in particular the footnote on p. 184. See also Louis-Albert Gaffre, *En Corse, au pays de la vendetta* (Montreal: Beauchemin & Fils, 1892).

52 For a general overview of Tarde's thought written in the era of the anarchist assaults see 'Foules et sectes au point de vue criminel', *La Revue des deux mondes*, 120 (1893), 349–87. For informative treatments of crowd psychology in the period see Susannah Barrows, *Distorting Mirrors: Visions of the Crowd in Late Nineteenth-Century France* (New Haven: Yale University Press, 1981) and Robert Nye, *The Origins of Crowd Psychology: Gustave LeBon and the Crisis of Mass Democracy in the Third Republic* (London and Beverly Hills; Sage Publications, 1975).

53 For Aubry's emotional statement on the violence of his era, see his *La Contagion du meurtre: étude d'anthropologie criminelle* (Paris: Alcan, 1896).

54 A. Hamon, *Psychologie de l'anarchiste-socialiste* (Paris: Stock, 1895), especially ch. 10.

9

Malingerers, the 'weakminded' criminal and the 'moral imbecile': how the English prison medical officer became an expert in mental deficiency, 1880–1930

STEPHEN WATSON

The Mental Deficiency Act of 1913 which followed the Report of the Royal Commission of Inquiry into the Care and Control of the Feeble-Minded (1904–8) contained a clause describing a type of mental deficiency called 'moral imbecility'. It stated that 'moral imbeciles' or 'persons who from an early age display some permanent mental defect coupled with strong vicious or criminal propensities on which punishment has had little or no deterrent effect' were now to be dealt with in special institutions to be created under the Act, rather than in prisons.[1] English prison medical officers (hereafter prison MOs) regarded themselves as experts in diagnosing such cases of moral defect,[2] and claimed that their expertise was based on their experience of observing prisoners in the normal course of their duties.[3] In this chapter, I shall argue that this knowledge of the mentally deficient criminal was a product of routine procedures for observing, classifying and segregating prisoners that had existed from approximately the mid-nineteenth century. To demonstrate this, I shall concentrate on three aspects of the prison MO's expertise: his duty to supervise punishment, his use of techniques of observation, and his use of criminal records in constructing case-histories of mentally deficient or 'weakminded' criminals.[4]

In structuring the essay in this way I am, of course, giving priority to a study of the relationship between techniques of control employed in the prison and the production of psychiatric and criminological knowledge. This approach is inspired by Michel Foucault's *Discipline and Punish*,[5] but it is also consistent with David Garland's more recent argument that 'the development of British criminology can best be understood by concentrating less upon the spread of ideas from abroad and more upon the ways in which penal and social institutions acted as a practical surface of emergence for this kind of knowledge'.[6] In describing the 'prehistory' of criminology (which was not established as an academic discipline in Britain until 1935), Garland is inevitably drawn to discuss the work of the prison

MO. The prison MO was a key element of the 'practical surface of emergence' that Garland describes. He functioned as part of a prison administration that needed psychiatric or criminological knowledge in order to function smoothly. Not only did the prison MO's duties result in a concern with cases of 'weakminded' or mentally defective criminals, but they also determined the particular form that a knowledge of the mentally defective habitual criminal would take. To substantiate this, it is not necessary to show that the term 'weakminded' was invented in the prison or that the prison was the only site that existed for the production of a knowledge of mental deficiency. On the contrary, I intend to show that the prison was only one of several institutions within which those labelled as weakminded, feebleminded or mentally deficient created similar problems of administration and control.

This study of the expertise of the prison MO is an attempt to replace 'social-control accounts of psychiatry' which see definitions of deviance as products of 'the socio-economic production relations of capitalist society'[7] by a study of the specific sites in which a knowledge of deviance is constituted. I will show how disciplinary techniques operated within the prison and how they led to the production of a knowledge of categories of deviance that was unique to the prison setting. It is important, however, to relate this analysis to developments in other institutional sites, such as schools, lunatic asylums, idiot asylums and poor-law institutions, during the late nineteenth and early twentieth centuries, because the type of knowledge generated within the prison took on a new significance when it came to be associated with wider national concerns about the problem of the 'feebleminded'.[8] The prison MO contributed to a growing public awareness of the problem of the mentally deficient, but also found (at least, until the 1920s) that the status of his expertise was enhanced by parallel developments in other institutional sites. The Eugenics Education Society (founded in 1907) was able to exploit existing concern with the problems of habitual recidivism, 'feebleminded' school children and pauper 'imbeciles', and link them with wider anxieties over differential fertility and 'national efficiency'.[9]

A knowledge of the habitual criminal that was peculiar to the prison may temporarily have gained in significance because of wider debates on the problem of the feebleminded in general, but by the 1920s it was clear that techniques that had developed in response to problems in schools were beginning to undermine the prison MO's claim to a unique expertise. The techniques of mental testing pioneered by the French psychologists Alfred Binet and Theodule Simon threatened to replace the techniques of observation and use of criminal records that were central to the English prison MO's expertise.[10] It was only in cases in which a moral, rather than an intellectual, defect was involved (such as cases of moral imbecility) that the prison MO's experience of supervising punishment and observing criminals could be held to facilitate accurate diagnosis. Thus the prison MOs' persistent concern with the category of moral imbecility during the 1920s reflected both their occupational concerns and their need to defend their expertise against the encroachment of rival techniques developed in other institutional settings.[11]

In order to appreciate the significance of the prison MO's expertise it is necessary to look both at the level of the prison, to see how the content of psychiatric knowledge was determined by institutional procedures, and at the broader development of psychiatry in Britain, to see how knowledge developed on a local level was integrated into a standard body of psychological literature. We shall begin by examining the ways in which the occupational duties of the prison MO determined the content of a knowledge of mental deficiency.

The supervision of punishment

In 1921 Sir Evelyn Ruggles-Brise, Chairman of the Prison Commissioners, gave this account of the prison MO's abilities:

> The prison medical officer has justly acquired a reputation as an expert in mental disease. Although a practical acquaintance with lunacy is expected of a candidate for the medical service, it is owing to the exceptional opportunities for the diagnosis of the varying and often peculiar mental states of prisoners that he is expected and is able to give an expert opinion, not only in the rare cases where sanity is in question, but also in those doubtful cases of mental defectiveness which are continually occurring in every mode and degree.[12]

This type of comment on the prison MO's abilities was not uncommon by the 1920s. It was echoed in the reports of the Prison Commissioners[13] and the representations of the British Medical Association to the Home Secretary concerning the pay of prison MOs from the 1890s,[14] while the prison MOs' interest in mental health generally and mental deficiency in particular is evident from the numerous articles which they published in journals such as the *Journal of Mental Science*.[15] What is especially interesting about Ruggles-Brise's account is the way he attributes the growth of the prison MO's expertise in mental health to his experience of dealing with 'the peculiar mental states of prisoners'. Ruggles-Brise does mention the prison MO's other duties, including visiting the sick, 'the sanitary condition of the buildings; ventilation; food; water; clothing and bedding',[16] but most of his chapter on the prison MO is about his expertise in 'mental disease'. The explanation Ruggles-Brise gives for the prison MO's interest in this area is simply that it arose as a natural consequence of his duties. Historians are usually right to be wary of taking such explanations for the growth of professional expertise at face value, but if we accept as a working hypothesis that the prison was one of the sites in which the discipline of psychiatry developed, then Ruggles-Brise's explanation may indeed bear further scrutiny.

Perhaps the most important duty of the prison MO was that established by the 1843 *Regulations for Local Gaols*, which stated that he should 'report to the Governor when discipline or treatment appeared to be injuriously affecting a prisoner's mind or body'.[17] In line with this duty, the prison MO was required to complete a form which read: 'I hereby certify that I have this day examined convict No.... and find him capable of undergoing the several descriptions of punishments as specified below [confinement in separate cells; flogging; reduced diet]. Also that he is fit for restraint of handcuffs, leg chains, or cross irons, body belt and canvas dress.'[18] By the turn of the century the Commissioners of Prisoners were willing to admit that the judgement as to whether a prisoner was *fit* for punishment implied a judgement as to whether he *deserved* punishment, and was thus 'of a mental capacity to be responsible for the misconduct he has committed'.[19] Thus an essentially administrative judgement – literally, whether a flogging would turn a prisoner into an invalid or not – became a judgement which involved an assessment of his or her mental state.

The prison MO's role in overseeing punishment is crucial to our understanding of the development of government policy towards mentally abnormal offenders. Within the nineteenth-century prison, a rigidly ordered regime of discipline operated. After the centralization of prison administration in the late 1870s, the prisoner's life was closely regulated and organized around a fixed routine.[20] Prison discipline was both a way of reforming the prisoner's behaviour and a means of detecting prisoners with mental disorders. It functioned like a grid against which any deviations in conduct could easily be monitored and assessed. As the prison MO was given the job of determining which inmates were unfit for discipline he had a key role within this kind of moral observatory and, starting in the 1840s, he was also responsible for organizing modified regimes for those 'weakminded' prisoners categorized as unfit for discipline on the grounds of mental disease.[21] Various Acts allowing the removal of criminal lunatics had existed since the first decade of the nineteenth century,[22] but from the 1840s onwards prison MOs became increasingly aware of a class of prisoners who, though not certifiably insane, were nevertheless 'unfit for discipline'.

It is clear from contemporary sources that the original meaning of 'weakminded' (as used in the prison) was literally 'unfit for discipline' on grounds of mental incapacity. From the autobiography of John Campbell, a prison MO at Woking and Dartmoor prisons in the 1850s, it appears that the term, as used in the 1860s, included cases of insanity.

> The term 'weakminded' does not give an exact idea of the class of which I am treating; for although some were merely eccentric and generally quiet and tractable, others evinced well marked indications of insanity – such as general insubordination, destructive and filthy habits, and sometimes serious attempts at suicide.[23]

It was not until the first decade of the twentieth century that 'weakmindedness' came to be associated specifically with mental deficiency, and as the following report from the Medical Inspector of the Prison Commission makes clear, 'unfitness for discipline' was still the criterion adopted in assessing the number of mentally deficient prisoners.

> As is well known, the term 'Weakminded', or as it now seems preferable to designate it, 'Feeblemindedness', has long been recognised in prison, and from time to time rules and regulations have been framed with the object of ensuring special care and treatment for these mentally deficient persons, who though not certifiably insane, were, in the opinion of the Medical Officer, unfit for ordinary penal discipline. This unfitness for ordinary penal discipline provides a test for arriving at a conclusion as to the number of these prisoners who are the worst, or the most obviously defective cases.[24]

What began as a pragmatic way of segregating those who were 'unfit for discipline' later provided a classification of a type of mentally abnormal prisoner that could be incorporated into a body of literature on mental deficiency, and was used by the Royal Commission on the Care and Control of the Feeble-Minded as evidence that special legislation was needed to deal with mentally deficient criminals. By the 1920s, prison MOs could claim with some justification that their experience in observing and classifying 'weakminded' criminals made them experts in mental deficiency.

Observation

A study of the works of prison MOs up to the 1920s reveals an almost obsessive preoccupation with the detection of malingerers. The autobiography of John Campbell has a whole chapter on the subject,[25] and by the late nineteenth century the detection of malingerers was such an important part of the prison MO's duties that it was invariably mentioned in pleas for better pay and conditions of service. In 1892, the Parliamentary Bills Committee of the BMA gave a dramatic account of this aspect of the prison MO's job: 'In discharging this part of his duties [apportioning labour and diet] he has to deal with a great amount of malingering, and has to match his professional acumen against the most cunning subterfuges of professional criminals seeking to evade the performance of their work.'[26]

The most common means of detecting malingerers was by means of the observation cell. This was simply an adaptation of the standard prison cell common in England from the 1840s, when fifty-four prisons were built on the 'Pentonville Plan'. These prisons were built on a radial plan with rows of prison cells projecting like spokes from a central hub. The design of each cell incorporated a 'small glass "spy-hole" for observation purposes'.[27] The observation cell was simply a modified cell, sometimes with an iron railing instead of a door, and sometimes padded or covered with rope and extra spy-holes. The warden in charge of the cell was instructed to observe his charges regularly and to enter in a book how they spent their time.[28] The use of observation cells as a matter of routine is first apparent at Millbank prison in the 1860s, and from the 1880s their use for diagnostic purposes became increasingly widespread as magistrates began sending cases to prison on remand 'for the state of their mind to be inquired into'.[29]

How was the observation cell used as a clinical tool? Unfortunately, prison MOs generally assumed that the merits of continuous observation were too self-evident to require any explanation. William Norwood East's *Introduction to Forensic Psychiatry in the Criminal Courts* (1927) is an exception in this respect, as it begins with a discussion of the virtues of observation in prison and its application to the detection of malingerers.

> In most cases an examination in prison presents advantages of its own, among which may be mentioned facilities for continuous observation, the notification of alteration in mood and variability of conduct, the presence of insomnia, refusal of food, dirty habits, or other symptoms suggestive of mental disease, and in certain cases anomalous manifestations which may suggest malingering.[30]

The use of the observation cell was in effect an extension of the normal disciplinary regime of the prison. Within the prison the prisoner was always observable, but if an inmate showed signs of mental disorder, the MO's response was to intensify surveillance and place the suspected malingerer in an observation cell. In Dartmoor prison during the 1920s the need to distinguish the malingerer from the truly insane or weakminded person was considered so urgent that the observation cell was further refined. The prison rules enabled the prison MO to 'apply any painful test to a prisoner to detect malingering or otherwise', and this principle was applied in a grotesque manner:

> Suppose a telephone box constructed of iron bars and enclosed in a huge glass coffin. Within the bars is just [enough] room for a man standing upright, who can be easily viewed from all directions through the bars and glass. A warder's explanation of this apparatus is as follows: A convict apparently becomes insane and is suspected of shamming. He is removed to hospital, stripped, and placed in the cage, which is guarded by a warder and inspected

> by the doctor. Above the convict's (supposed lunatic's) head is an ordinary shower bath apparatus, which is turned on, and left on if need be for 15 minutes (but not for more). Now the psychology of that test is as follows: if the man is only shamming madness, he will of course know why he has been removed to hospital. He will understand that he is supposed to be a lunatic, and having no other explanation for the shower bath without end, will suppose that it is the hospital treatment for his condition. Consequently, when the torture becomes unbearable, as is likely in less than five minutes (in view of the temperature of Dartmoor water, plus iron bars) he will confess to the doctor that he is shamming and so escape further treatment. But the man who is genuinely mad having no such internal key to the situation – no consciousness of pretence – will stand or collapse under the 15-minute shower bath without confession. The correctness of the psychology is only less admirable than the perfect adaptation of means to an end.[31]

Although this machine was apparently used only once,[32] it serves to highlight the unity of penal and diagnostic techniques in the prison setting. The machine combined the observation cell with a refinement of the diagnostic technique used to detect weakmindedness. It was the prisoner's reaction to penal discipline and his perceived inability to benefit from punishment that determined whether he was classed as 'weakminded'. The Dartmoor machine simply extended this principle further. What distinguished the malingerer from the 'genuinely mad' prisoner was an understanding of the system of rewards and punishments through which penal discipline operated. The malingerer understood this system and used it to his own advantage, and it was this understanding that betrayed him. The insane prisoner, however, had 'no such internal key to the situation'; he was literally 'unfit for discipline'.

The 'painful test' at Dartmoor is described as an autonomous machine that reduces the prison MO's role to that of inspecting the apparatus and then observing the prisoner's reaction to the icy 'shower bath without end'. Prison MOs often portrayed themselves as passive observers of the behaviour of prisoners, but they were careful to point out that observation was a skill that could only be acquired through experience. John Campbell commented that

> the utmost caution is required to discriminate between the really weak-minded and those cunning miscreants who feign mental peculiarities as a cloak for their misdeeds ... The cleverness and determination with which these impostures are carried out sometimes baffle the most experienced, but generally the close observation of them by those accustomed to such cases ultimately leads to detection.[33]

The portrayal of the prison MO as a passive observer of the effects of discipline upon weakminded cases and potential malingerers both underlines the importance of the prison MO's experience ('he will have better opportunities in prison than in any other institution for studying simulated insanity')[34] and assures the objectivity of his case histories. This dual function is very apparent in Norwood East's article 'A case of moral imbecility' published in the *Lancet* in 1921. The article begins, 'The subject of this sketch, a woman at one time under the prolonged observation of the writer, and then approaching middle age, presents in the ascertained incidents of her career features so distinctive of moral imbecility lasting over a period of many years . . . that some record may be of interest.'[35] Norwood East established right away that the subject was under his 'prolonged observation', and reinforces his account with a later section headed 'Characteristics noted when a prisoner under observation'. The case history is only a 'record' of events and behavioural characteristics observed by the prison MO. In Norwood East's description of moral imbecility, it is as if the prison MO is a passive observer of a process whereby the offender's interaction with the penal system (which produces a record of crimes and behaviours) automatically reveals the nature of her mental disease. The solution to problems of diagnosis and the detection of the malingerer is portrayed as architectural (the prison itself is a large observatory) and mechanical (the prison MO does not take an active part in the process of diagnosis, but merely observes the effects of prison discipline on the prisoner).

Although observation was often used to distinguish between malingerers and the mentally abnormal before 1880, Walker and McCabe have noted that after this date a period of remand in prison became increasingly popular with magistrates who were uncertain as to the state of mind of those brought before them on criminal charges.[36] By the 1920s, prison MOs at some English prisons could expect to provide many reports for cases placed on remand as well as to appear in court to give evidence. The 1922 report of the Stanhope Committee appointed to inquire into pay and conditions of service in the prison system found that medical officers at Brixton, Liverpool, Manchester, Birmingham and Leeds were receiving 'considerable' fees for giving evidence in court on the mental condition of prisoners. At Brixton, '700 to 800 reports on the mental condition of prisoners are rendered annually and 300 by the Medical Officer at Liverpool'.[37] In the 1920s, it was the prison MOs who worked at Brixton, Liverpool and Birmingham (William Norwood East, Maurice Ahern and M. Hamblin Smith respectively) who wrote books and published articles on insanity and mental deficiency and who found the moral imbecility category of particular interest. It is also significant that those prison MOs who were appointed to the position of Medical Inspector of Prisons all seem to have worked either in prisons with a large percentage of weakminded prisoners, or at prisons such as Brixton where a large number of psychiatric reports were required.[38]

The prison MO's role as an observer came to be acknowledged as a major part of his expertise, but not as a result of any concerted attempt to improve his status. The prison MO of the 1920s merely continued a practice that had begun in the mid-nineteenth century as a means of detecting malingerers. What had changed was not the practice itself but the way in which it was described. The parameters of an area that could be called 'psychological' had shifted to include not only the practice of doctors in lunatic asylums but the practice of those who dealt with a whole range of mental disorders such as 'feeblemindedness' and 'moral imbecility'. An explanation for this shift, which requires a broad overview of the development of psychological knowledge as a whole, will be sketched in the final part of this essay. But first, one other diagnostic tool employed by the prison MO requires examination: the case history.

The habitual criminal and the use of criminal records

The process of detecting, classifying and managing criminals requires detailed records. Such records were available in England after the 1869 Habitual Criminals Act required that a case history be kept of all second offenders.[39] By the 1890s, anthropometric measurements (based on measurement of bone size) were in widespread use for this purpose, while from 1901 onwards photographs replaced anthropometric measurements and fingerprinting became standard practice.[40]

It is significant that the work of Cesare Lombroso and other Italian criminal anthropologists appears to have had little impact on the practice of classifying mentally abnormal prisoners in England. It is well known that Charles Goring's study *The English Convict* (1913) effectively ended the credibility of Lombroso's theory of the existence of distinct criminal 'types', but it is also worth noting that earlier textbooks on psychiatry and mental deficiency by such authors as Charles Mercier and Alfred Tredgold had either ridiculed Lombroso's methods or denied the value of his theory of atavism. In England at least, observation of the prisoner's response to discipline and a case history based on a record of previous convictions carried more weight as diagnostic tools than a study of criminal physiognomy.[41]

From 1876 onwards there were excellent records of all those convicted of a second offence, including details of age, trade, appearance and previous convictions.[42] These were an important resource for prison MOs and were often used to support the contention that there was a close connection between habitual criminality and 'weakmindedness' or mental deficiency. For example, in their evidence to the Royal Commission on the Care and Control of the Feeble-Minded, several prison MOs provided case histories of convicts and cited a series of petty crimes and subsequent convictions as evidence that the 'weakminded' criminal and the habitual criminal were one and the same thing. Dr Treadwell, medical officer at Parkhurst prison in the Isle of Wight, where weakminded criminals had been concentrated since 1898, told the Commission that 'weakminded convicts have distinct criminal instincts – their instincts are criminal'. In several tables he listed the number of previous convictions of a hundred weakminded convicts, and provided some detailed case histories such as the following:

> J.S., age thirty-one on conviction in 1903 for stealing. No family history of insanity, epilepsy, alcohol or crime obtained. Lost his father and mother when young. Went to school for four or five years but attended very irregularly and states that at the age of twelve he started work in a foundry. Education very imperfect, reading and writing standard II, arithmetic standard I.
> Occupation: Labourer in a foundry but when work is slack he is always discharged with the first batch, then takes to travelling showman business or to thieving.
> Previous convictions:
> 1882 stealing (age about ten years).
> 1887 to 1902 eleven convictions for petty thefts, chiefly articles of clothing.
> Palate high and narrow; facial expression dull, heavy and unintelligent; memory poor, all mental faculties seem below the average for his class of life. Quiet, tractable and cheerful, and works under supervision. More than likely to continue criminal career unless supervised.[43]

A knowledge of the 'weakminded' criminal – the criminal who was 'unfit for discipline' – and an awareness of the problem of recidivism were the essential conditions for the belief expressed in textbooks such as Tredgold's *Mental Deficiency* (1908) that some habitual criminals formed a class characterized by a lack of moral sense. This class of habitual criminals was designated in the 1913 Mental Deficiency Act as comprising the 'moral imbeciles'. A record of petty crimes and convictions seemed to indicate an inability to recognize that the consequence of crime was punishment (in the official definition it was said that punishment had 'little or no deterrent effect' on moral imbeciles) and suggested a defective moral awareness. In the second (1914) edition of his *Mental Deficiency*, Tredgold divided moral imbeciles into three types: 'the morally perverse or habitual criminal type', 'the facile type' and 'the explosive type'. The adult 'habitual criminal type' was described as follows:

> In later years such persons are guilty of the more serious crimes of incendiarism, train-wrecking, criminal assaults upon little girls, and homicide ... Their whole lives consist of an almost unbroken series of offences, in many cases there being literally scores of convictions, whilst in some cases they

> amount to hundreds; they are the definitely mentally defective habitual criminals.[44]

Tredgold asserted that moral imbeciles not only suffered from a defect of the moral sense but that in the case of 'incorrigible, habitual criminals' their criminal careers indicated that they were also defective in 'judgement or volition', as they were 'quite incapable of foregoing a momentary satisfaction for a permanent advantage'.[45] The conduct of the moral imbecile as revealed by his criminal record was thus often taken as evidence of mental deficiency.

Prison MOs considered themselves to be experts in detecting such cases. Even after the introduction of mental tests to prisons in the 1920s,[46] observation of the prisoner's response to discipline and evidence of recidivism were regarded by some prison MOs as the only reliable means of detecting moral deficiency. The prison MO's claim to a unique understanding was a result of the close links between the moral imbecile definition and the concept of the habitual weakminded criminal, who was defined by his inability to respond to discipline. The effect of an extension of carceral power was the discovery of those who did not respond to the disciplinary techniques that operated within the prison. The solution was held to be the more subtle differentiation of types of mental defect, which could then be treated in institutions with regimes designed for particular behavioural abnormalities.[47]

Other settings, new techniques, different knowledges: the rise and fall of the moral imbecile category

In 1924 Maurice Hamblin Smith, prison MO for Birmingham, told the Prison Commissioners that:

> The whole question of the correct treatment of offenders is a purely psychological matter. No prison punishment ... can be inflicted without the concurrence of the medical officer. It is but a short and logical step to the position that no sentence of imprisonment should be awarded ... without due attention being paid to the finding of an adequate medical examination.[48]

A psychological knowledge of the offender was indeed a logical development of the prison MO's duties to supervise punishment, observe and classify prisoners, and provide reports for the courts. But prison MOs never made assertive claims for professional dominance within the prison because, at least until the 1920s, there was no conflict between the demands of clinical practice and the penal aims of deterrence, management and reform.

Between 1860 and 1920, the outcome of the prison MO's routine duties came to be regarded as part of a standard body of psychological knowledge. In order to explain how this occurred it is necessary to look beyond the confines of the prison to developments in schools, poor-law institutions, lunatic asylums and idiot asylums from the late nineteenth century. The prison was not the only institution to have its category of 'weakminded' cases. In schools, workhouses and asylums there was a growing awareness of a category of mental abnormality that caused problems of management but did not fit the simple classification of either lunatic or idiot, and presented problems of certification under existing lunacy law.[49] Existing studies of such institutions show that different institutional situations resulted in different ways of classifying weakminded inmates. Thus at Colney Hatch Asylum, Middlesex, in 1864 'idiots' and 'imbeciles' were classified according to the supposed cause of their defect, such as epilepsy or senility, whilst at Warwick Asylum in the 1870s and 1880s, definitions of idiocy were 'somewhat elastic'.[50] The records of the Royal Albert Idiot Asylum near Lancaster show that educational ability was the criterion of classification employed there in 1879.[51] This was hardly surprising, as the initial impetus for idiot asylums was educational, and educational aims were reflected in the use of the term 'weakminded' within such asylums to refer to a class intermediate between the idiot or imbecile class and the insane. 'Weakminded' in this context was synonymous with the 'feebleminded' class of pupils discovered in schools in the late nineteenth century.[52]

Another system of classification was employed within poor-law institutions. Under the 1847 General Consolidation Order, guardians were allowed to make special arrangements within workhouses for those labouring under diseases of the body or mind, but it was not until the late 1860s that separate wards were provided for what were described as 'imbeciles'. It appears that the classification employed in different workhouses varied considerably, ranging from a fine distinction between 'idiots', 'imbeciles' and the more educable 'weakminded' cases to a general lumping together of all cases as 'imbeciles'.[53]

The problem of the mentally deficient became a national issue, partly through the activities of the eugenics lobby but also because a number of institutions were finding that there was a class of inmates loosely described as 'weakminded' who posed special problems of management and needed care in separate institutions. The prison MO's knowledge of the 'weakminded' criminal became more important in this national context, but as we shall see, his expertise was also threatened.

The fact that various institutions had different ways of classifying their weakminded inmates was regarded as a problem by those who had the task of establishing a new administrative structure to cope with the problem of mental deficiency. The Royal Commission on the Care and Control of the Feeble-Minded, set up in 1904 to review existing methods of dealing with defectives, found that there were many divergences in diagnostic practices among the various institutions which they looked at, and that this resulted in a loose and equivocal use of the term 'mental defect'. The Commissioners also argued that in order to ensure a high standard of care, 'some system of classification of the mentally defective class from lunatics down to the feebleminded must be devised and generally accepted, so that each group of institutions shall fulfil a definite purpose and deal with a special section of the whole class'.[54] Such a system of classification could fulfil an administrative need, but precisely because it would need to be 'generally accepted' it was unlikely to satisfy those professionals whose claims to expertise in mental health rested on a close association with the particular institutions in which they worked. It was also the case that definitions of mental defectiveness produced within a particular institutional context did not necessarily make sense to professionals working in other kinds of institutions, and this was certainly true of the moral imbecile definition. Almost as soon as the Mental Deficiency Act began to take effect, the moral imbecile was revealed as something of a rarity, and the category became a bone of contention among prison MOs, school medical officers and medical superintendents of institutions such as Rampton.[55]

It appears that many doctors involved in the certification of mental deficiency under the 1913 Act either did not understand the definition of moral imbecility given in the Act, and thus tried to avoid using it, or they simply disagreed with it, and therefore refused to use it. As the report of the Royal Commission set up in 1954 to review the law relating to mental illness and mental deficiency noted, 'many doctors, probably the majority, never make a diagnosis of feebleminded[ness] or moral defectiveness, whether the patient's personality is predominantly aggressive or inadequate, unless the patient shows some limitation of intelligence or has a history of having been regarded as educationally subnormal or backward in childhood'.[56] The Commission's report of 1959 also noted that this interpretation of the moral imbecile clause (the term 'moral defective' had been substituted for 'moral imbecile' in 1927) was contrary to the intention of its predecessor of 1908, which had clearly been to make criminal or violent conduct itself a sign of defect: 'even slight limitation of intellect was not to be an essential criterion in determining whether a person could properly be described as a moral imbecile'.[57]

The moral imbecile definition quickly became an anomaly. The other definitions given in the 1913 Act of the terms 'idiot', 'imbecile' and 'feeble-minded' described categories that could be understood in terms of intellectual rather than moral defect. They could then be applied with the aid of modified versions of the Binet–Simon test which became widely available by the 1920s. Nikolas Rose has rightly emphasized the importance of the Binet–Simon test within schools. The definition of 'feebleminded' in the 1913 Act referred to those who 'may be capable of earning a living under favourable circumstances, but are incapable from mental defect existing from birth or from an early age (a) of competing on equal terms with their normal fellows; or (b) of managing themselves and their affairs with ordinary prudence'.[58] This legal definition was simply a gloss on the individual's social inadequacy. What the Binet–Simon test did was to turn this vague social definition into a test score by providing a measure of general intelligence that could readily be applied by professionals working in a variety of different institutional settings.[59] The moral imbecile definition, however, could not readily be absorbed into this trend towards easily quantifiable measures of mental defect. As several prominent prison MOs pointed out, moral defectiveness was betrayed by 'vicious' or 'criminal' behaviour and not by scores on intelligence tests.

The articles on the moral imbecile written in the 1920s by MOs at prisons such as Brixton and Liverpool can now be placed in context. They were simultaneously a defence of the moral imbecile category and of the prison MO's special expertise. Thus Dr Maurice Ahern argued in 1925 that 'the legal definition [of moral imbecility] seems to be singularly free from the original sin of obscurity'. According to Ahern, criminal conduct could 'reveal a deeper defect than can be plumbed by any measure at our disposal', and it was his opinion that 'in the estimation of this defect too much reliance and value is placed upon intelligence tests'.[60] Norwood East also denied that moral imbecility had to be linked to defects in intelligence and, as we have seen, placed great emphasis on the use of observation in the detection of moral imbecility.[61]

This link between the expertise of the prison MO and the moral imbecile category illustrates the importance of the prison in the production of a knowledge of weakminded habitual criminals. But the defensive tone of much of what prison MOs wrote about the definition and diagnosis of moral imbecility during the 1920s betrays a growing awareness that the techniques on which their claim to expertise in mental deficiency were based were beginning to lose credibility. The moral imbecile category was essentially the product of a unique set of relations between prison medicine, administration, and discipline. However, it was officially recognized in national legislation, and its apparent resonance with both lay and medical stereotypes of criminality and with a widely accepted set of social and political attitudes to the problem of the 'feebleminded' gave it a social and cultural authority which extended well beyond the walls of the prison. Once this political and social climate began to change, however, and prison MOs no longer enjoyed unrivalled opportunities of acquiring a knowledge of mental deficiency, the moral imbecile category, and with it, the prison MOs' claims to expertise, rapidly ceased to have any relevance.

The rise and fall of the moral imbecile category forms only a small part of the late nineteenth- and early twentieth-century history of mental deficiency. Although it played a crucial role in establishing prison MOs' claims to expertise in mental deficiency, its demise was by no means the only reason for their eventual loss of expert status. However, in a more general way the whole moral imbecile episode does illustrate graphically how local institutional settings and routines can give rise to very distinctive forms of expert knowledge and practice, and how this local, institutional knowledge can in turn interact with other, more general social-administrative, professional and political concerns to shape wider social definitions of deviance. It also reminds us how much the authority of experts depends not so much on the credibility of their methods as on a favourable social and political climate and a lack of serious competition for expert status. In doing so, the moral imbecile episode highlights the limitations of historical approaches which focus exclusively on either the 'micro' level of local power–knowledge relations or the 'macro' level of social control; and therein lies perhaps its greatest interest for both the history of psychiatry and that of legal medicine.

NOTES

1 *Public and General Acts 1913*, p. 136, *Mental Deficiency Act*, 3 and 4 Geo. V, c. 28, clause 1(d).

2 See G. Wilson, 'The moral imbecility of habitual criminals as exemplified by cranial measurement', *Transactions of the British Association for the Advancement of Science* (1869), title only, p. 129; W. N. East, 'A case of moral imbecility', *Lancet*, 2 (1921), 1052–6; I. D. Suttie, 'Moral imbecility', *Journal of Mental Science*, 70 (1924), 362–75; Suttie, 'Two cases illustrating the conception of moral imbecility', *Journal of Mental Science*, 70 (1924), 612–25; W. C. Sullivan, *Crime and Insanity* (London: Edwin Arnold, 1924); M. Ahern, 'Certification as a moral imbecile', *Journal of Mental Science*, 69 (1925), 264–7; M. H. Smith, 'The definition and diagnosis of moral imbecility III', *Journal of Medical Psychology*, 6 (1926), part 1, 47–54.

3 See J. Campbell, *Thirty Years' Experience as a Medical Officer in the English Convict Service* (London: T. Nelson, 1884), pp. 82–3; W. N. East, 'Some cases of mental disorder and defect seen in the criminal courts', *Journal of Mental Science*, 66 (1920), 422–37, p. 423; East, 'Case of moral imbecility', p. 1055; W. N. East, *An Introduction to Forensic Psychiatry in the Criminal Courts*, 2nd edn (London: J. Churchill, 1927), p. 7.

4 General accounts of the development of the prison MO's psychiatric expertise can be found in N. Walker and S. McCabe, *Crime and Insanity in England*, 2

vols. (Edinburgh: Edinburgh University Press, 1968, 1973), vol. I, pp. 84, 225–6, 231–2; vol. II, pp. 18–25, 38–43, 50–2 and J. Gunn, G. Robertson, S. Dell and C. Way, *Psychiatric Aspects of Imprisonment* (London: Academic Press, 1978), ch. 1. See also J. P. Eigen and G. Andoll, 'From mad doctor to forensic witness: the evolution of early English court psychiatry'. *International Journal of Law and Psychiatry*, 9 (1986), 159–69.

5 M. Foucault, *Discipline and Punish*, trans. A. Sheridan (London: Penguin, 1979).

6 D. Garland, 'British criminology before 1935', *British Journal of Criminology*, 28 (1988), 1–18, p. 1.

7 P. Miller, 'Critiques of psychiatry and critical sociologies of madness', in P. Miller and N. Rose, eds., *The Power of Psychiatry* (Cambridge: Polity Press, 1986), pp. 12–42, pp. 29 and 30.

8 N. Rose, *The Psychological Comple.:· Psychology, Politics and Society in England 1869–1939* (London: Routledg , .985), ch. 4.

9 For feebleminded children, see Rose, *Psychological Complex*, ch. 4 and G. Sutherland, *Ability, Merit and Measurement. Mental Testing and English Education 1880–1940* (Oxford: Oxford University Press, 1984), p. 25. For pauper imbeciles, see M. A. Crowther, *The Workhouse System 1834–1929. The History of an English Social Institution* (London: Batsford, 1981), p. 97 and K. Williams, *From Pauperism to Poverty* (London: Routledge, 1981), p. 116. For the concern over national efficiency, see G. R. Searle, *The Quest for National Efficiency* (Berkeley: University of California Press, 1971), p. 59.

10 S. Watson, 'The moral imbecile: a study of the relations between penal practice and psychiatric knowledge of the habitual offender', unpublished Ph.D thesis, University of Lancaster, 1988, pp. 196–7. See also Rose, *Psychological Complex*, p. 124 and W. C. Sullivan, 'Feeblemindedness and the measurement of the intelligence by the method of Simon and Binet', *Lancet*, 1 (1912), 777–80.

11 Watson, 'The moral imbecile', ch. 4. See East, *Introduction to Forensic Psychiatry*, p. 4; East, 'Some cases of mental disorder and defect', p. 423; and Ahern, 'Certification as a moral imbecile', p. 266.

12 E. Ruggles-Brise, *The English Prison System* (London: Macmillan, 1921), pp. 189–90.

13 *Report of the Commissioners of Prisons for 1904–1905* (London: HMSO, 1906), p. 9; *Report of the Commissioners of Prisons for 1925–26* (London: HMSO, 1927), p. 3.

14 Public Records Office (hereafter PRO), HO 45/11034, 'Prison M.O.s, Pay and Conditions of Service (1892–1920)', Memorandum on the duties, pay and prospects of the medical staff of the prison service from the BMA Parliamentary Bills Committee to the Home Secretary, 9 May 1892.

15 See the references to the *Journal of Mental Science* in note 2; also W. N. East, 'Physical and moral insensibility in the criminal', *Journal of Mental Science*, 47 (1901), 737–58 and East, 'Some cases of mental disorder and defect'. Other articles by prison MOs in medical journals inclue J. B. Thompson, 'The hereditary nature of crime', *Journal of Mental Science*, 15 (1870), 487–98; M. H. Smith, 'Notes on 100 mentally defective prisoners at Stafford', *Journal of Mental Science*, 59 (1913), 326–35; M. H. Smith, 'The medical examination of delinquents', *Journal of Mental Science*, 78 (1922), 254–62; Sullivan, 'Feeble-

mindedness and the measurement of the intelligence'; W. C. Sullivan, 'A lecture on crime and mental deficiency', *Lancet*, 2 (1921), 787–91; H. A. Grierson and C. H. L. Rixon, 'The intelligence of criminals', *Lancet*, 2 (1926), 277; and R. F. Jarrett, 'Some observations on social capacity; application of the Porteus Maze Tests to 100 Borstal lads', *Lancet*, 2 (1926), 59–60. For a more exhaustive list, see Watson, 'The moral imbecile'.

16 Ruggles-Brise, *English Prison System*, p. 185.

17 Quoted in Walker and McCabe, *Crime and Insanity in England*, vol. II, p. 50.

18 PRO, HO 144/170/A43422, 'Mathew Sampson, weakminded prisoner, (1897)', Standing Order 325.

19 PRO, HO 144/170/A43422, Home Office prison department to Commissioners of Prisons, 18 August 1897.

20 S. Hobhouse and F. Brockway, eds., *English Prisons Today, Being the Report of the Prison System Enquiry Committee* (London: special edition for subscribers, 1922), pp. 73–4; Gunn et al., *Psychiatric Aspects of Imprisonment*, p. 10.

21 Walker and McCabe, *Crime and Insanity in England*, vol. II, p. 50.

22 See R. Smith, *Trial by Medicine. Insanity and Responsibility in Victorian Trials* (Edinburgh: Edinburgh University Press, 1981), pp. 20–4, 229.

23 Campbell, *Thirty Years' Experience as a Medical Officer*, p. 78.

24 *Report of the Commissioners of Prisons for 1904–1905*, p. 38.

25 Campbell, *Thirty Years' Experience as a Medical Officer*, p. 65 *et seq*.

26 PRO, HO 45/11034, 'Prison M.O.s: Pay and Conditions of Service', BMA Parliamentary Bills Committee to Home Secretary, 9 May 1892.

27 United Nations Social Defence Research Institute, *Prison Architecture* (London: The Architectural Press, 1975), p. 22. The quotation is from Hobhouse and Brockway, eds., *English Prisons Today*, p. 96. See M. Ignatieff, *A Just Measure of Pain* (London: Macmillan, 1978), p. 198 for a description of Pentonville prison.

28 Hobhouse and Brockway, *English Prisons Today*, pp. 286–7.

29 Walker and McCabe, *Crime and Insanity in England*, vol. II, p. 51.

30 East, *Introduction to Forensic Psychiatry*, p. 7.

31 Hobhouse and Brockway, *English Prisons Today*, p. 290.

32 Ibid.

33 Campbell, *Thirty Years' Experience as a Medical Officer*, pp. 82–3.

34 East, 'Some cases of mental disorder and defect', pp. 424–5.

35 East, 'Case of moral imbecility', p. 1052.

36 Walker and McCabe, *Crime and Insanity in England*, vol. II, p. 51. See also J. Saunders, 'Magistrates and madmen: segregating the criminally insane in nineteenth-century Warwickshire', in V. Bailey, ed., *Policing and Punishment in Nineteenth-Century Britain* (London: Croom Helm, 1981), pp. 217–41, pp. 230–1.

37 *Report of the Committee Appointed to Inquire into the Pay and Conditions of Service at the Prisons and Borstal Institutions in England and Scotland and at Broadmoor Criminal Lunatic Asylum* (London: HMSO, 1923), p. 22.

38 Dr Oliver Treadwell, Medical Inspector of Prisons in 1913, had been the MO at Parkhurst prison, Isle of Wight, where mentally deficient cases were concentrated. See *Report of the Commissioners of Prisons for 1913–14* (London: HMSO, 1914), p. 25. Dr G. B. Griffiths, Medical Inspector in 1919, had formerly

been MO at both Brixton and Parkhurst prisons (*Report of the Commissioners of Prisons for 1919–20* (London: HMSO, 1920), p. 26). Norwood East, formerly MO at Brixton, in turn became Medical Inspector in 1923 (*Report of the Commissioners of Prisons for 1923–4* (London: HMSO, 1924), p. 32).

39 *Public and General Acts 1869*, p. 576, *Habitual Criminals Act*, 32 and 33 Vict., c. 99.

40 *Report of the Committee Appointed by the Secretary of State on the Best Means Available of Identifying Habitual Criminals* (London: HMSO, 1894), p. 7; PRO, P.Com. 7/250/7332/286, 'Circular 9th July 1901'.

41 See C. Goring, *The English Convict* (London: HMSO for the Home Office Prisons Commission, 1913), reprinted by N. J. Patterson Smith (Montclair, NJ: Patterson Smith, 1972), and D. Garland, *Punishment and Welfare: A History of Penal Strategies* (Aldershot: Gower, 1985), p. 173. For other contemporary reactions to Lombroso, see A. Tredgold, *Mental Deficiency (Amentia)*, 2nd edn (London: Baillière, Tindall and Cox, 1914), p. 7, C. Mercier, *Crime and Criminals: Being the Jurisprudence of Crime, Medical, Biological and Psychological* (London: University of London Press, 1918), pp. 208–10.

42 PRO, P.Com. 7/250/7332/286: 'On identification: measurements by the anthropometrical system ceased and superseded by photographs and fingerprints, 1900–1901'.

43 *Report of the Royal Commission on the Care and Control of the Feeble-Minded* (the Radnor Commission), *Minutes of Evidence*, vol. I (London: HMSO 1908), p. 249, reply to question 4301.

44 Tredgold, *Mental Deficiency*, p. 327. See also A. Tredgold, 'Moral imbecility', *The Practitioner*, 99 (1917), 43–56. For other descriptions of the relationship between moral imbecility and crime, see H. Ellis, *The Criminal*, 2nd edn (London: Walter Scott, 1901), p. 37; C. Mercier, 'Moral imbecility', *The Practitioner*, 99 (1977), 301–8; and Sullivan, *Crime and Insanity*, p. 195.

45 Tredgold, *Mental Deficiency*, p. 321.

46 See East, *Introduction to Forensic Psychiatry*, pp. 4–5, and M. H. Smith, *The Psychology of the Criminal*, 2nd edn (London: Methuen, 1933), pp. 34–5.

47 One such institution was Rampton, which was used from 1920 for 'violent and dangerous' defectives. See Watson, 'The moral imbecile', p. 251.

48 *Report of the Commissioners of Prisons for the year 1924–5* (London: HMSO, 1926), Appendix 2, p. 41.

49 See Rose, *Psychological Complex*, p. 99; M. A. Barrett, 'From education to segregation: an inquiry into the changing character of special provision for the retarded in England, c.1846–1918', unpublished Ph.D thesis, University of Lancaster, 1986, pp. 155–6, 160–1; and Watson, 'The moral imbecile', pp. 53, 57–8, 61–3.

50 R. Hunter and I. Macalpine, *Psychiatry for the Poor – 1851 Colney Hatch Asylum, Friern Hospital 1973 – a Medical and Social History* (Folkestone: Dawsons', 1974), p. 234; J. Saunders, 'Quarantining the weak-minded: psychiatric definitions of degeneracy and the late-Victorian asylum', in W. F. Bynum, R. Porter and M. Shepherd, eds., *The Anatomy of Madness: Essays in the History of Psychiatry*, vol. III (London: Routledge, 1988), pp. 273–97, p. 281.

51 Barrett, 'From education to segregation', pp. 172, 178.

52 See Williams, *From Pauperism to Poverty*, p. 116; Rose, *Psychological Complex*, ch. 4.
53 Saunders, 'Quarantining the weak-minded', pp. 282–3.
54 *Report of the Royal Commission on the Care and Control of the Feeble-Minded* (1908), part 6, section 543 and part 1, ch. 4, section 191.
55 See the papers by F. C. Shrubshall (Senior MO with the London County Council, and Lecturer in Mental Deficiency at the Maudsley Hospital, London), M. Hamblin Smith (prison MO at Birmingham), R. W. Thomas (Medical Superintendent of Rampton) and Cyril Burt, given to a symposium entitled 'The definition and diagnosis of moral imbecility' at a joint meeting of the Educational and Medical Sections of the British Psychological Society, in *Journal of Medical Psychology*, 6 (1926), 10–83. See also H. Herd (Assistant School Medical Inspector in Manchester), 'The diagnosis of moral imbecility', *Lancet*, 2 (1922), 741–2; Herd, *The Diagnosis of Mental Deficiency* (London: Hodder & Stoughton, 1930), pp. 9, 193–200.
56 *Report of the Royal Commission on the Law Relating to Mental Illness and Mental Deficiency* (the Percy Commission) (London: HMSO, 1959), p. 57, para. 177.
57 Ibid.
58 Ibid.
59 See Rose, *The Psychological Complex*, p. 129 and Sullivan, 'Feeblemindedness and the measurement of the intelligence', p. 777.
60 Ahern, 'Certification as a moral imbecile', pp. 189, 190.
61 East, 'Some cases of mental disorder and defect', p. 423; W. N. East, 'Delinquency and mental defect (1)', *Journal of Medical Psychology*, 3 (1923), 153–67, p. 165.

IV

The politics of post-mortems

10

The magistrate of the poor? Coroners and deaths in custody in nineteenth-century England

JOE SIM and TONY WARD

The coroner's inquest, long regarded as a quiet and curious backwater of the English legal system, has been the subject of considerable controversy in recent years; controversy which has often centred on the investigation of deaths in custody.[1] There is an interesting parallel between the current debates and those that raged during the mid-nineteenth century. Then, as now, the issue of the proper role (if any) of the coroner's inquest was closely linked to the question of political and legal accountability for deaths in custodial institutions. Present-day critics of the coroner are often accused of seeking to politicize what should be a neutral process of scientific and legal inquiry. As Lindsay Prior has argued, however, the de-politicization of death is itself a relatively recent phenomenon.[2] As we aim to show in this chapter, the leading coroners of the Victorian period were fully aware of the political dimension of their work, and exploited it to ensure the survival of their office.

It was in the 1830s that coroners, after several centuries as a rather unimportant appendage of the criminal law,[3] began to find a new role for themselves alongside the growing apparatus of governmental fact-finding and inspection. The creation of the Inspectorates of Anatomy (1832), Factories (1833) and Prisons (1835), together with the Births and Deaths Registration Act (1836), and the various inquiries initiated by the public health reformers, marked a new form of governmental involvement in what Foucault has termed the 'bio-politics of population', the investigation and regulation of the conditions affecting human life and death.[4] At the same time, the new Poor Law of 1834 replaced outdoor relief by the 'workhouse test', and the harsh logic of 'less eligibility' became a central principle in both workhouse and prison administration. The Prisons Inspectorate and the Poor Law Commission strove, with limited powers, to enforce both hygiene and discipline in institutions controlled by often recalcitrant local authorities.[5] Although coroners were local officials, their investigations complemented those of central government agencies. But the pressure to expose abuses came not only from above, but also from below. With its coroner elected (in most districts)[6] by the county freeholders, its jury of local people and its relatively informal proceedings (inquests were often convened in public houses), the coroner's inquest could take on a distinctly 'popular' flavour[7] and in some cases it provided, as we shall see, a forum in which the poor could challenge the powerful.

This complex dialectic has been largely neglected in the historical and sociological literature. We shall concentrate here on the role of coroners in investigating deaths in prisons and workhouses, and on the conflict between coroners and magistrates in which these deaths were a central issue. By approaching inquests in this way, we will also be able to shed some light on another important aspect of nineteenth-century legal medicine: the role of medical men in prisons.

Coroners and prisoners, 1800–34

A number of historians and social theorists have pointed to the disciplinary strategies which emerged at the end of the eighteenth century in relation to the prison system.[8] These strategies built on power, domination and subordination were designed to regulate and discipline the behaviour of those who fell outside, or rejected, the parameters of individualism and utilitarianism. Within the prisons (and later, the workhouses), the screw of penal discipline was tightened as the confined were subjected to institutional regimes designed to develop habits of sobriety and industry and to instil ideologies of acquiescence and respectability. These developments had a significant impact on the medical care that the confined received. Ill-health was not blamed on the structure of social institutions but was understood as 'the outward sign of [the poor's] inward want of discipline, morality and honour'.[9] Medical care inside and outside prisons and workhouses was therefore caught up in and reflected the wider concerns of discipline, individual deterrence and collective punishment.[10]

These changes were to prolong and intensify debates about sickness and death in prisons. From the end of the eighteenth century there was controversy about deaths behind the walls of the penitentiary. Although from the earliest days of the coroner's office inquests had been mandatory on all prison deaths, they rarely criticized institutional policies.[11] Thomas Forbes examined the inquests on the 376 prisoners, including 85 women, who died in Coldbath Fields prison between 1795 and 1829. Close scrutiny of these cases reveals:

> an apparent lack of official interest in determining why prisoners died. Indeed one wonders whether the vagueness of the record represents an effort to conceal actual causes of death – a state of affairs which would not be

surprising in a prison in utter disrepute. No cause was recorded for almost one third of the deaths. Almost one-fifth were piously ascribed to a 'visitation of God', a whitewashing phrase that also was frequently used by coroners' juries of the time for deaths in prison; it was as nonspecific as it was unassailable. 'Decay of nature' referred to a decline in physical vigour and must have been nearly synonymous with 'debility'. 'Dropsy' of course we would regard as a symptom rather than a disease. These six [*sic*] listed causes account for 85% of the deaths; what actual diseases were responsible we can only guess.[12]

The 158 inquests on deaths in the King's Bench debtors' prison from 1825 to April 1832 were even less informative. In all but eight cases the verdict was either 'visitation of God' or 'natural death'; only in six cases of cholera were the causes of the 'natural deaths' specified. On the other hand, two deaths, one by falling from a window, the other from heart and liver disease, were attributed to mental 'derangement' or 'irritation' caused by imprisonment. The coroner claimed that it often took eight or nine hours to arrive at these conclusions, for which he received a fee of one guinea per inquest, payable by the relations or friends of the deceased prisoner.[13] In view of the results, however, it is little wonder that Dr William Farr, the statistician responsible for compiling the Registrar-General's reports, complained in 1837 that 'the inquest in gaols is at present very much a matter of form ... The causes of death registered as the result of a solemn, juridical, investigation are the most unintelligible in the register.'[14]

Margaret de Lacy, in her study of prison reform in Lancashire, describes the inquest on a controversial death in Lancaster Castle in 1812 as 'a mere pro-forma proceeding ... The jury was simply left in the room with the body, which was covered with a sheet, and informed that anyone who wished could have it uncovered. Not unnaturally, no-one did ... They rapidly came to the conclusion that Rawlinson had committed suicide and disbanded. The coroner did not even keep minutes.' Following a practice which was to be abolished by the Gaols Act of 1823, half the jurors were inmates of the gaol; the others were workmen employed at the Castle, which according to the gaoler was customary at Lancaster.[15] Another inquest in the same year, on a prisoner who died in Dartmoor, led to allegations in Parliament that the jurors were 'under the influence of the governor of the prison' and that they were swayed by the coroner's 'improper' summing-up:

He told the jurors there was no alternative between bringing in a verdict of 'Murder' or 'Died by the visitation of God' which induced the jurors to bring in the latter verdict, though three of them afterwards said, they thought it would have been more proper to declare, that the prisoner died through the negligence of the gaoler or his servant.[16]

Twelve prisoners made statements to the MP who raised the issue. They were particularly critical of the prison surgeon, who before the inquest had 'given a very different account of the transaction from what he thought proper to give afterwards'.[17]

The packing of coroners' juries with the gaoler's tradesmen was denounced in 1830 by Colonel Blenner Lasser Fairman, writing in the *Lancet*; he also claimed that the lawyers acting at inquests were 'more or less' connected with the governors of prisons. He concluded:

> 'Died by the visitation of God' is the return nine times out of ten when the verdict ought to be 'of a broken heart through persecution of the most relentless and unjust kind' – 'of disease brought on by a removal from a bed of sickness to a place of incarceration' – 'of abstinence and starvation through the absolute want of the necessities of life' – or perhaps 'from excessive drinking brought on by anxiety and dejection of mind, through a long confinement'.[18]

The confinement of the orator and activist Henry Hunt at Ilchester prison led to a number of debates in the Commons and Lords throughout 1822. MPs in particular argued that there was no control in the prison; 'the gaoler was not checked by the surgeon, the surgeon by the coroner nor the coroner by the magistrates'.[19] Of 600 prisoners, 400 were said to be ill due to the conditions. At the inquest into the death of James Bryant, the jury heard that the gaol was flooded six times in as many weeks. Furthermore:

> there was no room in which the deceased could sit with a fire in it during his last illness, that was not at least six inches deep in water. The jury, upon hearing the evidence, declared that the deceased had died by the visitation of God; but added that the event had been accelerated by the damp state of the prison.[20]

These cases from the first three decades of the nineteenth century indicate some of the dimensions of the debate concerning coroners and, from the prisoners' perspective, the unwillingness and inability of the courts to examine critically the complex reasons behind the ill-health and deaths of the confined. Although it was not only in relation to prisons that coroners were accused of conducting inquests as 'a mere matter of course' – an MP's description in 1816 of inquests on paupers and people without relatives or friends[21] – the investigation of prison deaths was particularly open to this kind of criticism, both because they were the only deaths where the law unambiguously required an inquest even where there was no suspicion of homicide, and because of the politically sensitive nature of these deaths at a time when the new penitentiaries were under frequent attack. The passing of the 1834 Poor Law Amendment Act, with its requirement that workhouses be 'less eligible' than the living standards of the poorest labourers, intensified the discipline of institutional regimes still further and sharpened the debate about deaths in custody and the role of coroners' courts in dealing with them. The career of the radical surgeon Thomas Wakley (1795–1862), who became the most famous of Victorian coroners, illustrates how closely these issues were connected.

Wakley and the workhouse

As founder and editor of the *Lancet*, and later as an MP, Wakley campaigned against the harshness of the new Poor Law, as well as the class bias of the Anatomy Act which delivered up the bodies of workhouse inmates for dissection.[22] He used 'statistical science' to demonstrate the high mortality rates of the workhouses – those 'ante-chambers of the grave'[23] – and also the prisons.[24] the *Lancet* called for inquests to be held on all deaths in public hospitals, to expose 'the ignorance, negligence or misconduct of public functionaries',[25] but it also inveighed against 'the imbecility and ignorance of coroners', which it blamed on their predominantly legal background:

> A lawyer in the shape of a coroner! A man who could not apply a plaster to a sore finger but who will explain to you the anatomy and physiology of the brain and the surgical treatment of its various antecedents in 3 or 4 brief sentences. Here, also, let us hope for a speedy and effectual reform.[26]

Wakley decided in 1830 to hasten such reform by himself standing for election as coroner for the Eastern District of Middlesex. After an immensely expensive contest,[27] he was narrowly beaten by William Baker, a solicitor. This setback did nothing to soften the *Lancet*'s attitude to legal coroners. In 1831 it referred to a number of recent inquests in which coroners had been 'unchecked in their dark course of ignorance and iniquity' and where the public were 'deluded by the mockery of legal technicalities and almost robbed by the extortion of office fees'.[28]

Wakley was elected to Parliament in 1835. He seconded a motion to repeal the Poor Law Amendment Act[29] and sponsored a crucial reform of coroners' law, the Remuneration of Medical Witnesses Act of 1836. This empowered coroners to pay doctors to conduct post-mortems, and also gave coroners' juries power to insist that medical evidence be called. Then, in 1839, the coronership for the Western District of Middlesex fell vacant. This time Wakley was elected.

One of Wakley's first acts as coroner was to issue instructions that all deaths in custody – including workshops, asylums and police stations – were to be reported to him. When a pauper in the Hendon workhouse died after falling into a vat and was buried without an inquest, Wakley was informed by the local registrar and had the body exhumed. His jury found that the pauper had died by scalding, and that the workhouse authorities had contributed to his death by neglecting to place a rail around the vat. When the Master of the workhouse raised the technical objection that the jury had not identified the body, Wakley retorted: 'If this is not the pauper who was killed in your vat, pray, sir, how many paupers have you boiled?'[30]

This inquest earned Wakley the enmity of the local vicar, Rev. Theodore Williams, who was chairman of the guardians of the workhouse and also a magistrate. As well as being *ex-officio* poor-law guardians in rural districts,[31] magistrates were responsible for paying the coroners' fees, and claimed the power to withhold the fee if an inquest had not been 'duly held'.[32] As the magistrates interpreted the law, an inquest (other than one on a prisoner) was 'duly held' only if the coroner had reason to suspect a crime. Rev. Williams accordingly instigated an inquiry by the Middlesex justices into the fees of the county's coroners and the number of 'unnecessary' inquests they conducted. It turned out, however, that Wakley, by instructing parish officials to make careful inquiries when a death was reported, had reduced the number of inquests in his district. It was his colleague and former opponent, William Baker, who bore the brunt of the justices' criticism over the number of inquests in his district.[33]

The strained relations between the Middlesex justices and their coroners were further investigated in 1839 by a Parliamentary committee of which Wakley was himself a member. The central issue argued before the committee was that of the justices' power to veto the coroners' fees, an issue that was to remain unresolved for more than twenty years. In arguing that the office of coroner must be financially independent of the magistracy, Wakley focused (as did Baker in his evidence) on deaths in custody and the effects of the Poor Law:

> The justices of the peace are the controlling authorities in gaols and in lunatic asylums; they are sometimes concerned in cases where life is lost in conflicts between the people and the civil power; the magistrates are the persons to whom the poor apply in cases of urgent necessity, when the requisite aid is refused to them by the parochial officers; in the whole of these cases the coroners may be brought into conflicts with the magistrates in the discharge of the most solemn and important portions of their public duties. If coroners be subject to the control of persons who are thus engaged, seeing the tyranny that might be exercised over them in relation to their accounts, they might shrink from the performance of their duty at a time when their most powerful energies should be called into action in the public service.[34]

The office of coroner was, Wakley asserted, 'a very peculiar one', standing 'between all persons in authority and the people'; and 'it would be as well to abolish the office' as to allow the magistrates the power they claimed.[35] The

Select Committee's report made some detailed criticisms of the justices, but expressed no 'opinion on the general subject of the office of coroner'.

It was not long before Hendon workhouse was again a centre of conflict. In November 1840 one of the inmates, James Lisney, died from diabetes. His daughter alleged that his death had been hastened by his confinement in a damp room as a punishment for impertinence. Wakley proceeded to hold an inquest, which took place in the workhouse itself. In his opening remarks, he told the jury that 'the allegation of the daughter was of a very serious import; and it is quite clear that, if allegations of this kind get forth without inquiries being instituted, and investigations too, somewhat of a searching nature, the poor would very soon believe, whether rightly or wrongly, that the inquest afforded them no protection whatever'. Referring to the 'annoyances' to which he had been subjected after his previous inquest at the workhouse, he threatened to resign his office unless the justices' powers were changed.[36]

Although Wakley had ordered the jury to be summoned from the neighbouring village of Edgware, rather than from Hendon itself, it soon became evident that a number of jurors knew some of the protagonists, and had strong opinions about the workhouse. When Rev. Williams stated that it was useless to call Lisney's widow, as 'her senses are quite gone', one of the jurymen intervened to confirm that she was 'little better than an idiot'. Another juror suggested the reason: 'Two years ago she was a fine sprightly woman; her insanity lies at that man's door' – meaning Rev. Williams. And when the workhouse porter said that he 'never saw any inhumanity here yet':

A JUROR: There is plenty talked about.
CORONER: Hush! Nothing can be more irregular than these remarks.[37]

When paupers were called as witnesses, Wakley ordered the court to be cleared, since they might otherwise 'consider themselves to be under some kind of coercion'.[38] Rev. Williams energetically defended his conduct, arguing that firm action was necessary in view of the 'spirit of insubordination' in the workhouse at the time (one inmate had gone so far as to say 'that he had rights in that house and those rights they were determined to maintain'); and that the room where Lisney had been confined was 'more comfortable than 99 cottages out of every 100 in Hendon'. In his summing-up, Wakley was careful to present both sides of the ambiguous medical evidence, but could not resist pointing out that the workhouse guardians had shown 'as much impertinence' to him in the course of the inquest as the deceased had shown towards them. 'How', he asked, 'would any of the gentlemen who interfered like to be sentenced to 24 hours of bread and water, and 24 hours' confinement, for what they said?' After deliberating for an hour and a half, the jury determined that this 'inhumane' treatment of a man 'in an infirm state of health' had brought about his death.[39]

Lisney's inquest was doubtless far from typical of workhouse inquests in general. Within weeks of the verdict, *The Times* (which campaigned relentlessly against the new Poor Law and carried frequent reports of workhouse inquests)[40] published a long letter from Jonathan Toogood highlighting a number of issues concerning 'that hard-hearted law, commonly called "The Poor Law Amendment Act"'. One of these issues was the conduct of inquests on the poor:

> Men are often elected to the office of coroner who are so totally unfit for its duties, as to be quite unequal to conduct an inquiry themselves, or direct a jury. Of this I have seen many lamentable instances. In this part of the country the evidence of a medical man is generally dispensed with, and a post-mortem examination is a matter of very rare occurrence; so that unless the cause of death be obvious and visible, it is scarcely ever ascertained, and the coroner directs the jury to find a verdict of 'death by the visitation of God', which they return accordingly.[41]

Toogood went on, however, to acknowledge 'the obligations which the public are under to those [coroners] who discreetly and fearlessly perform their duties, particularly in the innumerable cases of death under the New Poor-law, where every effort is made to shield abuses and obstruct the course of justice'.[42]

The difference in attitudes between Wakley and some of his colleagues was illustrated by the deaths of 180 pauper children in the Tooting child farm (run by a private contractor, Mr Drouet) during the cholera epidemic of 1848–9.[43] As Charles Dickens noted in the *Examiner*, 'The learned coroner for the county of Surrey deemed it quite unnecessary to hold any inquests on these dead children', and but for the fact that 'certain of these miserable little creatures happened to die within Mr Wakley's jurisdiction', the conditions at the Farm might never have come to light.

> Mr Wakley, however, being of little faith, holds inquests, and even manifests a disposition to institute a very searching inquiry . . . Remembering that there is a public institution called the 'Board of Health', Mr Wakley summons before him Dr Grainger, an inspector acting under that board, who has examined Mr Drouet's Elysium, and has drawn up a report concerning it.[44]

Grainger's report was damning, and Wakley's jury brought in a verdict of manslaughter; but Drouet, much to Dickens's disgust, was acquitted at his trial by direction of the judge.[45]

The Board of Health was indebted to coroners such as Wakley and Baker who, unlike their colleagues in Surrey, saw upholding the Board's 'stringent orders and regulations'[46] as an important part of their duties. As R. A.

Lewis points out, 'The Board had little control over the [Poor Law] Guardians, and it was only through the uncertain result of a coroner's inquest' that it could bring pressure to bear.[47] The Board of Health considered that inquests should be held 'almost without exception' on paupers who died from epidemic disease,[48] and instructed its officials to notify coroners of all 'deaths suspected to be from violence, accident, neglect or carelessness'.[49] This was one manifestation of the alliance between 'populist' coroners and the sanitarian movement, which Olive Anderson has rightly noted as being an important factor in the coroners' struggle with the magistrates.[50]

Coroners and magistrates

A lively account of the struggle between the coroners and the magistrates has been provided by J. D. J. Havard in his book *The Detection of Secret Homicide*. Havard's view of the conflict is a simple one: the magistrates, motivated partly by a 'misguided zeal for economy' and partly by resentment of the coroners' powers, 'entered upon a vicious campaign of obstructing the medico-legal investigation of sudden deaths',[51] by withholding fees for inquests they considered unnecessary and by instructing the county police forces which they controlled that certain categories of deaths were not to be reported to coroners. This account does less than justice to the magistrates' side of the case, as Anderson points out.[52] It also misses the most interesting question about the conflict, which is not how the magistrates were able to delay the advance of legal medicine for so long, but rather why the advance of legal medicine did not cause the coroners to be swept aside.

When the English system of coroners' inquests was compared to the medico-legal systems of countries like France and Austria, as it was by the Scottish surgeon James Craig in 1855, it was easy to portray it as an anachronism: 'a good, a useful, a necessary law, but probably the clumsiest and most complicated ... that the world has ever seen ... It is lauded by a few and condemned by many. It is a relic of a bygone age.'[53] A similar case was argued in the most detailed and influential statement of the magistrates' case, the report prepared by a committee of Middlesex justices in 1851, and circulated to their colleagues throughout the country.

The Committee acknowledged that its deliberations were inspired by a concern about the cost of inquests, 'which is certainly not unnatural, seeing that in the course of no more than 20 years, the item of expenditure in question has been multiplied nearly sixfold ... from £1,284 in 1828 to £7,557 in 1848'.[54] Over the same period, the number of inquests held in Wakley's and Baker's jurisdictions had increased by 127 per cent and 146 per cent respectively, which the Committee calculated as being about four times the increase in population, while the number of committals for trial for murder or manslaughter had decreased.[55] Little more than one per cent of inquests resulted in murder or manslaughter verdicts, and in the great majority of these cases, argued the Committee, the inquest expensively and inconveniently duplicated the investigations conducted by the police and in the magistrates' court. The Committee concluded that the growth in the number of inquests could not be justified by the coroners' role in the detection of crime.

The Committee's strongest criticisms were reserved for the coroners' juries, with their 'misplaced interference and irrelevant questions'.[56] Coroners' juries were easy targets; since there was, uniquely, no property qualification for this form of jury service, the jurors were often poor, and sometimes illiterate (although in Middlesex, unlike some other counties, only a tiny proportion were unable to sign their verdicts).[57] Their selection, the Committee complained, was 'commonly left in the hands of such incompetent functionaries as the parish constables',[58] (although Wakley employed a servant of his own for this purpose).[59] On the other hand, 'to compel the more competent and better educated classes to serve as jurymen on these occasions would be attended with great public inconvenience'.[60] The Committee had 'no hesitation' in recommending that coroners' juries should be abolished. Not only that, but it proposed the abolition of the office of coroner itself. Once the present coroners retired, their powers should be transferred to the magistracy. In the meantime, they should normally act only on information received from the police.[61]

The Committee did not question the need for medico-legal investigation of unexplained sudden death. Its argument was that such investigations should be carried out by the police, by the registrars of deaths, and by two proposed new agencies, a Public Prosecutor and one or more medically qualified professional post-mortem examiners. When inquests were held, medical witnesses would contribute the necessary expert knowledge, which the magistrates could evaluate by applying their 'judicial habits of mind'.[62]

While the Committee dealt in considerable depth with the procedures for investigating sudden death, it completely ignored the coroners' argument that the investigators needed to be independent of the magistrates and the police. This was one of the main points made by *The Times* in criticizing the Middlesex justices' vetting of the coroners' fees:

> But again it is to be said that the coroner is eminently the magistrate of the poor. In all the inquiries he is called upon to conduct, in either the workhouse or in the prison, he absolutely appears as the judge of the men who have now voted that they will subsequently constitute themselves judges, in turn, of the propriety of his entering upon the inquiry at all. Such an absurdity is too patent to pass current for a moment.[63]

The Committee also ignored the obvious point, advanced repeatedly by William Baker,[64] that making the police the coroners' sole source of information would allow them to conceal deaths for which they were themselves responsible.[65]

These arguments were forcefully restated in a report by the officer of health for the City of London, Henry Letheby, who was also Professor of Chemistry and Legal Medicine at the College of the London Hospital. Stipendiary or police magistrates were appointed by the Home Secretary, and 'it has been truly said, that the Police Magistrate has no will of his own, when his opinions differ from those of the government'.[66] What likelihood was there, then, that a police magistrate would vigorously inquire into the fatal consequences of military flogging, as Wakley had in a famous case in 1846?[67] 'Or suppose that a death took place at a police station, or in a prison, from the violence or neglect of those who had authority there, who is to investigate the facts of such a case? Or who is likely to have the hardihood to make the truth of it public?' Like the justices, Letheby advocated the appointment of professional officers to conduct preliminary inquiries and to perform or superintend post-mortems. But unlike the Scottish procurators-fiscal or their continental equivalents, these officers should have 'no power of pronouncing judgement; for the whole duty of publicly investigating the facts would rest, as now, with the Coroner and his jury'.[68] Letheby claimed the support of the City coroner (who was also a Middlesex JP)[69] and of the leading sanitary reformer Edwin Chadwick for this suggestion.

The Middlesex justices' report was coupled with a resolution 'that no inquest ought to be held upon a dead body, except where the Coroner has received information affording reasonable ground for suspecting that the death has been occasioned, – or at least for doubting whether it may not have been occasioned – by some criminal act or omission'.[70] Similar resolutions were adopted in a number of other counties after the Middlesex report was circulated.[71] What they meant in practice was that the coroners would receive no fees unless the justices were satisfied that the resolution was complied with. As Baker pointed out, the resolution was inconsistent with the body of the report, which acknowledged that inquests were often necessary to expose negligence falling short of a criminal offence.[72] An equally telling objection was made by Wakley, who argued that the resolution would defeat the inquest's object of allaying unjustified suspicion, since the very fact that an inquest was held would brand a death as suspicious.[73] The coroners campaigned fiercely against this restriction, with a degree of success which one of their leading opponents, the Chairman of the Gloucestershire Bench, ruefully acknowledged:

> The coroners being elected by the freeholders, are generally popular. They are fluent in speeches adapted to their juries, whose signatures they obtain to memorials in favour of particular inquests, and to declarations against the exercise of the quarter sessional veto. They avail themselves also of opportunities of descanting, through the medium of the county press, upon evils which they assume to have proceeded, or expect to arise, from magisterial interference, producing the effect which they desire upon a considerable portion of the public.[74]

Such local tactics probably had more impact than the efforts of the few active members of the Coroners' Society to organize their brethren on a national basis.[75] But the coroners also benefited from the sheer ineptitude of the magistrates' tactics. At a time when the sanitary movement was fanning political concern about infanticide, it seems extraordinary that the West Yorkshire justices (on the advice of counsel) should instruct their constabulary that coroners need not be informed of 'infants overlaid in bed'[76] – a type of accident notoriously difficult to distinguish from deliberate suffocation – or that the Middlesex justices should save a few pounds in 1859 by disallowing the fees for nine inquests on children who had plainly died unnatural deaths. Such decisions played into the hands of critics who accused the justices of 'holding out a premium on murder';[77] but they did not deter the Middlesex coroners from recording a dramatic increase in suffocation, 'found dead' and murder verdicts on infants the following year.[78]

The trial and execution of Dr William Palmer in 1856 did even more than the infanticide issue to bring the magistrates' instructions into disrepute. Palmer was thought to have fatally poisoned as many as thirteen people at Rugeley in Staffordshire, a county where the magistrates were particularly aggressive in curbing the coroners' activities.[79] In his contribution to the Registrar-General's report for the year, William Farr blamed Palmer's crimes, and other 'homicidal eruptions' in Essex and Norfolk, on the magistrates' interference with coroners. 'The utility of the inquest', he wrote, 'is not to be proved by the number of *crimes committed* but by the number of *crimes prevented*.'[80] This was the keynote of the evidence which a deputation of coroners, led by Wakley, gave to the Royal Commission appointed in 1858 to examine 'The costs of prosecutions and the expenses of inquests'. Palmer's case was referred to repeatedly in the evidence before the Commissioners. The Commission proposed a compromise: coroners should be paid by salaries rather than fees, but should hold inquests only when requested to do so by the police.

The coroners strongly criticized this recommendation when the whole subject of coroners' inquests was investigated by a Parliamentary Select Committee in 1860. Again, the point was made that the police would be able to conceal their own misconduct,[81] but it was now the issues of poisoning and infanticide that dominated the debate. The Hampshire coroner J. H. Todd complained bitterly of being 'obstructed and kept back' by the police. 'I used to take a number of inquests on children found dead, some of these were from criminal causes; but now I scarcely ever take an inquest of this kind ... [N]o notice is sent to me; the police dispose of them'.[82]

The report of the 1860 Select Committee marked a decisive victory for the coroners. The Royal Commission's proposal that their inquiries should be initiated by the police was rejected. The recommendation that they should be paid by salary rather than by fee was enacted almost immediately, and in a way that was deliberately designed to encourage rather than restrain the holding of inquests: coroners' salaries were to be revised periodically according to the average number of inquests they had held over the previous five years.[83] The Committee accepted the view of the coroners and sanitarians that inquests should be held in all cases of sudden or accidental death, on the grounds elegantly summarized by Farr: 'for the denunciation of the guilty, for the comfort of the innocent, and for the information of the public, who should be taught the nature and extent of the dangers that surround them'.[84] This view was not, however, given legislative effect until 1887, and in the meantime there continued to be wide variations in the way coroners interpreted their duties.[85] Another recommendation of the 1860 Committee, that coroners' juries should be selected on the same basis as those in other courts, was finally implemented in 1983![86]

One objective which the coroners failed to gain was the extension of the medieval requirement for inquests on prison deaths to other forms of custody, such as the workhouse. This point was strongly argued in the learned treatise which the barrister Joshua Toulmin Smith submitted to the Royal Commission on the coroners' behalf,[87] and was also raised before the Commission by Wakley,[88] but the coroners who appeared before the 1860 Select Committee did not press it.[89] By this time the workhouses were, in F. B. Smith's phrase, 'effectively barracks for the infirm and closets for the dying',[90] and to inquire into every inmate's death would surely have taxed the energies of the most industrious coroner. But despite their relative lack of prominence in this crucial report, both prison and workhouse inquests would continue to arouse controversy in the latter part of the nineteenth century.

Coroners, prisoners and paupers, 1850–87

The impact of the new Poor Law upon institutional regimes was felt in the prison as well as the workhouse. The belief that the new law had 'inadvertently made the condition of the pauper less eligible than that of the criminal'[91] gave added momentum to the 'constant seesaw between the desire of the authorities, both central and local, to cut the diet in the interest of making it less attractive and their need to keep prisoners in good health' – or at least keep them alive.[92] From 1843, following recommendations made by Sir James Graham (then Home Secretary), dietary scales could be up- or down-graded by the prison authorities. Because of the demands of discipline it was usually the latter course that was adopted; and as Philip Priestley has noted, some prisoners 'became the subjects of deliberate experiments designed to test the limits' to which the diet could be reduced.[93] Hunger and ill-health were constant factors in prisoners' lives. As the Howard Association commented: 'A man goes to bed hungry and gets up hungry, in fact he is always hungry; and this lasts for not weeks, not months, but for years.'[94]

The punitive thrust of the regime, the will to discipline, could have severe consequences for prisoners, as was shown by one of the most notorious Victorian prison deaths, that of Edward Andrews in 1853. At the age of fifteen, Andrews was committed to Birmingham prison for stealing four pounds of beef. He was placed on the crank, which was to be turned 10,000 times a day: 2,000 turns before breakfast, 4,000 between breakfast and dinner, another 4,000 between dinner and supper. If the task was incomplete he was placed on bread and water. The shortfall had to be made up and he was not permitted to go to bed until an hour and a half after the other prisoners. The boy hanged himself; two other prisoners attempted suicide at the same time. Though the coroner's jury returned a verdict of 'suicide in a state of insanity', the evidence given by the prison chaplain led to the establishment of a commission of inquiry which found that the governor and surgeon had been 'guilty of acts not only illegal but grossly cruel'.[95] Both were prosecuted; the governor, who had had Andrews placed in a straitjacket fastened to the wall, was gaoled for three months.[96] The commission strongly criticized the magistrates, as well as the medical inspector of prisons, for failing to detect and prevent these abuses. For the coroners' supporters, the case proved the value of inquests in revealing what the magistrates would prefer to conceal.[97]

From the perspective of the confined, life in the mid-Victorian penal system was hard, uncompromising and often brutal. A number of books were published in the mid-to-late nineteenth century which detailed the lives and the circumstances of death of individual prisoners. As Priestly has pointed out, 'there was no shortage of men in prison who when they heard of any sudden death in the hospital were "ready to swear 'his light has been put out by the doctor'"'.[98] The anonymous 'One Who has Tried Them [the prisons]' described the death of a prisoner who

> complained that he was subject to heart complaint: but the doctor and Old Bob [the hospital warder] had got it into their heads that he was shamming and the former certified him fit for first class labour. It was very hot summer weather; the man was placed upon the wheel, and used to puff and blow and exhibit signs of intense distress while at work; but this was looked upon as a dodge, and no notice was taken of it, and the man continued at wheel work. A few nights later the warder, going round to lock up cell-doors at bedtime, heard a strange gurgling noise in this man's cell, and looking in, saw him stretched upon his bed gasping for breath ... There was the usual inquest on the body, and the verdict of course was 'Death from natural causes'.[99]

These conditions were aggravated by the recommendations of a Select Committee of the House of Lords chaired by Lord Carnarvon in 1862–3. It recommended a more punitive regime, and while not actually prepared to recommend that the diet be reduced, the Committee suggested that experiments might be conducted in order to ascertain how far this could safely be done.[100] In 1864, a Departmental Committee was established, chaired by Dr William Guy, the medical superintendent of Millbank prison and Professor of Forensic Medicine at King's College, London. He was assisted by Dr Maitland of Gosport military prison and Dr Clark of Dartmoor. The Committee gave 'cautious approval' to a 'limited reduction in the separate prisons' dietaries'.[101]

The reduction in diet was directly linked to a number of deaths in custody. In April 1868, the Howard Association published a pamphlet calling attention to recent inquests on those who had died in prison or shortly after their release apparently because of lack of food. The *Lancet* made a similar point in the same month when it described the case of 18-year-old Edward Barrett who had died after a stint in Coldbath Fields prison. It was said that he went to prison in robust health, but when released he could hardly walk. The inquest heard of other cases where prisoners had been 'reduced to shadows and shorn of their strength' by the hard labour and meagre diet of the prison:

> The penance of the treadmill begins at 6.30 a.m. and lasts until 8 a.m. when there is a short interval for breakfast, which consists of one pint of gruel and six ounces of bread. When this is over, the treadmill is resumed till dinner; when the prisoners get, on Mondays, Thursdays, and Fridays, one pint of gruel and six ounces of bread, varied on Tuesdays and Saturdays by eight ounces of potatoes, four of meat, and six of bread; and on Sundays by one pint of soup and six ounces of bread. At 5 p.m. the work of the mill ceases, and the prisoners then get half-a-pint of gruel and six ounces of bread. The Coroner justly observed that this fare was quite insufficient for the amount of work exacted from the prisoners, not only in quantity, but (we may add) in quality, the due proportion of tissue-forming constituents being hardly represented at all on three days of the week, and totally absent on the other four.[102]

Prisoners' accounts were important in describing a different reality from the increasingly circumscribed official reports. *Six Years in the Convict Prisons of England* published in 1869, *Five Years' Penal Servitude* by the anonymous 'One Who Has Endured It' published in 1877 and *Her Majesty's Prisons: Their Effects and Defects* by 'One Who Has Tried Them' all catalogued cases of medical abuse and the decline and deaths of prisoners.[103] Prisoners also used the coroners' inquests as forums for providing alternative accounts to official discourse. It was here that the statements of prison managers and medical officers were severely challenged. Juries were often sceptical of official accounts from whatever source they came. As Dr Quinton, the prison surgeon at Glasgow, commented in 1910, the inquests were

> frequently embarrassing, if not annoying, to the prison witnesses, especially medical officers. A fixed idea seemed to possess the minds of jurymen that prisoners were either starved, or done to death under the new management. The examination of witnesses often assumed an aggressive or offensive tone on matters related to hospital and general treatment, the sufficiency of diets, the use of stimulants, and so on – questions which had not aroused any similar attention when prisoners were being maintained out of the rates ... popular distrust of the system, judging from press comments, seemed to exist in no uncertain degree. So captious and unreasonable were some juries that an intelligent onlooker remarked that 'medical officers were practically tried for manslaughter at every inquest'.[104]

While prison doctors could publicly disagree over the precise interpretation of mortality rates, as Drs Rendle and Nicolson did in the columns of the *British Medical Journal* between April and June 1871,[105] the medical press was increasingly concerned about the fatal effects that the prison diet could have on the confined. Margaret Girvan's death in Armagh prison in August 1879 was one example given by the *Lancet* where the inquest jury's verdict that the deceased had died of 'hectic fever in a shattered constitution' was coupled with a rider that the 'very low scale of diet which she received in the prison from the day of her commital had a great deal to do with the result'.[106]

In February of that year, the report was published of an inquiry into the death of John Nolan in Coldbath Fields. The prisoner's death caused both the medical and popular press to call for changes in the system of discipline and diet. According to the inquest jury, Nolan died in the prison infirmary from 'the mortal effects of acute inflammation of the lungs' and his death was 'accelerated by the repeated and excessive punishment of bread-and-water diet, which was ordered by the governor and sanctioned by the surgeon. The jury are of the opinion that it is impossible for the medical officer properly or effectually to attend to his duties at the prison without being resident.'[107] One member of the jury stated that 'he did not believe a word of the doctor's evidence. It was full of contradictions.'[108] The doctor defended the discipline of the prison before the coroner. He provided a detailed account of the prisoner's life inside. He said that he examined fifty or sixty prisoners each day; when he examined the deceased 'he had a slight cold and I kept him in the convalescent ward for two days'. His view of the deceased focused on his ill-discipline; his bed-wetting was put down to laziness; and the doctor considered a cold cell better to sleep in than a warm one. Prisoners were 'legitimately punished if they do not do their work. I believe the deceased wilfully neglected his work and that it was not inability from weakness. If the deceased had stated that he could not do his work, and had showed sufficient reason, I should have lessened his amount of work.'[109]

The official inquiry exonerated the surgeon and the governor and did not endorse the opinion of the coroner's jury 'that the duties of the medical officer cannot be properly performed without residence'.[110] The surgeon himself argued that the inquest had been unfairly conducted, that public meetings had been held on Clerkenwell Green and in public houses 'to influence the jury', that discharged prisoners were admitted 'to prompt the coroner with questions' and that he had

> distinctly stated to the coroner and jury . . . that I was responsible entirely for all the punishments being carried out and that no prisoner was ever punished without my certifying that he was fit to bear it. I do not in this case believe that the punishment had anything to do with the prisoner's illness and death . . . The sudden change in the weather was quite sufficient to account for his illness.[111]

The *Lancet* was less sanguine and argued that the jury's verdict was fully justified by the 'extraordinary facts disclosed by the inquest. It is impossible for the matter to rest here and the question of prison mortality, discipline and diet with special reference to Nolan's case must be brought for early discussion in the House of Commons.'[112] In January 1882 its writers argued that short terms of imprisonment were 'destructive to health, and consequently dangerous to life'.[113]

In April 1882 there was 'another prison scandal' at Chester gaol. When James Fry was admitted to the prison he was found to be suffering from bronchial cough and angina pectoris, with disease of the mitral valve. He was not prescribed medicine, nor was his food increased to any noticeable degree. At the inquest the jury returned a verdict of death by natural causes, but considered that his death was accelerated 'by the want of a more nutritious and generous diet than that allowed the deceased while in prison; they also blamed the medical officer for not having him treated as a patient in the prison hospital'.[114]

Coroners' juries thus played an important part in raising popular discontents about the disciplinary orientation of the prisons. This extended to deaths in other institutions. In 1877 Fred Chalkley died in Clerkenwell House of Detention after being taken there by the police. The inquest jury was scathing in its indictment of the police's behaviour, as were the people from his local area who wrote to the Home Office about this death. The jury stated that 'the treatment of the deceased as a prisoner whilst in the hands of the police authorities was calculated to retard his recovery'.[115]

We have not looked in detail at workhouse inquests after 1850, but F. B. Smith's account of workhouse medical care indicates that there were numerous inquests which revealed 'a harrowing compound of neglect and mindless cruelty'.[116] Some juries and coroners continued to criticize the medical profession's neglect of the poor, both inside and outside workhouses;[117] but such criticisms received less support from within the profession as its radical element declined.[118] In February 1884 *The Lancet* noted that coroners' juries were 'increasingly prone to censure the medical officers of workhouses and poor-law districts', and showed an 'insolent' attitude towards the way poor-law medical officers discharged their obligations. [119] Thomas Wakley must have turned in his grave.

Conclusion

The *Lancet*'s change of attitude illustrates how tangled and contradictory were the politics of coroners' inquests in the nineteenth century. This is not a story of enlightened doctors furthering the cause of progress in the teeth of opposition from benighted lawyers and magistrates. It is certainly true that much of the impetus for reform came from those who were anxious to improve the recording of causes of death, to promote more effective investigation of crime, and to advance the cause of public health. On the face of it, these aims could have been as well or better served by a professional system of medico-legal investigation on the lines proposed by the Middlesex justices. But this would have transferred many of the coroners' powers to the magistrates who, in their administrative capacities, were frequently at odds with central government agencies over questions of public health and institutional management. For the magistrates, preserving their local autonomy could mean hiding some of the abuses we have described.

The coroner's court in the nineteenth century was a site of conflict on a number of different levels. First and most obviously, there was the dispute between the legal and medical professions whose rivalry continued through the nineteenth century and beyond.[120] Second, there was conflict between an increasingly centralized state bureaucracy and some of those who held power in and over local communities. Third, there was also conflict between the locally powerful. Thus, a coroner like Baker who inveighed against the 'spirit of centralization' and defended the traditional prerogatives of the parish could make common cause with the centralized General Board of Health against the local poor-law guardians.[121]

At the same time, the coroner's court was a forum where some of the most marginalized groups in Victorian society, such as prisoners, paupers and their relatives, could challenge the practices of disciplinary institutions and the medical profession. It was also the only court in which working-class people could participate as jurors. While there were many inquests in which juries tamely recorded 'visitation of God' verdicts as instructed by the coroner, there were others in which their verdicts reflected a form of popular justice. The coroners' claim to be the 'magistrates of the poor' was not entirely unfounded.

The Victorian debate about coroners also involved a conflict between two fundamentally different conceptions of the investigation of sudden death. The Middlesex justices' report evokes a picture of medico-legal investigation as a scientific enterprise in which doctors, lawyers and policemen would combine their respective professional skills to arrive at some objective truth. The few but prominent populist coroners insisted that many deaths raised questions not only of physical causation – which was indeed the province of medical science – but of moral and political responsibility, and that these questions should be examined by a popular tribunal. This conflict persists today. Critics have pointed to the continuing problems associated with coroners' courts, and the inability of such courts to challenge official accounts of deaths in custody.[122] For coroners, these critics are seeking to politicize an apolitical process of inquiry. For the critics, while the coroner's court sometimes exposes abuses of institutional power, like its nineteenth-century predecessor it more often fails to live up to its full potential to represent the interests of the powerless against those of state institutions.

NOTES

Thanks to Anette Ballinger for her help with this chapter, and to Mick Ryan for his constructive criticisms.

1 P. Scraton and K. Chadwick, *In the Arms of the Law: Coroners' Inquests and Deaths in Custody* (London: Pluto, 1986); M. Benn and K. Worpole, *Death in the City* (London: Canary, 1986); J. Tweedie and T. Ward, 'The Gibraltar shootings and the politics of inquests', *Journal of Law and Society*, 16 (1989), 464–76.

2 L. Prior, *The Social Organization of Death: Medical Discourse and Social Practices in Belfast* (Basingstoke and London: Macmillan, 1989).

3 J. M. Beattie, *Crime and the Courts in England 1660–1800* (Oxford: Clarendon, 1986), pp. 80–1; J. D. J. Havard, *The Detection of Secret Homicide* (London: Macmillan, 1960), pp. 35–7.

4 M. Foucault, *The History of Sexuality: An Introduction* (London: Penguin, 1984), pp. 139–41.

5 M. A. Crowther, *The Workhouse System 1834–1929* (London: Methuen, 1983); S. McConville, *A History of English Prison Administration, Vol. I, 1750–1877* (London: Routledge, 1981).

6 County coroners were elected; borough coroners were appointed by town councils; franchise coroners were appointed by individual landowners.

7 O. Anderson, *Suicide in Victorian and Edwardian England* (Oxford: Clarendon, 1987), pp. 33–5.

8 J. Sim, *Medical Power in Prisons: The Prison Medical Service in England 1774–1989* (Milton Keynes and Philadelphia: Open University Press, 1990), ch. 3. For an overview of the various positions, see M. Ignatieff, 'State, civil society and total institutions: a critique of recent social histories of punishment', in S. Cohen and A. Scull, eds., *Social Control and the State* (Oxford: Martin Robertson, 1983).

9 M. Ignatieff, *A Just Measure of Pain* (London: Macmillan, 1978), p. 60.

10 Sim, *Medical Power*, chs. 2 and 3.

11 R. Hunnisett, *The Mediaeval Coroner* (Cambridge: Cambridge University Press, 1961), pp. 35–6; T. R. Forbes, 'London coroners' inquests for 1590', *Journal of the History of Medicine*, 28 (1973), 332–4; T. R. Forbes, 'Crowner's quest', *Transactions of the American Philosophical Society*, 68: 1 (1978), 1–52, at p. 33.

12 T. R. Forbes, 'A mortality record for Cold Bath Fields', *Bulletin of the New York Academy of Medicine*, 53 (1977), 668–9.

13 Parliamentary Papers (hereafter PP), (1831–1912), XXXV, p. 61.

14 'Letter from William Farr', in Registrar-General, *First Annual Report*, PP, 1839, XVI, p. 1.

15 M. de Lacy, *Prison Reform in Lancashire, 1700–1850* (Manchester: Manchester University Press, 1986), p. 126.

16 *Parliamentary Reports*, 1812, III, p. 418.

17 Ibid., p. 145.

18 *Lancet*, 2 (1830–1), 144.

19 *Parliamentary Debates*, 1822, VI, Col. 862.

20 Ibid., Col. 1079.

21 *Parliamentary Debates*, 1816, XXXIII, Col. 545.

22 R. Richardson, *Death, Dissection and the Destitute* (Harmondsworth: Penguin, 1989), pp. 155, 207–9, 212.

23 Cited in C. Brook, *Thomas Wakley* (London: Socialist Medical Association, 1962), p. 19.

24 *Lancet*, 2 (1837–8), 779; 2 (1839–40), 428, 530.

25 *Lancet*, 2 (1827–8), 532.

26 *Lancet*, 2 (1828–9), 754.

27 Wakley and Baker estimated their expenses at £7,000 and £4,000 respectively: S. S. Sprigge, *The Life and Times of Thomas Wakley* (London: Longmans, 1897), p. 373; Middlesex Quarter Sessions, *Report ... as to the Duties and Remuneration of Coroners* (London: J. T. Norris, 1851), p. 31.

28 *Lancet*, 2 (1831), 630.
29 Sprigge, *Wakley*, p. 308.
30 Ibid., p. 384.During the 1840s, Wakley was also very zealous in taking inquests on occupational deaths due to industrial 'accidents'. For a time, this use of inquests to publicize employers' neglect of health and safety at work was as politically controversial as Wakley's exposure of abuses of custodial power in workhouses and prisons. See Elizabeth Cawthon, 'Thomas Wakley and the medical coronership – occupational death and the judicial process', *Medical History*, 30 (1986), 191–202.
31 Crowther, *The Workhouse System*, p. 36.
32 Havard, *Secret Homicide*, pp. 38–43.
33 PP, 1840, XIV, p. 339, question 81.
34 Ibid., question 1492.
35 Ibid., question 1494.
36 *Papers Relating to an Inquest Held Before Mr Wakley* ... [an apparently verbatim transcript made for the Poor Law commission], PP, 1841, XXI, pp. 3–4.
37 Ibid., pp. 5, 25.
38 Ibid., p. 2.
39 Ibid., pp. 45–6.
40 G. Himmelfarb, *The Idea of Poverty* (London: Faber & Faber, 1984), pp. 177–9, 184–5; G. Thurston, 'A queer sort of thing', *Medico-Legal Journal*, 37 (1969), 165–71, at pp. 168–9.
41 *The Times*, 26 January 1841, reprinted in *Provincial Medical and Surgical Journal*, 1 (1840–1), 309.
42 Ibid.
43 R. A. Lewis, *Edwin Chadwick and the Public Health Movement* (London: Longmans, 1952), pp. 205–6.
44 C. Dickens, 'The paradise at Tooting', *Examiner*, 20 January 1849.
45 C. Dickens, 'The Tooting Farm' and 'The verdict for Drouet', *Examiner*, 27 January 1849 and 21 April 1849.
46 W. Baker, *A Practical Compendium of the Recent Statutes, Cases and Decisions Affecting the Office of Coroner* (London: Butterworths, 1851), p. iv.
47 Lewis, *Edwin Chadwick*, p. 207.
48 Cited in Baker, *Practical Compendium*, pp. 196–7.
49 'Letter of statement on duties of officers of health' (1851), reprinted in C. F. Brockington, *Public Health in the Nineteenth Century* (London: E. & S. Livingstone, 1965), p. 182.
50 Anderson, *Suicide in Victorian England*, p. 15.
51 Havard, *Secret Homicide*, p. 51.
52 Anderson, *Suicide in Victorian England*, p. 17n.
53 J. Craig, *The Law of the Coroner* (Edinburgh: Sutherland & Knox, 1855), p. 16.
54 Middlesex Quarter Sessions, *Duties of Coroners*, p. 8.
55 Ibid., pp. 10–12.
56 Ibid., p. 26.
57 PP, 1854–55, XLV, p. 639.
58 Middlesex Quarter Sessions, *Duties of Coroners*, p. 26.
59 Sprigge, *Wakley*, p. 378.

60 Middlesex Quarter Sessions, *Duties of Coroners*, p. 26.
61 Ibid., pp. 25, 29.
62 Ibid., pp. 33, 36–7.
63 *The Times*, 29 January 1850.
64 W. Baker, *A Letter to H. M. Justices of the Peace for Middlesex* (London: Homans, 1839), p. 27; Baker, *Practical Compendium*, p. 33; Royal Commission, *The Costs of Prosecutions and the Expenses of Inquests*, PP, 1859 (Sess. 2), XIII, p. 13, Appendix 14D.
65 For more on relations between coroners and the police, see T. Ward, 'Coroners, police, and deaths in custody in England: a historical perspective', *Working Papers in European Criminology*, 6 (1985), 186–215.
66 H. Letheby, *Report ... on Certain Imperfect Mortality Returns Relating to the Verdicts of Coroners' Juries* (London: M. Lowndes, 1856), p. 11.
67 See H. Hopkins, *The Strange Death of Private White* (London: Weidenfeld & Nicolson, 1977).
68 Letheby, *Report*, pp. 14–15.
69 PP, 1860, LVII, p. 331 ('Orders and Regulations Made, and Resolutions Passed, by County Magistrates in England and Wales, since 1850, Relating to the Expenses of Holding Coroner's Inquests').
70 Middlesex Quarter Sessions, *Duties of Coroners*, p. 58.
71 PP, 1860, LVII, p. 313 ('Return on the Number of Coroners' Inquests Held in England and Wales, 1849 to 1859; Number on which Coroners' Fees were Not Allowed').
72 Royal Commission, *Costs of Prosecutions*, p. 130.
73 Ibid., p. 79, question 1658.
74 P. B. Purnell, letter to the Home Secretary, in PP, 1860, LVII, at p. 374.
75 Some rather desperate appeals to coroners to take an active part in the Society's activities are preserved in the East Sussex Record Office, Lewes (file A 1689). In Middlesex, the Coroners' Society presented a petition opposing the magistrates' report: *The Times*, 13 June 1851.
76 PP, 1857 (Sess. 2), XXXII, p. 419.
77 J. Toulmin Smith, *The Right Holding of the Coroner's Court, and Some Recent Interferences Therewith: Being a Report Laid Before the Royal Commissioners* (London: Henry Sweet, 1859), p. 48 (using the nine children's cases as examples).
78 L. Rose, *The Massacre of the Innocents: Infanticide in Britain 1800–1939* (London: Routledge, 1986), p. 64. Rose seems to take it for granted that murder or manslaughter verdicts on infants were 'frank' and accident verdicts were 'shallow and uninformed'. However, the timing of the outbreak of 'frankness' in Middlesex does seem remarkably convenient from the coroners' point of view. See also Havard, *Secret Homicide*, pp. 51–7; and, for a more sceptical view of infanticide, A. S. Wohl, *Endangered Lives* (London: Methuen, 1984), pp. 33–4.
79 Royal Commission, *Costs of Prosecutions*, question 1658; Baker, *Practical Compendium*, p. 11.
80 Registrar-General, *Nineteenth Annual Report*, PP, 1857–8, XXIII, 1, p. 198.
81 Select Committee of the Office of Coroner, PP, 1860, XXII, 257, question 566.
82 Ibid., questions 624–6.
83 Coroners Act 1860 (23 and 24 Vict., c. 116), s. 4.

84 Registrar-General, *Nineteenth Annual Report*, p. 198.
85 Anon., 'Responsibility and discretion of coroners', *Lancet*, 1 (1881), 147–8.
86 Coroners' Juries Act, 1983.
87 Toulmin Smith, *The Coroner's Court*, p. 32.
88 Royal Commission, *Costs of Prosecutions*, question 1659.
89 See particularly Select Committee on Coroners, *Minutes* (1860), question 465 (on lunatic asylums).
90 F. B. Smith, *The People's Health 1830–1910* (London: Croom Helm, 1979), p. 383.
91 Himmelfarb, *Idea of Poverty*, p. 381.
92 De Lacy, *Prison Reform*, p. 180.
93 P. Priestley, *Victorian Prison Lives* (London: Methuen, 1985), p. 151.
94 Ibid., p. 157.
95 PP, 1854, XXXI, p. 1.
96 M. D. Hill, *Suggestions for the Repression of Crime* (London: Parker & Son, 1857), p. 232.
97 J. Toulmin Smith, *The Parish. Its Obligations and Powers: Its Officers and their Duties*, 2nd edn (London: Henry Sweet, 1857), p. 376.
98 Priestley, *Prison Lives*, p. 188.
99 Ibid., pp. 188–9.
100 McConville, *History of English Prison Administration*, vol. I, p. 418.
101 Ibid.
102 *Lancet*, 2 (1854), 107.
103 Sim, *Medical Power*, ch. 3.
104 R. F. Quinton, *Crime and Criminals* (London: Longmans, Green, 1910), pp. 188–9.
105 *British Medical Journal*, 8 April, 22 April, 27 May, 17 June 1871.
106 *Lancet*, 2 (1879), 373.
107 PP, 1878–9, LIX, p. 539.
108 Press report of the case in Public Record Office, HO 45/947/79161.
109 PP, 1878–9, LIX, 501, p. 12.
110 Ibid., p. 12.
111 Ibid., p. 36.
112 *Lancet*, 2 (1878), 823.
113 *Lancet*, 1 (1882), 120.
114 *Lancet*, 1 (1882), 616.
115 Public Record Office, HO 45/9444/67290.
116 Smith, *People's Health*, pp. 387–8.
117 For example, *The Times*, 1 January 1850; J. H. Todd, *A Letter to the Rev. George Deane* (Winchester, Jacob & Johnson, 1856); Public Record Office, HO 45/9962/X8246 (Letter from Deputy Coroner for Middlesex, 1886).
118 Smith, *People's Health*, p. 382.
119 *Lancet*, 1 (1884), 308.
120 In 1926 the Coroners (Amendment) Act laid down that coroners must be *either* legally or medically qualified, a compromise which remains in force today.
121 Baker, *Letter*, p. 37; *Practical Compendium*, pp. 47–8.
122 See above, note 1.

11

Coroners, corruption and the politics of death: forensic pathology in the United States

JULIE JOHNSON

The complexity and decentralization of the United States' legal system presents an intriguing intellectual puzzle to the historian of American legal medicine. Not only are there federal, state and local laws, but also city, county, and township jurisdictions, and English, French, and Spanish legal traditions. The varying levels of legal and medical education and practice, both within and between regions, are additional factors demanding study and consideration.[1] Social historians have recently begun to examine the creation of national medico-legal institutions and issues and their change over time, viewing local differences as clues to historical understanding, rather than as obstacles.[2] This essay contributes to this effort by examining the development of forensic pathology in the United States, paying particular attention to its institutional locus, the coroner's office. This office, where the application of forensic pathological knowledge legitimized social policy, was the site of confrontation for the professions of law, medicine, and politics.

The office of coroner is an inheritance from English common law. In the colonial and early federal eras it was a minor political office, whose occupant was usually appointed by the governor. Whereas English coroners were often physicians, attorneys, or local magistrates, American coroners usually had no professional qualifications, and were typically farmers, carters, or undertakers. This was due in part to the less metropolitan and class-conscious nature of American society, but the low population density and the geographical dispersal of the population also played a part. In many places, possession of a wagon suitable for hauling away bodies was a major recommendation for the job of coroner.[3]

The Jacksonian era had a profound effect on American society and politics. In this period (the 1820s through the 1840s), the suffrage was extended beyond the land-owning class to the growing urban working class, creating the conditions necessary for the rise of the urban political machine. Many formerly appointive public offices became elective, the coroner's among them. Jacksonian Democrats celebrated the intelligence and integrity of the common man while belittling the attainments of the social and professional elite. Thus, as the western territories were settled and the number of coroners grew, there was no accompanying demand that they possess medical or legal credentials. Political, not professional skills were what was demanded of potential coroners.[4]

By the mid-nineteenth century, the coroner's office had become an obscure but integral part of the government bureaucracy. Its powers varied from jurisdiction to jurisdiction. In some, the coroner was empowered to investigate all sudden deaths, and was enabled, though not obliged, to order autopsies; in others, only deaths that were obviously suspicious or violent could be investigated and autopsied. In all jurisdictions, the coroner's main responsibility was to convene and preside over a juried inquest, whose function was to determine whether the death in question was the result of accident, suicide, murder, or natural causes.[5] The coroner and his jury heard evidence from family, neighbours, friends, doctors, the police, and whoever else might have information to offer, and returned a verdict on the cause, manner, and, sometimes, author of the death. The coroner's inquest was thus often the first step in a murder investigation, determining whether a crime meriting prosecution had been committed.

Medical testimony often figured prominently in inquests, but it was seldom authoritative until the late nineteenth century. There was little scope for the pursuit of forensic pathology as anything more than an avocation in the US until the turn of the twentieth century; few physicians saw more than a handful of obviously suspicious deaths in the course of their practice, though many may have gone unrecognized. Those physicians fortunate enough to have attended medical school might have received some brief instruction on medico-legal autopsies as part of their course in medical jurisprudence. Others might have had access to textbooks, more or less up-to-date depending on their circumstances, which outlined the post-mortem signs of violent death.[6] But even if a physician had never before performed a post-mortem examination, American law nevertheless considered him an expert in any aspect of medicine, regardless of his actual experience or training.[7]

As the United States grew from a primarily rural, agricultural society to an urban, industrial one, continued medico-legal ignorance and apathy seemed increasingly to place the preservation of the law and social order at risk. Forensic pathology's emergence as a specific occupation coincides with a time of tremendous social upheaval in the United States. During the last quarter of the nineteenth century, hundreds of thousands of immigrants arrived in American cities each year, crowding into the burgeoning manufacturing districts where single rooms often housed entire families.

Native-born Americans, generally of English or German Protestant stock, were appalled by the conditions of immigrant life. The sheer numbers of immigrants seemed overwhelming, and the sense of difference which many felt towards the polyglot, swarthy, often Catholic or Jewish newcomers often turned to fear. Although the poverty and misery of urban workers seemed to some to reflect the dark side of progress, most Americans, revelling in their growing industrial prowess, were slow to criticize the capitalist system on which it was based and found fault instead with the newcomers themselves. As Michael Katz has pointed out, to be poor in America was and is essentially to be labelled criminal – the miserable conditions of the slums were simply a just punishment.[8]

Crime was very much on the minds of urban Americans in the late nineteenth century. The numbers of murders and suicides rose dramatically in the late nineteenth and early twentieth centuries.[9] Crimes also became more difficult to solve. In a small town, there was seldom much difficulty in identifying a victim, and once that was known, in identifying his or her family, friends, and business partners – always the most likely suspects. But a death in a city tenement block housing thousands was another matter. The anarchy that bearded Slavic foreigners preached on street corners seemed an increasingly frightening possibility. Solutions were sought from new sources, particularly the medical and social sciences.[10] The anthropometric approach of criminologists such as Cesare Lombroso was enthusiastically embraced by a society that increasingly defined itself in terms of racial and ethnic difference.[11] While some laboured to identify potential criminals and thus prevent crime, others turned their attention to the problem of identifying and prosecuting actual criminals.

Forensic pathology seemed to offer assurances that justice would be served and the social order preserved. Its scientific practitioners would identify unknown victims and determine the cause of their deaths and the manner in which they occurred: homicide, suicide, or accident. In cases of homicide, the forensic expert could identify the type of weapon used or measure the angle of its entry, thus giving the police clues to aid them in apprehending the criminal. Finally, in the court of law, the full weight of scientific (and therefore, in the prevailing positivistic atmosphere, irrefutable) evidence would be brought to bear, ensuring conviction by all but the most stupid or obdurate jury.

Nor was the state the only party interested in the accurate determination of causes of death: the thriving insurance industry had a significant stake in it as well. Life insurance policies were sold that were void in the event of suicide, or which paid double for accidental deaths. And as the rate of industrial accidents rose and workmen's compensation lawsuits were less frequently decided by the 'fellow servant' rule that absolved owners from liability, medical testimony played a greater role in apportioning blame and therefore compensation.[12]

Improvement in forensic pathological practice was one of many diverse institutional reforms of the Progressive era devised in response to the chaotic social and business conditions of late nineteenth-century America. But the growth of forensic pathology has often been hampered by its association with corruption – the physical corruption of long-dead bodies and the moral corruption of crime – and in the US, a third sort of corruption figured prominently: the political corruption of municipal bureaucracies. Calls for the expansion of forensic pathological knowledge and its application in the United States centred on reform of its practice in the coroner's office. In urban areas by the second half of the nineteenth century the coronership had become a well-established part of the patronage and spoils system that characterized much of American municipal government.[13]

America's large cities were politically in the control of what were termed 'machines'. New York City's Tammany Hall was one of the oldest and most infamous, but nearly every major city, and many smaller ones, had party-dominated political networks running the government. Native-born wealth usually condemned the machines, but they served their immigrant and working-class constituencies well and proved difficult to overthrow. To its critics, the machine's awarding of jobs and municipal contracts to supporters was corrupt and inefficient; but machine adherents charged critics with sour grapes and challenged them to develop a better way of ensuring political participation. To be sure, the machines did indulge in egregious acts of pocket-lining and vote-stealing from time to time, but seldom without public outcry and legislative reform that curtailed, though it did not destroy, the power of political leaders. Because the continued growth of American cities so visibly depended upon machine-controlled municipal services such as gas, water, electricity, and street paving, urban political reform became a rallying point for Progressive reformers at the end of the nineteenth century.[14]

Under political machines, urban coroners possessed great legal and political power. Many urban coroners possessed detective forces comparable to those of the police, and some had prosecutorial powers rivalling those of the district attorney. Coroner's Deputies – the men in charge of claiming bodies and transporting them to the morgue – routinely collected bribes from undertakers whose services they recommended to the families of the dead and were often accused of looting the deceased's effects. Embezzlement was also common: in Philadelphia, for example, the coroner's office was responsible for the administration of the estates of those whose deaths came under its jurisdiction, and its stewardship seldom bore close examination.[15] The fees coroners and their juries earned per inquest provided further opportunity for graft and political patronage. Coroners enjoyed great discretion in the choice and presentation of evidence and the direction of the jury's verdict, and were known to mediate or negotiate causes of death. For the price of a campaign contribution or the return of a favour, details of the death of a respected businessman who died in embarrassing circumstances could be suppressed, abortion-related deaths among the wealthy could be overlooked, and even where the deceased was poor, a word from a ward politician might change a suicide verdict to one of death by natural causes.[16]

Few jurisdictions required the coroner to have professional qualifications of any kind; nor was any specialized training or expertise required of his staff, all of whom were political appointees. Coroner's physicians, who performed the autopsies, were usually only required to be medical doctors, not pathologists. Most were from the lower and middle ranks of the profession, and were granted the part-time position as a reward for faithful service as ward leaders or political organizers.[17]

Middle-class reformers, however, regarded the *quid pro quo* operations of the coroner's office as outrageous perversions of justice. They saw coroners as furthering the breakdown of law and order by allowing crime to go unpunished, whether because of the inexperience of the coroner's physicians or simple cupidity. Physicians in particular vilified coroners for their errors in post-mortem diagnosis and regularly lambasted them in the medical press for their ignorance and venality.[18] Socially and professionally elite urban physicians often led attempts to reform the coroner's office, which took two forms. The simpler expedient was to demand the election of a physician to the office, in the belief that medical science would be better served – or at least acknowledged – by a medical practitioner. The more thoroughgoing approach was to seek abolition of the coroner's office and its replacement by a medical examiner system.

Though the scientific prestige of a medical examiner might be great, his political power was considerably less than that of most coroners. Under the model system promoted by the American Medical Association as early as the 1850s, the physician–medical examiner was empowered to investigate all sudden or suspicious deaths, but the inquest was to be abolished, thereby eliminating opportunities for both corruption and scientific error. The medical examiner alone would have the power to state the cause and manner of death, with investigation of any crimes being the sole province of the police, and prosecution that of the district attorney.[19] The first medical examiner system was established in 1877 in Massachusetts, but it remained an anomaly for nearly four decades.

Abolishing the coroner's office was a difficult process to initiate; often it required a state constitutional amendment, a process which pitted urban interests against rural ones in the state legislature, and reformers against entrenched political and economic interests.[20] Like the crime that prompted it, medico-legal reform was (erroneously) seen as only an urban problem.

The medical profession itself lacked the unity to lobby effectively for such reforms. Until the twentieth century the practice of medicine in the United States was often an insecure means of earning a living for all but a small urban elite. Orthodox medicine had little to offer to distinguish it from its sectarian competitors until the rise of bacteriology. Standards of education at even the best medical schools were lax until the 1890s, and diploma mills and the nostrum industry flourished. The opening in 1893 of the Johns Hopkins School of Medicine, whose structure and curriculum reflected the influence of German science and medicine, constituted the most visible sign of a new era of medical professionalism. During the next twenty years, the medical elite worked together to raise educational standards, re-enact licensing laws, and expose sectarian and patent medicine 'quackery'. Such reforms had both an economic and a scientific motivation: the quality of medical care was improved for some, but the supply of physicians was reduced as well, resulting in greater earning power for those who were able to meet the demands of the new medical curriculum.[21] Gross mistakes in diagnosis perpetrated by coroners in this era, ranging from labelling bludgeoning deaths as suicides to denying the existence of rabies as a disease entity, seemed to strike at the heart of the new scientific medicine, and hence at the basis for American physicians' claims to power and prestige. The coroner's office was therefore a prime target for Progressive, professionalizing medical men's reforming zeal.[22]

There was, however, little recognition among physicians of the specific knowledge that was required for proper post-mortem diagnosis of traumatic death. As an academic discipline in the US, pathology itself was barely two decades old at the turn of the century, and was changing its clinical emphasis from gross morbid anatomy to laboratory-based microscopic analysis.[23] Both clinical and forensic pathology were moving from being part-time to full-time occupations, the former based in the hospital laboratory, the latter in the municipal morgue. Forensic pathological knowledge was burgeoning, but the site of its acquisition was far removed from that of ordinary medical practice.

New York City's Charles Norris, Boston's George Burgess Magrath, and Philadelphia's William Scott Wadsworth were the first generation of American physicians employed full-time in medico-legal practice. The three men worked under very different systems, however. The governor of Massachusetts appointed Magrath as medical examiner of Suffolk County

(Boston) in 1906, the first in a series of seven-year terms. Although he was a Harvard-trained pathologist, Magrath was appointed under the 1877 law that only required medical examiners to be physicians, as the specialty of pathology barely existed in the US at the time of the law's enactment.[24] Norris was selected New York City's first medical examiner in 1918 after a rigorous Civil Service Examination for which only those with forensic pathological expertise were allowed to sit. He experienced the best conditions for medico-legal practice that existed in the US, although even he complained of inadequate funding and was forced to accept political appointees among his staff.[25] Wadsworth, who was appointed coroner's physician in Philadelphia in 1899, worked under conditions more familiar to most American forensic pathologists. His bosses were usually lay coroners, and though Wadsworth achieved an international reputation as an expert in forensic pathology, toxicology, and ballistics, scarcely one of his five decades with the Philadelphia coroner's office was free from scandal involving fiscal mismanagement by some member of the administrative staff. Most of the other medical staff simply passed through the coroner's office on their way to another politically connected appointment, whether at Philadelphia General Hospital or one of the state hospitals.[26]

Aside from the usual course in medical jurisprudence that most medical schools offered, covering psychiatric evaluations, malpractice, expert testimony and medical ethics in addition to a cursory introduction to medico-legal autopsies, no instruction in forensic pathology was offered in American medical schools at the turn of the century.[27] Regular physicians, therefore, had little understanding of and even less regard for forensic pathological expertise. In part, this reflected the low status of pathological anatomy in the American medical hierarchy. American physicians linked their claims to social prestige explicitly to their new ability to cure and control infection. The old days of managing death were gone; now the physician was expected to fight it, and win. Bacteriologists, and later immunologists – the 'Microbe Hunters' – were the heroes of the laboratory, while surgeons, who with anaesthesia and asepsis could now explore and excise parts of the body hitherto dangerously inaccessible, were the champions of health against disease.[28] Interventionist medicine was becoming the new model of practice. Against this background, the role of the pathologist was diminished. He had little to do with the living. His job was to examine biopsy tissue and body fluids for disease that someone else would then treat, or to perform post-mortems. In an institutional structure in which control of access to patients, and eventually, of the entire hospital, was becoming increasingly important and conferred great power, pathologists were anomalous.[29]

Forensic pathologists, of course, were entirely excluded from the hospital, but the problem of institutional control affected them nevertheless. Under the coroner system, the coroner's office, inquest, and morgue were controlled by politicians. The medical examiner system sought to redress this, but continued to allow the lawyers to control the courts – indeed, even surrendering the coroner's prosecutorial powers. Neither system presented an institutional structure that recognized the special role of medico-legal knowledge in mediating between scientific and legal standards of proof; both allowed the old antagonism between medicine and the law to continue.

The adversarial relationship which the law imposed on expert witnesses and the necessity of proving scientific points to a lay audience – the judge and jury – galled the medical profession. Legal procedure not only offered an affront to their expertise, but also provided a public forum for dissent which, many physicians felt, harmed the profession's efforts to forge a collective identity and enhance its economic position and social status. The medical profession continually tried to have courtroom procedures and evidentiary rules changed to its advantage, attempting to privilege medical testimony over that of lay witnesses and to exempt physicians from cross-examination. Doctors met with fierce opposition from the legal profession, however, which was adamant about retaining control of the courtroom.[30]

American legal procedure has two ways of treating evidence. If the issue in question is considered to be generally acknowledged to be true, i.e. a matter of common sense or general knowledge, the judge may take judicial notice of the issue and declare it 'law for the court'. No testimony controverting the issue may then be presented. Most medical evidence, however, falls into the category of 'fact for the jury'. In this instance, opposing views of the issue may be presented by defence and prosecution, leaving the jury to make up its own mind on the matter. A fact may therefore be sufficiently proven to the medical and scientific community without meeting legal requirements for judicial notice. The result was often a battle of experts, with the term 'expert' loosely defined. In the eyes of the law, and often of the jury as well, a graduate of Harvard or Hopkins was no more expert than one whose education had been obtained at a diploma mill. Some men made careers as expert witnesses, often, because of their court experience, acquitting themselves better on the stand than acclaimed clinicians. Juries, faced with conflicting testimony and perhaps swayed more than they ought to have been by a smooth courtroom manner, often discounted scientific evidence in their decisions, to the chagrin of the scientists.[31]

Forensic pathologists often seem to have found a middle ground between the professions of law and medicine. Although not insisting on any special status in the courtroom, the circumscription of their practice often worked in their favour. The number of medico-legal autopsies they had performed and other indices of their experience were included as part of their testimony; the idea that a man who had already seen several score close-range gunshot wounds (for example) would easily recognize another appealed strongly to a jury's common sense. Moreover, forensic pathologists' experience in court allowed them to evade the traps of cross-examination that too often ensnared the unwary clinician. Forensic pathologists played the game according to the rules of the law; they let their testimony be guided by the requirements of the attorney's case, and their knowledge and acceptance of legal procedure tended to spare them the annoyance and humiliation that many more combative clinicians experienced.[32]

In their efforts to extend the jurisdiction of the profession as a whole, however, physicians ignored the essential differences between clinical and forensic pathological practice. Their calls for reform of the coroner's office placed the need for forensic medical expertise second in importance to control of the office by a general medical authority. Most reformers, in fact, declared that the work of the coroner's office was purely medical, denying the legal component altogether.[33] Although this stance strengthened the argument for medical control of the office, it had unanticipated consequences.

In most jurisdictions, the kinds of physicians who were elected to the post of coroner in the first half of the twentieth century were seldom scientific or professional standard bearers of medicine. Rather, in keeping with the realities of urban government, they were men whose local political credentials outweighed their medical ones. Philadelphia's first physician-coroner, Herbert Goddard, elected in 1940 (after four decades of effort by the city's medical elite to put a doctor in office), was not a pathologist but an otolaryngologist who was chiefly famous for having removed Al Capone's tonsils during the gangster's stay at Philadelphia's Eastern State Penitentiary.[34] Goddard had been active in local politics for decades, and had served as the city's assistant director of public health until his election as coroner. Upon taking office, rather than rectifying William Scott Wadsworth's demotion from the post of chief coroner's physician by the previous administration, the new coroner instead appointed a friend to the post.[35] Matthew Roth, another old friend of Goddard's whom he made his chief deputy, was later found guilty of embezzlement during his tenure in the coroner's office.[36] Philadelphia's story is not anomalous; medical control of the coroner's office was not the panacea it was represented to be. Local political bosses continually outmanoeuvered medico-legal reformers.

Opponents of strict medical orientation and control of the coroner's office argued, often convincingly, that the job of coroner was primarily an administrative one, and that as long as the office-holder employed qualified forensic pathologists as coroner's physicians, he need possess no medical qualifications himself.[37] The availability of trained men and women was limited, however; as municipal employees, forensic pathologists were paid far less than private practitioners. The popular conception of the coroner's physician was of a broken-down, alcoholic wreck unfit to treat the living, or a sociopathic personality who preferred the company of the dead. It was hardly the company a talented young physician would care to join.[38]

Several major US cities undertook investigations of their coroners' offices in the 1910s and 1920s, and in 1924 the problems surrounding American medico-legal investigation came to the attention of the National Research Council. The NRC was a quintessential Progressive organization. Founded in 1916 at the request of President Woodrow Wilson, it functioned as a think tank, bringing the skills and knowledge of the nation's foremost scientific experts to bear on issues of public policy.[39] Its Division of Medicine created a Committee on Medicolegal Problems in 1924, headed by Ludwig Hektoen, a leading pathologist who, as head of the John McCormick Institute of Infectious Diseases, was connected with the Rockefeller Foundation.[40] Other members of the committee were equally prominent: Adolf Meyer of Johns Hopkins was America's foremost psychiatrist, and Victor Vaughan was former Dean of the University of Michigan Medical School and one of the architects of American medical educational reform.[41] Concerned with homicide from the beginning, they first considered a criminological examination of the link between ethnicity and murder, but Hektoen, a former coroner's pathologist himself, switched the committee's attention to the medico-legal investigation of homicide at the urging of fellow members of the Institute of Medicine of Chicago.[42] Hektoen persuaded Abraham Flexner and the Rockefeller Foundation's General Education Board to underwrite a study of the nation's medico-legal investigative system. Legal luminaries Roscoe Pound of Harvard University and John Wigmore of Northwestern University were added to the committee, as was William C. Woodward, the head of the American Medical Association's Bureau of Legal Medicine.[43]

The committee's first publication, *The Coroner and the Medical Examiner*, was issued in 1928 and brought national attention to bear on the issue of forensic pathological practice. It used case studies of five cities – Boston, New York, Chicago, New Orleans, and San Francisco – but presented the problems of each city as symptomatic of the coroner system as a whole, rather than merely local and idiosyncratic. The report argued for wholesale abolition of the coroner's office and the nationwide replication of New York's medical examiner system, which was considered 'practically immune from politics' though hampered by lack of funds.[44] Although the NRC sent letters concerning the report to every state governor and attorney general, there was little immediate response, and for a time the committee considered abandoning coroners to their fate. However, the American Bar Association began to show some interest in the subject in 1929, leading the committee to commission digests of laws concerning medico-legal investigation and dead bodies.[45] By the early 1930s, it was evident to the committee that national reform would continue to be slow until sufficient numbers of forensic pathologists had been trained, and in 1932 the committee published its recommendations for educational reform and expansion.[46]

In response, both New York University and Harvard University moved to institute medico-legal education at the university level. A Department of Forensic Medicine was established in the NYU School of Medicine, with the city's chief medical examiner, Charles Norris, as professor and chair. The faculty included other members of his staff as well as the chief medical examiner of nearby Newark, New Jersey, Harrison S. Martland.[47] In the same year, Frances Glessner Lee, an International Harvester Company heiress, endowed a chair of legal medicine at Harvard Medical School, with the stipulation that Suffolk County medical examiner, George B. Magrath, her late brother's best friend from his Harvard days, be appointed to the position.[48] A few years later, Mrs Lee helped persuade the Rockefeller Foundation to expand the chair into an entire department.[49]

Although the Rockefeller Foundation had previously funded research at the New York medical examiner's office and was well acquainted with the high calibre of expertise to be found there, it chose to throw the full weight of its financial backing behind Harvard's programme for several reasons. The most obvious were Harvard's reputation as America's most elite university and the high standing of its medical school. Harvard also offered an approach to teaching legal medicine that was more in keeping with traditional methods of imparting medical knowledge, and the Rockefeller Foundation's General Education Board had been a major force in the establishment of that tradition in the early twentieth century, having given 78 million dollars for medical educational reform by 1929, predominantly to top schools like Harvard.[50] Harvard's teaching staff were, like those at most other medical schools, full-time academics and only part-time practitioners, whereas the NYU staff's primary professional identity came from their positions at the medical examiner's office. Harvard's planners even failed at first to comprehend the absolute necessity of a direct link to the medical examiner's office, envisaging only a loose connection that would ensure the supply of what was still called 'clinical material'.[51] In short, the NYU department was organized by forensic experts themselves, with the special requirements of training for the field clearly in mind, whereas Harvard's was designed to conform to the expectations of the academic medical backgrounds of the school's administrators and the physician board-members of the Rockefeller Foundation.[52]

Alan Moritz, a young academic pathologist from Cleveland, was chosen in 1937 to be the Harvard department's first head and promptly embarked on a two-year tour of European legal medicine institutes at Rockefeller expense.[53] The autonomy and respect that European medico-legal experts enjoyed focused Moritz's attention on the issue of institutional control. The medical examiner system was clearly the desired institutional model; not only did it place a forensic pathologist in overall administrative charge, but it also created subordinate salaried positions under civil service rules for junior forensic pathologists, thereby expanding opportunities for employment and training in the field. Moritz, and his successor in 1949, Richard Ford, therefore lobbied extensively for the establishment of medical examiner systems, lecturing professional and civic audiences nationwide and testifying before state and local legislatures and grand juries.[54] In addition, they welcomed popular efforts to educate the public about the need to reform forensic pathological practice. The Institute of Medicine of Chicago had led the way in 1934 with an exhibition at the Century of Progress World's Fair which extolled the medical examiner system.[55] In the late 1940s, Harvard cooperated with Metro-Goldwyn-Mayer on *Mystery Street*, a movie thriller about the Department of Legal Medicine. The exploits of medical examiners were detailed in books and newspaper accounts of trials, while magazine articles with titles like 'The Coroner Racket: A National Scandal' and 'How Murderers Beat the Law' were written about the faults of the coroner system.[56] The prolific mystery writer and attorney Erle Stanley Gardner also took up the cause, dedicating several of his Perry Mason mysteries to particular members and alumni of the Harvard Department of Legal Medicine.[57]

Despite all the favourable publicity for the medical examiner system, change was slow. The Depression and the Second World War diverted funds to more immediate problems than changing the institutional structure of forensic pathology. Politicians often staved off attacks on the coroner's office by agreeing to employ forensic pathologists, and Harvard could hardly refuse to place its graduates in these positions, as the continuation of the department – and its funding from the Rockefeller Foundation – hinged upon its graduates being able to practise the specialty for which they had been trained.

In addition to raising the public's consciousness (Ford estimated that he travelled 20,000 miles in one year promoting the medical examiner system), Moritz and Ford also struggled to gain recognition for forensic pathology within the medical profession itself.[58] In 1954, the American Medical Association's (AMA) Committee on Medicolegal Problems formed a sub-committee, headed by Ford, to examine the possibility of obtaining subspecialty certification for forensic pathology from the American Board of Pathology (ABP).[59] Efforts made a few years earlier to form a separate Board of Legal Medicine had been frowned on by the AMA, which was attempting to stem the postwar proliferation of specialty boards. Boards of Specialty had been established in the United States from the 1910s as a means of defining and limiting areas of interest, of setting standards of training and practice, and of maintaining an elite.[60] By the 1950s, there were boards for nineteen specialties, and it had reached the point where general practitioners, weary of being considered the dinosaurs of the medical profession, were threatening to form their own specialty board. Specialization was threatening to fragment the profession, causing the AMA to cast a cold eye on aspiring new disciplines.[61]

The ABP had been founded in 1936 at a time of great crisis for the discipline of pathology. Because of the service role of pathology in relation to other specialties, and because of its reliance on laboratory technology, pathologists found their status as physicians challenged within the growing hospital hierarchy. The hospital administrators wished to employ pathologists on a salaried basis, but pathologists felt that this degraded their work to the level of technician, and insisted that pathology be recompensed on the usual fee-for-service basis.[62] Moreover, when pathology had first established itself as a discipline in the 1880s, it had seemed natural to include bacteriology within its purview; by the 1920s, however, as bacteriology fragmented into microbiology and physiological chemistry, such an association no longer seemed appropriate.[63] Bacteriology was not the only subspecialty threatening to secede from pathology, however. In the next two decades, haematologists, neuropathologists, clinical microbiologists and clinical chemists exacted permission to receive subspecialty certification from the ABP without first being required to show competence in pathological anatomy or clinical pathology as the price for remaining in the discipline.[64] Pathologists in the 1950s, therefore, would hardly have been cheered by the prospect of yet another subspecialty asserting itself.

Furthermore, although demand for full-time forensic pathologists existed in urban centres, in smaller towns and rural areas hospital pathologists were usually called upon by coroners to perform any necessary medico-legal post-mortems. This part-time duty represented additional income and, more importantly, access to clinical material for isolated practitioners. Many held that certification in pathological anatomy and an unspecified amount of experience in medico-legal autopsy work was sufficient to create expertise in forensic pathology.[65] Ford felt differently. He believed that subspecialty certification was necessary for the creation and maintenance of standards, and that forensic pathology had to be recognized officially as a distinct medical specialty in order to attract practitioners to the field. Moreover, he did not want certification in pathological anatomy to be a prerequisite to certification in forensic pathology, not because of any disciplinary conflict, but simply because the extra training time demanded would present an obstacle to entering the field.[66]

This was not the only issue to be negotiated with the ABP. Approval of training centres also caused contention, as training centres based in medical examiner offices rather than academic departments of medicine looked suspiciously like 'trade schools' to regular pathologists.[67] In the end, a compromise was reached: certification in pathological anatomy as a prerequisite for certification in forensic pathology in return for designation of medical examiners' offices as training centres.[68] By 1957, all the details had been worked out and the ABP had advertised its approval to the Advisory Board of Medical Specialties of the American Medical Association, which had the final say. But the Advisory Board, faced with approving forensic pathology and another mainly urban medical specialty, traumatic surgery, deferred approval of both for a year. It was February 1958 before official approval was at last received, and 1959 before the first examinations were held.[69]

Achievement of official professional recognition had little effect on the practice of forensic pathology, however. Although most jurisdictions today recognize the need for forensic pathological expertise, the measurement of that expertise remains problematic. The compromises effected during the campaign for certification allowed physicians with only a small portion of their practice in forensic pathology to become certified. This became a matter of concern in 1963, when President Kennedy's autopsy was performed, and in the opinion of many, botched, by a team of military surgeons who had received only cursory training in medico-legal post-mortem technique.[70] Forensic pathologists remain ill-paid by American medical standards, and share with public health officials the difficulties of depending on legislatures for their funding.

The prestige that was expected to accompany the establishment of professional standards for forensic pathology has never materialized. Forensic pathologists sought to abandon the tainted political power of the coroner and exchange it for the greater cultural power of science. Instead, forensic pathologists in the United States are regarded as a cadre of expert technicians, with very little real professional power outside their own sphere.[71] Although medicine was the most powerful professional model available in twentieth-century America, the power of medicine alone was unable to overcome the influences of both politics and the law on the development of forensic pathology. From the first, forensic pathology was relegated to an inferior position in the medical hierarchy, for it had no place in the hospital and was not aimed at treatment of the living. The Rockefeller Foundation's support of forensic medical training reinforced an inappropriate academic model of education, one which emphasized traditional clinical standards that were inapplicable to forensic pathological practice.

Moreover, in choosing to follow the professional model of medicine, American forensic pathologists have ignored the legal component of their specialty. Although lawyers did not resist the introduction of forensic pathology into the courtroom (as they did attempts to introduce forensic psychiatry and psychology) they did little to encourage the development of a truly interdisciplinary specialty.[72] Lawyers were content for forensic pathologists to remain useful but non-threatening contributors to the legal process.

Finally, the medical examiner system, American physicians' preferred institutional model for medico-legal practice, failed to deliver forensic pathologists the degree of autonomy and respect they sought. Its emphasis on medical credentials and control further obscured the legal component of the work, and its advocates' insistence that political considerations would be completely exorcized was extraordinarily ingenuous. Moreover, the medical examiner system proved very difficult to implement; criticisms of the coroner system could be easily silenced by the simple act of hiring forensic pathologists to fill the subordinate position of autopsy physician, obviating the need to replace the political figure of the coroner with the scientific figure of the medical examiner. In taking on politicians, American physicians found themselves confronting a group that exercised power in an entirely different manner. The abstract value system of science means little in the practical world of municipal bureaucracy, and positivism does not lend itself well to political compromise.

NOTES

Abbreviations employed:

JAMA	*Journal of the American Medical Association*
DLM	Department of Legal Medicine Files, Harvard Medical Archives, Countway Library
NRC	National Research Council, DIV MED: Committee on Medicolegal Problems
RAC	Rockefeller Foundation Archives, R.G. 1.1 200A Harvard University – Legal Medicine, Box 87
DAB	*Dictionary of American Biography*

1 For the history of American legal education, see Lawrence Friedman, *A History of American Law*, 2nd edn (New York: Simon & Schuster, 1985), especially

pp. 606–32, and Robert Bocking Stevens, *Law School: Legal Education in America from the 1850s to the 1980s* (Chapel Hill: University of North Carolina Press, 1983). For medical education, see Ronald L. Numbers, ed., *The Education of American Physicians* (Berkeley: University of California Press, 1980) and Paul W. Starr, *The Social Transformation of American Medicine* (New York: Basic Books, 1982), pp. 30–59, 112–44. George Rosen's *The Structure of American Medical Practice, 1875–1941* (Philadelphia: University of Pennsylvania Press, 1973) is an excellent introduction to the history of non-elite medical practice in the United States.

2 See Janet A. Tighe, 'A question of responsibility: the development of American forensic psychiatry, 1830–1930', unpublished Ph.D dissertation, University of Pennsylvania, 1984; James C. Mohr, *Abortion in America: The Origins and Evolution of National Policy, 1800–1900* (New York: Oxford University Press, 1978); and Mohr, *Doctors and the Law: Medical Jurisprudence in Nineteenth-Century America* (New York and Oxford: Oxford University Press, 1993). See also Leslie Reagan, '"About to meet her maker": women, doctors, dying declarations, and the state's investigation of abortion, Chicago, 1867–1940', *Journal of American History*, 77 (1991), 1240–64 and Kenneth Allen De Ville, *Medical Malpractice in Nineteenth-Century America: Origins and Legacy* (New York: New York University Press, 1990).

3 S. W. Abbott, 'The coroner system in the United States at the end of the nineteenth century', *Boston Medical and Surgical Journal*, 143 (1900), 418–20; Paul F. Mellen, 'Coroner's inquests in colonial Massachusetts', *Journal of the History of Medicine and Allied Sciences*, 40 (1985), 462–72; Oscar T. Schultz and E. M. Morgan, *The Coroner and the Medical Examiner* (*Bulletin of the National Research Council* No. 64) (Washington, DC, 1928); Dorothy I. Lansing, 'The coroner system and some of its coroners in early Pennsylvania', *Transactions and Studies of the College of Physicians of Philadelphia*, 44 (1977), 135–40; E. Donald Shapiro and Anthony David, 'Law and pathology throughout the ages: the coroner and his descendants – legitimate and illegitimate', *New York State Journal of Medicine*, 72 (1972), 805–9; William G. Eckert, 'The development of American forensic pathology, part I: colonial days to the early twentieth century', *Pathologist*, 31 (1977), 646–9.

4 See, for example, Arthur M. Schlesinger, *The Age of Jackson* (Boston: Little, Brown, 1953).

5 Abbott, 'Coroner system'; Schultz and Morgan, *The Coroner and the Medical Examiner*; George H. Weinmann, *A Compendium of the Statute Law of Coroners and Medical Examiners in the United States* (*Bulletin of the National Research Council* No. 83) (Washington, DC, 1931).

6 Chester R. Burns, 'Medical ethics and jurisprudence', in Numbers, ed., *Education of American Physicians*, pp. 273–89 gives an overview of the growth and extent of medico-legal education in American medical schools from the early nineteenth century to the present. Medical jurisprudence encompassed a variety of subjects, of which forensic pathology and toxicology formed only a part. It should always be kept in mind, however, that many American physicians failed to receive (or seek) an academic medical education. See also Russell C. Maulitz, 'Pathology', in the same volume, pp. 122–42. The classic American texts include Theodore R. Beck, *Elements of Medical Jurisprudence* (Albany:

Webster & Skinner, 1823); John Ordronaux, *The Jurisprudence of Medicine* (Philadelphia: T. & J. W. Johnson, 1869); and Francis Wharton and Alfred Stillé, *A Treatise on Medical Jurisprudence* (Philadelphia: Key Bros., 1855), which went through five editions by 1905. Many of the standard English texts also circulated in the United States.

7 Learned Hand, 'Historical and practical considerations regarding expert testimony', *Harvard Law Review*, 15 (1901–2), 40–58; Hubert Winston Smith, 'Cooperation between law and science in scientific proof', *Texas Law Review*, 19 (1941), 414–35 and Smith, 'Scientific proof and the relations of law and medicine', *Clinics*, 1 (1943), 1353–404; John A. Maguire, 'Expert testimony', in Edwin R. A. Seligman, ed., *Encyclopedia of the Social Sciences* (New York: MacMillan, 1931), pp. 13–15.

8 Michael B. Katz, *In the Shadow of the Poorhouse: A Social History of Welfare in America* (New York: Basic Books, 1986) and Katz, *The Undeserving Poor: From the War on Poverty to the War on Welfare* (New York: Pantheon, 1989).

9 There is disagreement among scholars as to whether crime rose in the nineteenth century at a rate greater than that of the population, but there was certainly a rise in the total numbers of crimes committed which served to inflate fears of the city and its poorer inhabitants. See Roger Lane, *Violent Death in the City: Murder, Suicide and Accident in Nineteenth Century Philadelphia* (Cambridge, MA: Harvard University Press, 1979); H. C. Brearley, *Homicide in the United States* (Montclair, NJ: Patterson Smith, 1969); and Frederick L. Hoffman, *The Homicide Problem* (Newark, NJ: The Prudential Press, 1925).

10 Robert H. Wiebe, *The Search for Order, 1877–1920* (New York: Hill & Wang, 1967); Charles E. Rosenberg, 'Science, society, and social thought', in Rosenberg, *No Other Gods: On Science and American Social Thought* (Baltimore: Johns Hopkins Press, 1976), pp. 1–21.

11 See, for example, American Academy of Medicine, *Physical Bases of Crime: A Symposium* (Easton, PA: American Academy of Medicine Press, 1914); Alphonse Bertillon, *Identification of the Criminal Classes by the Anthropometric Method* (London: Spottiswood & Co., 1889); Bernaldo de Quiros y Perez, *Modern Theories of Criminality* (Boston: Little, Brown, 1911); Arthur E. Fink, *Causes of Crime: Biological Theories in the United States, 1800–1915* (New York: A. S. Barnes & Company, 1962); Cesare Lombroso, *Les Applications de l'anthropologie criminelle* (Paris: F. Alcan, 1891); and Lombroso, *L'Homme criminel: étude anthropologique et médico-légale* (Paris: Alcan, 1876).

12 Vivianna Zelizer, *Morals and Markets: The Development of Life Insurance in the United States* (New York: Columbia University Press, 1979); Crystal Eastman, *Work, Accidents, and the Law* (New York: Charities Publication Committee, 1910); Charles C. Norris, 'The medical examiner versus the coroner', *National Municipal Review*, 9 (1920), 498–504; Louis R. Padberg, 'The relation of the physician to the coroner's office', *Missouri State Medical Association Journal*, 10 (1914), 361–5.

13 Schultz and Morgan, *The Coroner and the Medical Examiner*, pp. 13–14.

14 The classic article is Samuel P. Hays, 'The politics of municipal reform in the Progressive era', *Pacific Northwest Quarterly*, 55 (October 1965), 157–69. See also Steven P. Erie, *Rainbow's End: Irish-Americans and the Dilemmas of Urban Machine Politics, 1840–1985* (Berkeley: University of California Press, 1988)

and for a contemporary view, Lincoln Steffens, *The Shame of the Cities* (New York: Hill & Wang, 1957).

15 'Stenographer's notes of testimony before the September 1951 grand jury', Philadelphia City Archives (hereafter cited as Philadelphia Testimony), pp. 1012–25.

16 Philadelphia Testimony, passim; Leonard Michael Wallstein, *Report on the Special Examination of the Accounts and Methods of the Office of Coroner in the City of New York* (New York: Office of the Commissioner of Accounts, 1915); Ludwig Hektoen, 'The coroner (in Cook County)', in Illinois Association for Criminal Justice, *Illinois Crime Survey* (Montclair, NJ: Patterson Smith, 1968; first published in 1929), pp. 377–88; Raymond Moley, 'The sheriff and the coroner', in *The Missouri Crime Survey* (Montclair, NJ: Patterson Smith, 1968; first published in 1926), pp. 77–108 (hereafter cited as *Missouri Survey*); *The Coroner's Office: Report of the Investigation Made by the Coroner's Committee of the Municipal Association in the Interest of Economy and Efficiency* (Cleveland, Ohio: Municipal Association of Cleveland Efficiency Series Report No. 2, 1912, hereafter cited as *Cleveland Report*); Harrison S. Martland, 'Recent progress in the medicolegal field in the United States', *Proceedings of the Institute of Medicine of Chicago*, 9 (1933), 261–78; 'The reformation of the coroner's office', *JAMA*, 91 (1928), 963.

17 Weinmann, *Compendium of the Statute Law*, passim; Wallstein, *Report*; *Missouri Survey*; Hektoen, 'The coroner'; Schultz and Morgan, *The Coroner and the Medical Examiner*; *Cleveland Report*; Philadelphia Testimony.

18 Julie Johnson, 'William Scott Wadsworth: an appreciation of an anomalous career', *Transactions and Studies of the College of Physicians of Philadelphia*, Series 5, 12 (1990), 335–46; Samuel Warren Abbott, 'The coroner's inquest a medieval relic', *Philadelphia Medical Journal* (1898), 121–2; 'Coroner's science', *Philadelphia Medical Journal* (1902), 767; F. W. Searle, 'Coroner or medical examiner, which?', *Journal of Medicine and Science* (1903), 42–5; David I. Macht, 'The ancient office of coroner', *Johns Hopkins Hospital Bulletin*, 24 (1913), 148–53; 'Coroner's jury verdicts', *JAMA*, 36 (1901), 1709; 'The useless coroner', *JAMA*, 39 (1902), 1529; 'Abolish the coroner's office', *JAMA*, 40 (1903), 103; 'The necessity for better provision for legal medicine in this country', *JAMA*, 47 (1906), 585–7; 'The office of the coroner', *JAMA*, 60 (1913), 1644–5; 'The office of coroner', *JAMA*, 62 (1914), 1099; R. B. H. Gradwohl, 'The office of coroner: its past, its present, and the advisability of its abolishment in the commonwealth of Missouri', *JAMA*, 54 (1910), 842–6. Rosemary Stevens discusses *JAMA*'s role as medical muckraker in *American Medicine and the Public Interest* (New Haven: Yale University Press, 1971), p. 58.

19 American Medical Association, *Digest of Official Actions, 1846–1958* (Chicago: American Medical Association, 1958), pp. 24–5.

20 Schultz and Morgan, *The Coroner and the Medical Examiner*, pp. 50–90.

21 Starr, *Social Transformation*, pp. 79–145.

22 Raymond Moley, *An Outline of the Cleveland Crime Survey* (Cleveland, Ohio: The Cleveland Foundation, 1922), p. 50; 'Coroner's science', *Philadelphia Medical Journal* (1902), 767; Hektoen, 'The coroner', pp. 384–6; Wallstein, *Report*, passim; *Missouri Survey*, passim.

23 Maulitz, 'Pathology', and Esmond Long, *A History of Pathology* (New York: Dover Publications, Inc., 1965).
24 William F. Boos, *The Poison Trail* (Boston: Hale, Cushman and Flint, 1939), especially pp. 39–42; Jürgen Thorwald, *Dead Men Tell Tales* (London: Thames & Hudson, 1964), p. 120; 'George Burgess Magrath', *American Journal of Medical Jurisprudence*, 2 (1939), 52–3.
25 Edward D. Radin, *12 Against Crime* (New York: G. P. Putnam's Sons, 1950), pp. 3–24; Thorwald, *Dead Men Tell Tales*, pp. 122–5; Marshall Houts, *Where Death Delights: The Story of Dr. Milton Helpern and Forensic Medicine* (New York: Coward-McCann, 1967), p. 124.
26 Johnson, 'William Scott Wadsworth', 335–46.
27 Maulitz, 'Pathology', and Burns, 'Medical ethics and jurisprudence'.
28 Paul De Kruif, *The Microbe Hunters* (New York: Harcourt, Brace & Company, 1926); Starr, *Social Transformation*, pp. 156–7.
29 Stevens, *American Medicine*, pp. 226–8; Russell Maulitz, 'Pathologists, clinicians, and the role of pathophysiology', in Gerald Geison, ed., *Physiology in the American Context, 1850–1940* (Baltimore: American Physiological Society, 1987), pp. 210–33; William McKee German, *Doctors Anonymous: The Story of Laboratory Medicine* (New York: Duell, Sloan & Pearce, 1941).
30 Tighe, 'A question of responsibility', passim; Alfred Koerner, 'Diagnosis and treatment of legal congestion', *American Journal of Medical Jurisprudence*, 1 (1938), 34; Smith, 'Cooperation between law and science' and 'Scientific proof'; William L. Foster, 'Expert testimony: prevalent complaints and proposed remedies', *Harvard Law Review*, 11 (1897), 169–86; Edmund D. Morgan, 'Suggested remedy for obstruction to expert testimony by rules of evidence', *Clinics*, 1 (1943), 1627–43; Roscoe Pound, 'A ministry of justice as a means of making progress in medicine available for courts and legislatures', *Clinics*, 1 (1943), 1644–57; Catherine Crawford, 'A scientific profession: medical reform and forensic medicine in British periodicals of the early nineteenth century', in Roger French and Andrew Wear, eds., *British Medicine in an Age of Reform* (London: Routledge, 1991), pp. 201–30.
31 John Evarts Tracy, *Handbook of the Law of Evidence* (New York: Prentice-Hall, 1952), pp. 79–85; M. A. Barwise, 'Scientific proof and legal proof', *Maine Law Review*, 8 (1914–15), 67–86; Smith, 'Scientific proof' and 'Cooperation'; Hand, 'Historical and practical considerations'.
32 Milton Helpern and Bernard Knight, *Autopsy: The Memoirs of Milton Helpern, the World's Greatest Medical Detective* (New York: St Martin's Press, 1977), pp. 61–5; Koerner, 'Diagnosis and treatment', p. 34; Foster, 'Expert testimony'; Morgan, 'Suggested remedy'; Pound, 'A ministry of justice'.
33 See, for example, Editorial, *Philadelphia Medical Journal*, 29 November 1902, 814–15.
34 Johnson, 'William Scott Wadsworth', p. 344.
35 Ibid.
36 Ibid., p. 345.
37 William Scott Wadsworth, 'The coroner and the physician', *New York Medical Journal*, 103 (1916), 400–2; National Association of Coroners, 'First Annual Meeting, 1937–1938', DLM.
38 Michael M. Baden and Judith Adler Hennessee, *Unnatural Death: Confessions*

of a Medical Examiner (New York: Random House, 1989), p. 24; Richard Ford's notes for American Board of Pathology meeting, Chicago, October 1955, DLM.

39 *A History of the National Research Council, 1919–1933.* (Washington, DC, 1933).

40 William K. Beatty, 'Ludwig Hektoen: scientist and counsellor', *Proceedings of the Institute of Medicine of Chicago*, 35 (1982), 7–9.

41 Beatty, 'Ludwig Hektoen', pp. 7–9; Edwin F. Hirsch, 'The growth of forensic pathology in Illinois', *Proceedings of the Institute of Medicine of Chicago*, 26 (1967), 314–21; Paul R. Cannon, 'Ludwig Hektoen, 1863–1951', *Biographical Memoirs*, vol. XXVIII (Washington, DC: National Academy of Sciences, 1954), pp. 163–97; Henry Sewell, 'Victor Clarence Vaughan', *DAB* (New York: Charles Scribner's Sons, 1936), vol. XIX, pp. 236–7; Lucille B. Ritvo, 'Adolf Meyer', *DAB*, Supplement 4, pp. 569–72.

42 Victor Vaughan to George E. Vincent, 31 October 1924; Ludwig Hektoen to Herman Adler, 5 January 1925; Victor Vaughan to Vernon Kellogg, 2 June 1925 (NRC, 1924–6, General).

43 Ludwig Hektoen to R. M. Pearce, 14 January 1925 (NRC, 1924–6, General); Abraham Flexner to Ludwig Hektoen, 2 June 1925; memo, Victor Vaughan to Vernon Kellogg, 8 February 1926; Victor Vaughan to John Wigmore, 18 January 1926 (NRC, 1925–7, Surveys: Medicolegal Problems, General); Stephen Botein, 'John Henry Wigmore', *DAB*, Supplement 3, pp. 820–3; G. Edward White, '(Nathan) Roscoe Pound', *DAB*, Supplement 7, pp. 624–8. The American Medical Association established its Bureau of Legal Medicine in 1922 to serve as a clearinghouse for legal information and legislation of interest to the medical profession. It was not a specialty board or certifying agency, and should not be confused with the short-lived American Board of Legal Medicine of the 1930s. See J. W. Holloway, 'The Bureau of Legal Medicine and Legislation', in Morris Fishbein, *A History of the American Medical Association 1847–1947* (Philadelphia: W. B. Saunders Company, 1947), pp. 1010–33.

44 Schultz and Morgan, *The Coroner and the Medical Examiner*, pp. 58–77.

45 George H. Weinmann, *A Survey of the Law Concerning Dead Human Bodies* (*Bulletin of the National Research Council* No. 73) (Washington, DC, 1929) and Weinmann, *Compendium of the Statute Law*.

46 Minutes of the Committee on Medicolegal Problems, 2 November 1929, NRC; Oscar T. Schultz, *Possibilities and Need for Development of Legal Medicine in the United States* (*Bulletin of the National Research Council* No. 87) (Washington, DC, 1932).

47 Milton Helpern, 'The organization and founding of the department of forensic medicine of New York University', New York University Medical Archives; New York University College of Medicine, *Reports of Officers* (1932–3), p. 73.

48 C. Sidney Burwell to Alan Gregg, 5 January 1939, DLM.

49 Alan Gregg's Diary, 14 March 1935; Alan Gregg, memorandum of interview with Frances Glessner Lee, 19 March 1943, RAC.

50 E. Richard Brown, *Rockefeller Medicine Men: Medicine and Capitalism in America* (Berkeley: University of California Press, 1979), p. 155; Raymond Fosdick, *The Story of the Rockefeller Foundation* (New York: Harper & Brothers, 1952), p. 100; C. Sidney Burwell to Alan Gregg, 1 January 1939, RAC.

51 Alan R. Moritz to Robert A. Lambert, 11 January 1940, RAC.
52 Burwell to Gregg, 1 January 1939; George W. Gray, 'The medical sciences and the law', report to the Rockefeller Trustees, April 1945, RAC.
53 Rockefeller Foundation Resolution RF 39029, 17 March 1939; Frances Glessner Lee to Alan Gregg, 4 June 1942; Robert A. Lambert, memorandum of interview with Francis Glessner Lee, 21 May 1935, RAC.
54 Alan Moritz to Alan Gregg, 23 May 1947, RAC; Richard Ford to George Berry, 1 April 1952, Rockefeller Foundation Correspondence, DLM.
55 Century of Progress archives, University of Illinois at Chicago, Special Collections.
56 Radin, *12 Against Crime*, especially pp. 225–42; Ted Collins, ed., *New York Murders* (New York: Duell, Sloan and Pearce, 1944), p. xiii; Thomas C. Desmond, 'The coroner racket: A national scandal', *Coronet*, 28 (1950), 60–4; Peter Martin, 'How murderers beat the law', *Saturday Evening Post*, 10 December 1949, pp. 32–66.
57 In keeping with the defence orientation of his protagonist's practice, Gardner stressed forensic medicine's role in clearing the innocent, rather than convicting the guilty. *The Case of the Glamorous Ghost* (1955) was dedicated to the memory of George Burgess Magrath; *The Case of the Demure Defendant* (1956) to Dr Daniel J. Condon, the Maricopa County (Phoenix) Arizona medical examiner and Department of Legal Medicine alumnus; *The Case of the Long-Legged Models* (1957) to Michael Anthony Luongo of Harvard; *The Case of the Footloose Doll* (1958) to Dr Theodore J. Curphey, Los Angeles Coroner/Medical Examiner; *The Case of the Moth-Eaten Mink* (1952) to Russell S. Fisher, Chief Medical Examiner of Maryland and a graduate of the Harvard Department of Legal Medicine.
58 Richard Ford to George Berry, 1 April 1952, DLM.
59 Richard Ford to Lester Adelson, 8 December 1954, DLM.
60 William B. Wartman to Charles P. Larson, 13 December 1954, DLM and Stevens, *American Medicine*, pp. 204–5, 212–7.
61 Stevens, *American Medicine*, pp. 318–47.
62 Ibid., pp. 226–8.
63 Maulitz, 'Pathologists, clinicians, and the role of pathophysiology', pp. 210–33.
64 Lester Adelson to Richard Ford, 13 January 1954; Charles Larson to Shields Warren, 5 April 1955; James McNaught to Charles Larson, 13 April 1955, DLM.
65 Richard Ford to Lester Adelson, 8 January 1954, DLM.
66 Ibid.; Richard Ford to James Kernohan, 29 March 1955, DLM.
67 Richard Ford to Shields Warren, 26 April 1955; undated memo, Forensic Pathology Committee of the College of American Pathologists and the AMA Subcommittee on Forensic Pathology to the American Board of Pathology, DLM.
68 Richard Ford to Charles Larson, 28 November 1956; Shields Warren to Richard Ford, 28 January 1957, DLM.
69 Richard Ford to Charles Larson, 26 March 1957; Edward B. Smith to Richard Ford, 25 February 1958, DLM; American Board of Pathology, 'Requirements for certification in the special field of forensic pathology', memo, 21 May 1958.
70 The protocol and results of the autopsy on John Fitzgerald Kennedy are just

two of the many points of contention in the history of the assassination and its aftermath. Forensic pathologists, like their fellow citizens, are divided in their opinion as to whether Lee Harvey Oswald fired the fatal bullet. What is undisputed, however, is that the chief autopsy surgeon was not certified in forensic pathology, and had never before performed a post-mortem on a gunshot victim. One of his assistants was certified in forensic pathology, but he too lacked practical experience. Their failure to follow standard protocol in recording their findings has rendered the latter unreliable in the eyes of many, and the question of admissibility in court would certainly have arisen had Jack Ruby not assassinated Oswald before he could come to trial. For a detailed critique of the flaws in President Kennedy's autopsy, see Houts, *Where Death Delights*, pp. 26–73 and Baden and Hennessee, *Unnatural Death*, pp. 6–22.

71 Roger Smith 'Forensic pathology, scientific expertise, and the criminal law', in Roger Smith and Brian Wynne, eds., *Expert Evidence: Interpreting Science in the Law* (New York: Routledge, 1989), pp. 56–92 is an acute analysis of the role of the British forensic pathologist, which has many parallels to the American situation. Although the institutional structures of their practices differ, the common tradition of American and British legal procedure renders the *application* of forensic scientists' knowledge in the courts very similar.

72 Tighe, 'A question of responsibility'; Matthew Hale, *Human Science and Social Order: Hugo S. Munsterberg and the Origins of Applied Psychology* (Philadelphia: Temple University Press, 1980); John H. Wigmore, 'Professor Munsterberg and the psychology of testimony', *Illinois Law Review*, 3 (1909), 399–445.

V

Medical authority in question

12

Unbuilt Bloomsbury: medico-legal institutes and forensic science laboratories in England between the wars

NORMAN AMBAGE and MICHAEL CLARK

Introduction

During the half-century following 1870, state- or municipally-sponsored institutes of forensic medicine were established in Paris, Berlin, Vienna, Budapest and many other principal cities of Europe. Usually associated with university medical faculties, they served the dual purpose of teaching and research in forensic medicine and conducting medico-legal investigations, usually on behalf of the authorities.[1] The late nineteenth and early twentieth centuries also saw the creation of a number of laboratories specially devoted to 'criminalistics' or 'police science', a somewhat ill-defined field which may, however, roughly be equated with what was later to become known as 'forensic science'. These laboratories were sometimes associated with or even formed part of local medico-legal institutes, as in the case of Lyon, but were more often attached to government chemical or toxicological laboratories, as in the Swedish case, or else were exclusively under police control.[2] By 1930, almost every European capital and many other principal cities had its own medico-legal institute (France, for example, had three by 1933, in Paris, Lyon and Lille), while France, Italy, Germany, Switzerland, Sweden and even Finland all had at least one 'police science' laboratory.[3] Similar institutions also existed in Egypt, a country under overall British control but with its own, largely French-inspired internal administration and system of justice, while Ceylon had developed a rudimentary but apparently quite effective forensic science service run by the government chemist C. T. Symons.[4]

Among materially advanced European states and jurisdictions, only Great Britain and especially England stood out. While Scotland had the large and highly reputable regius professor's department of forensic medicine in Glasgow, and was busy developing another in Edinburgh,[5] England had no comparable institutions either in the sphere of forensic medicine or in that of forensic science. Although attendance for two terms at a course of lectures on 'medical jurisprudence' had been a compulsory part of the medical curriculum in England as in Scotland since the 1860s, there was no standard course of studies, the quality of instruction often left much to be desired, and there were scarcely any opportunities for students to gain practical experience in the conduct of medico-legal post-mortems. Examinations in medical jurisprudence were generally perfunctory, and there were no opportunities for postgraduate study.[6] By the 1920s, senior medico-legal practitioners and a few would-be reformers of legal education had become seriously concerned about the defects of English medico-legal education and practice, while during the 1930s, the Home Office was similarly to become aware of the inadequate provision for scientific aids to the detection of crime. This essay traces the origins and development of the professional and public agitation for the establishment of an English medico-legal institute during the interwar years and follows the steps taken by the Home Office in the 1930s to create a national network of forensic science laboratories for England and Wales. It also examines the relations between these two developments, and seeks to explain why the second was so much more successful than the first. Finally, it assesses the long-term consequences for English forensic medicine of the failure to establish a 'National Institute of Forensic Medicine', on the one hand, and the growth of an autonomous forensic science service, on the other.

The campaign to establish a medico-legal institute in London down to 1934

The beginnings of the campaign to establish a central medico-legal institute in association with the University of London may be traced at least as far back as 1902 when, in his presidential address to the newly-formed Medico-Legal Society, Sir William Job Collins (1859–1946) drew attention to the many defects in the existing provision for medico-legal education in London, and hoped that 'under the wing of the reconstituted University of London, a study so essentially academic [as medical jurisprudence] may find some congenial encouragement.'[7] In March 1907, while leading a joint deputation of the Medico-Legal Society and the London County Council to the Lord Chancellor on the subjects of death certification and coroners' law reform, Collins took advantage of the opportunity to impress upon Lord Loreburn 'the advantage[s] that should arise ... from the development of a school of medical jurisprudence in London worthy of the Metropolis and associated with its University',[8] while in July 1907, during a discussion of the dermatologist George Pernet's 'Remarks on the teaching of medical jurisprudence in Paris and London' at the Medico-Legal Society, several speakers agreed 'that a large practical and official school of medical jurisprudence was necessary [in London]'.[9] Some years later, in

1915, Professor Harvey Littlejohn of Edinburgh University more explicitly advocated 'the institution of a Medico-Legal Institute for London, closely associated with the Home Office ... [which] would be a centre of activity in this special branch of medicine', and suggested that 'It might be utilized largely by coroners in their work, and its officials be the Home Office experts in all medico-legal matters.'[10] The idea of a central medico-legal institute as part of a more general reform of medico-legal education in London was thus not unfamiliar or uncongenial to medico-legalists before the 1920s. However, it was not until the mid-1920s, when Lord Atkin of Aberdovey (1867–1944) became President of the Medico-Legal Society as well as Chairman of the Council of Legal Education, that detailed proposals for the creation of such an institute were first put forward.[11]

In May 1925, at Atkin's suggestion, the Council of the Medico-Legal Society formed a special committee, consisting of the Home Office pathologists Sir Bernard Spilsbury and Sir William Willcox, the barrister Frederick Danford Thomas, Mr Roland Burrows, KC, and Dr John Webster, the 'junior' Home Office Analyst, to consider 'the establishment in London of a central medico-legal institute for England and Wales',[12] and in June 1925 Atkin, Willcox and Spilsbury presented the committee's outline proposals to the Society's annual general meeting.[13] The committee recommended the establishment of a central medico-legal institute, together with a chair of medical jurisprudence, 'for the investigation of medico-legal cases, and for the control of the teaching of medical jurisprudence' in London. The institute would be under the joint control of the Home Office as regards medico-legal investigation and research, and of the Board of Education, the University of London and the Royal Colleges of Physicians and Surgeons as regards the teaching of forensic medicine. Its staff would be 'available for carrying out ... medico-legal investigations for the whole of England and Wales if required', until such time as similar institutes were established in provincial universities. The institute's staff was to consist of 'a number of full-time experts', including the Professor of Medical Jurisprudence, a 'Director of Investigations', a bacteriologist, a toxicologist and several part-time pathologists and laboratory assistants. They were to liaise with other senior members of the University's science and medical faculties, and to be responsible for postgraduate as well as undergraduate teaching in forensic medicine. Finally, in addition to the facilities for the post-mortem examination of bodies sent to the institute, there was to be a library and a museum of medico-legal and pathological specimens – this latter being a favourite idea of Spilsbury's.[14]

Not without some criticisms, these suggestions were formally adopted by the Society,[15] and subsequently met with general approval from the medical press, although both the *Lancet* and the *British Medical Journal* stressed 'the many [practical] difficulties – financial, statutory and otherwise' – which stood in the way of their realization.[16] However, Atkin felt sufficiently encouraged to suggest that his committee should continue to seek support from such interested parties as the Home Office, the Department of Public Prosecutions, the London County Council and the London medical schools, and begin to consider more concrete proposals for setting up the institute.[17] However, just as the movement in favour of the institute thus seemed to be gathering momentum, for reasons which are still not entirely clear it began to peter out instead. In December 1925, at the Medico-Legal Society's annual dinner, Earl Russell (presiding) confirmed 'that it was hoped in the next year or two to advance the scheme of a medico-legal institution for London',[18] but in fact no further progress had been made by the time Atkin handed over the presidency of the Society to Willcox in June 1927, and very little more was heard publicly of the scheme for the next two years. In June 1929 Willcox and Spilsbury told the Society that Atkin's scheme had had to be abandoned for want of financial support, but they also cited several other formidable obstacles to its realization, including problems of planning and organization, the vested interests of the London medical schools, conflicts of jurisdiction inherent in the existing state of coroners' law and practice, and what Spilsbury later described as 'a lack of Government encouragement, apart from words'.[19]

Between 1927 and 1934, the medico-legal institute proposals were never wholly lost sight of. Indeed, the general features of the scheme and the principal obstacles to its realization were discussed at length by the Medico-Legal Society in June 1929 and again in June 1931, while in December 1933 Atkin made a direct appeal for support to the presidents of the Royal Colleges of Physicians and Surgeons.[20] However, it was not until 1934–5 that circumstances were to change in such a way as not only to bring the question of the institute into the foreground of official (and, to a lesser extent, public) attention, but to open up the whole question of the place of science and medicine in the institutional organization and practice of police work and the administration of justice.

Origins and early development of the forensic science service in England and Wales

The interwar years saw the police forces of England and Wales struggling to adapt to rapidly changing economic and social conditions and new operational requirements. Reported crime figures rose sharply during the immediate postwar years and failed subsequently to return to their pre-1914 levels, while the economic and political upheavals of the immediate postwar years were accompanied by widespread public criticism of the police and a wave of industrial unrest among the rank-and-file.[21] The Desborough Committee, set up to review the organization of the police service throughout Great Britain in the aftermath of the police strikes of 1919, recommended the amalgamation of many small, inefficient local forces into larger, more efficient units,[22] but despite widespread public concern about the apparent inability of the detective branch to stem the rise of crime, by the early 1930s little had been done either to reorganize local police forces or to modernize police methods. However, in May 1933, a Home Office Departmental Committee on Detective Work and Procedure was appointed under the chairmanship of Arthur Dixon (1881–1969), former secretary to the Desborough Committee and, since 1922, Assistant Under-Secretary of State in charge of the Home Office Police Department, 'to enquire and report upon the organization and procedure of the police forces of England and Wales for the purpose of the detection of crime'.[23] In his official capacity, Dixon had long been convinced of the need for rationalization of the police forces, while in his leisure hours, he was a keen amateur scientist fascinated by the possibilities of applying science to police detective work.[24] As chairman of the Detective Committee, one of Dixon's first acts was to create a sub-committee (Sub-Committee D) to examine scientific aids to criminal investigation in England and Wales. The Detective Committee's findings, together with the roving reports of C. T. Symons, whom Dixon appointed Home Office Forensic Science Advisor on his return to England from Ceylon in 1934, were greatly to strengthen Dixon's belief that the police forces of England and Wales were in need of wholesale reorganization and modernization, and that the existing provision for 'scientific aids' to the detection of crime was quite inadequate.

On paper at least, a considerable body of forensic-scientific technique was already available to the police by the early 1930s.[25] Toxicology, in particular, had existed as a distinct specialty since the 1850s and was firmly established in several of the London teaching hospitals.[26] Blood-grouping techniques had begun to flourish after the discovery of the ABO blood-group system at the turn of the century and the sub-groups M and N in the 1920s. By the 1930s, the importance of blood-grouping in paternity cases had come to be recognized, and similar techniques had begun to be applied to the investigation of bloodstains.[27] In optical physics, considerable progress had been made in the use of ultra-violet and infra-red spectroscopy to detect removed or altered markings and semen and urine stains,[28] and interest was growing in the use of X-rays to examine fingerprints and ammunition.[29] Forgery, too, had come within the scientist's range of expertise. Chemical tests could now determine the age and constituents of ink, microscopic examinations could distinguish between old hand-made paper and linen and wood-pulp paper, detailed examinations of watermarks could be made, and research into 'graphometry', the scientific analysis of handwriting, was under way.[30] In the field of ballistics, it was now possible to examine spent bullet cases, to isolate rifling marks on fired projectiles, to discover the composition of the gunpowder used, and to produce comparison photomicrographs.[31] Thus without exaggerating the sensitivity and precision of some of the techniques employed or the degree of specialization which had been attained, scientific crime detection had clearly undergone rapid technical progress since the turn of the century, and now required substantial investment in laboratory equipment and technical support.

What concerned Dixon and the Detective Committee most, however, was not so much the extent and sophistication of available forensic techniques as their uptake by police detective forces. As Dixon noted:

> The application of science to detective purposes is a branch of police work in which this country is definitely backward. Very useful work has been done in a few forces, but this has been a matter of local and individual enterprise ... the possibilities of laboratory work for day to day purposes and as an aid to the detection of commonplace crimes like burglary and house-breaking (in which present day detection is making such a poor show) are unknown to, or at any rate quite unexplored by, most detectives in the country.[32]

Such 'forensic science' as did exist was organized on a largely *ad hoc* basis. Those who assisted the police in scientific investigations were, by and large, either public analysts or academic scientists who dabbled in forensic problems, such as Professors W. H. Roberts of Liverpool and F. G. Tryhorn of Hull, or else members of specialized occupations not normally connected with the police, such as the London gunsmith Robert Churchill, who was regularly called in by Scotland Yard to advise them on ballistics problems.[33] In addition, occasional use was made of the services of the Home Office Analysts, the Government Chemist's Laboratory and the National Physical Laboratory.[34]

Dixon wanted to bring science to bear upon everyday police problems and to make detectives aware of the ways in which science could help them; he wanted to develop scientific aids to the detection of crime on a 'comprehensive scale'.[35] He therefore decided upon a general plan of action. First, policemen were to be instructed in the benefits of scientific aids. Second, local police forces were to be provided with simple apparatus to stimulate their interest in scientific analyses. Third, regional laboratories, which were to be provided with 'all-round equipment' and well-qualified 'all-round staff[s]', were to be established throughout the country. The bulk of day-to-day examinations were to take place in these establishments. In addition, Dixon proposed that a central laboratory should be created to act as a clearing-house for information, to coordinate research, and to house a central library and museum of specimens. Finally, 'supplementary arrangements' were to be made to ensure that local police forces could call upon independent scientific and medical expertise should a particularly difficult problem arise. To this end, the new regional laboratories were to be located in university towns where the assistance of academic scientists could readily be obtained.[36]

The first of the new Home Office regional forensic science laboratories was established at Nottingham in 1936. Nottingham was chosen for a number of reasons. The local chief constable, Captain Athelstan Popkess, was enthusiastic about scientific aids to the detection of crime and had taken the trouble personally to visit police laboratories in Prague, Paris, Berlin and Dresden to obtain information and advice on scientific police work. There was already a small, vigorous scientific department within the Nottingham police force, which employed a full-time physicist and retained a consultant botanist, while the local Watch Committee was eager to support the chief constable in this new venture. The new laboratory was to carry out chemical, physical and biological examinations. Chemically, the scientists were to identify blood as such and to analyse oil, paint, dyes, inks, poisons and drugs. On the physical side, suspect documents were to be examined for erasure marks, fraud and handwriting peculiarities, and research into tool-marks and ballistics problems carried out. As for biology, analyses were to be made of blood species, blood groups and sperm; hairs, feathers and fur; textiles, wood and leather; and animal and vegetable debris and dust.[37]

Meanwhile Lord Trenchard (1873–1956), who had already launched a wide range of reforms since his appointment as Commissioner of the Metropolitan Police in 1931 and had kept in close touch with the work of the Detective Committee, had decided to establish a forensic science laboratory alongide his new Metropolitan Police College at Hendon in north London.[38] Trenchard was convinced that 'a Force like the Metropolitan ... cannot be regarded as fully efficient without its own scientific department', and saw the creation of a forensic science laboratory or, better still, a national medico-legal institute as one way of restoring the Metropolitan Police to its traditional primacy among British police forces.[39] On the recommendation of Spilsbury and Lord Dawson of Penn, President of the Royal College of Physicians, Trenchard consulted Scotland's two most senior medico-legal experts, Professors John Glaister, Jr of Glasgow and Sydney Smith of Edinburgh, both of whom unhesitatingly recommended that a doctor should be put in charge of any new police laboratory.[40] However, as neither of them was willing to come to London for the comparatively modest salary on offer, Dr James Davidson, an Edinburgh pathologist and colleague of Smith's, was appointed first Director of the

Laboratory instead. The chemists L. C. Nickolls and C. G. Daubney were seconded to the Laboratory from the Government Chemist's Laboratory, and Detective-Sergeant C. R. M. Cuthbert of Scotland Yard was appointed police liaison officer.[41]

The new Metropolitan Police Laboratory was opened at Hendon by the Home Secretary, Sir John Gilmour, on 10 April 1935. But Trenchard already had a much more ambitious project in mind. On his advice, Gilmour simultaneously announced the creation of an Advisory Committee to oversee the development of the new Laboratory and to keep 'in close and effective touch on the one hand with other police institutions ... and on the other hand with any Medico-Legal or Scientific Institute that may be constituted for teaching and research work in forensic medicine or other relevant sciences'.[42] Of the Committee's eventual twelve members, five, including Lord Dawson of Penn, Sir Arthur MacNalty, chief medical officer of the Ministry of Health, the Home Office pathologist Sir Bernard Spilsbury and Sir Frederick Menzies, chief medical officer to the London County Council, were medical men.[43]

Dixon was alarmed by the apparent medical bias of Trenchard's plans. Although forensic medicine had, by and large, hitherto dominated the field of scientific crime investigation, Dixon's plan was to bring science, rather than medicine, to the assistance of the police. It was clear to Dixon that, in relation to the perceived growth in crime, those offences causing most concern were, as Trenchard himelf had pointed out in his annual reports, break-ins and larcenies rather than the most serious crimes of violence. According to Home Office statistics, 95 per cent of all reported indictable offences were crimes against property, that is, offences more susceptible to scientific than to medical investigation, while of the mere 2.5 per cent which were crimes of violence against the person, cases of rape and indecent assault outnumbered homicides of all descriptions by more than 50 per cent.[44] Dixon and Symons believed that established forensic pathologists such as Spilsbury were more interested in obscure or suspicious cases of sudden death than in common offences such as rape, indecent assault and drunken driving, whose investigation normally involved police surgeons and, later, forensic chemists and biologists rather than forensic pathologists. Dixon did not exclude the possibility of a medico-legal institute being established alongside his own planned network of regional forensic science laboratories, but he believed that the provision of medico-legal expertise was best organized locally rather than nationally, and was horrified by Trenchard's casual assumption that all the regional laboratories would be placed under the direction of the proposed central medico-legal institute. As time passed, the differences between Trenchard's plan for a central 'Medico-Legal or Scientific Institute' and Dixon's scheme for a national forensic science service with local 'supplementary arrangements' for medico-legal expertise became steadily more apparent, and the conventional niceties of official communication barely sufficed to conceal the growing tension and hostility between them.[45]

Forensic medicine and science in England in the 1930s

Before the 1930s, in England as in Scotland, the field of scientific crime investigation had been virtually indistinguishable from that of forensic medicine. Although in many other parts of Europe separate provision was made for forensic examinations involving chemistry, biology and physics, in England most such investigations were carried out either by medically qualified chemists such as the Home Office Analysts Gerald Roche Lynch and John Webster, or by freelance experts working under the direction of forensic pathologists. Continuing in the Victorian tradition of all-round forensic 'expertise', medico-legal experts such as Sir Bernard Spilsbury performed many of their own forensic-chemical, biological and bacteriological investigations, and were responsible for presenting and interpreting the results of analyses made by non-medically qualified chemists in court.[46] Unlike forensic medicine, 'forensic science' had few independent practitioners, no institutional base or professional organization of its own, and for all practical purposes was subsumed under forensic medicine.

However, despite this apparently strong position, English forensic medicine was in many respects unprepared to meet the challenge presented by an institutionally and professionally autonomous forensic science. The fact that no English institution featured in the Rockefeller Foundation's world-wide survey of *Institutes of Legal Medicine* (1928) highlighted the grave deficiencies of the existing provision for medico-legal education and research in England and Wales compared with Scotland and most other European countries. Great divisions existed within legal medicine between metropolitan and provincial practitioners, on the one hand, and between senior pathologists and police surgeons, on the other. Hardworking, experienced police surgeons such as Morgan Finnucane bitterly resented attempts by largely self-certifying expert pathologists to secure a virtual monopoly of medico-legal work, while non-medically qualified chemists such as C. Ainsworth Mitchell were equally resentful of their treatment by medical experts as forensic 'also rans'.[47] The Ministry of Health had failed to make any adequate provision for forensic medicine in the new London Postgraduate Medical School, while the Home Office refused to initiate or consent to any positive scheme of medico-legal reform. In these circumstances, the idea of a medico-legal institute closely connected with the University of London, whose well-paid and experienced staff would constitute an authoritative source of medico-legal expertise for the whole country, served as a powerful focus for more general aspirations towards a reform of English forensic medicine which would harmonize its internal divisions, enhance the prestige of its leading practitioners and reaffirm its traditional dominance of the field of scientific crime investigation. Yet the renewed agitation for medico-legal reform in the mid-1930s was instead to expose many of the underlying conflicts of interest and opinion within forensic medicine, the isolation and political impotence of its leading spokesmen, and the growing irrelevance of traditional conceptions of medically-dominated and directed 'scientific jurisprudence' to the newly emerging pattern of forensic science.

The contrasting fortunes of the Detective Committee and the Home Office Advisory Committee on the Scientific Investigation of Crime

In June 1936, the Advisory Committee on the Scientific Investigation of Crime, which had been established to oversee the development of Trenchard's new Metropolitan Police Laboratory, issued an interim report which noted that although the laboratory was still at an experimental stage, it was founded upon sound principles and predicted that its development would 'follow naturally upon an increasing realisation of its value as part of the crime-fighting machinery'.[48] Accordingly, even before the publication of its report, the Committee recommended an increase in the laboratory's staff – ironically, the only one of its recommendations which was to be accepted.[49] As regards the use of science generally in the detection of crime, the Committee concluded that the laboratory was 'a development of immense value which should be pressed forward without delay'.[50]

At this point, however, the Committee's interest in forensic science and in the Hendon laboratory itself abruptly ceased. Instead, attention shifted to the question of a medico-legal institute. The Committee:

> made no excuse for having concentrated upon this general problem ... We recognise, of course, that in doing so we may be regarded as having gone beyond the strict limitations of our Terms of Reference, since the recommendations we propose cover a wider field than that of any organisation related solely to police requirements.[51]

The Committee considered that the 'provision made in this country for the teaching and practice of forensic medicine [was] on the whole inadequate'.[52] It therefore recommended the establishment of a central medico-legal institute, preferably to be located in the Bloomsbury precinct of the University of London, to carry out teaching and research in forensic medicine and perform routine post-mortem examinations for coroners and the police. In order that the institute might be academically recognized, it was to be established 'as a School of the University of London in the Faculty of Medicine' and its director to be given a chair in forensic medicine.[53] The Committee concluded that its report was a 'brief outline of a scheme which ... is long overdue and should be pressed forward as a matter of definite public importance'.[54]

Like the proposals made by Lord Atkin's sub-committee more than a decade earlier, the Advisory Committee's report was well received by the medical press.[55] Doubtless encouraged by this reception and apparently convinced that his Committee's proposals enjoyed the full support of the University of London, Trenchard promptly began to seek financial backing for the institute from a variety of potential benefactors, including Lords Austin and Nuffield, Sir Henry Wellcome and the Rockefeller Foundation.[56] The Home Office, however, took a much less sanguine view, as did the Treasury. The official members of the Advisory Committee had repeatedly, though unsuccessfully, tried to steer the Committee away from its preoccupation with the medico-legal institute scheme back to its brief to oversee the development of the 'almost forgotten' Hendon laboratory,[57] and even before the publication of the interim report, Sir Russell Scott (1877–1960), Permanent Under-Secretary of State at the Home Office and a close ally of Dixon's on the Committee, had decided to hand over all responsibility for the Committee's proposals to the Ministry of Health, on the grounds that the 'proposed scheme [was] primarily concerned not with the scientific investigation of crime but with medical education'.[58] The Ministry of Health's reaction to this move was highly ambivalent. While Sir Arthur MacNalty, chief medical officer to the Ministry and himself a member of the Advisory Committee, conceded that there was a strong case for establishing a medico-legal institute, he and his colleagues were well aware of Dixon and Scott's lack of enthusiasm for the scheme, and strongly resented being made to do the Home Office's dirty work for it. During the latter part of 1936 and the early months of 1937, they discussed the Advisory Committee's proposals at great length, but although generally convinced of the merits of the medico-legal institute scheme, they were ultimately no more willing to accept responsibility for its implementation than the Home Office had been. Once it became apparent that the University of London was no longer wholeheartedly in favour of the proposal, the Ministry of Health's own interest rapidly declined.[59] After almost a year, a question was asked in the House of Commons about the fate of the Advisory Committee's report. Sir John Simon, Gilmour's successor at the Home Office, replied that he was still 'in consultation on the matter'.[60] In June 1938, Trenchard wrote to the Home Office saying that if nothing was done about the proposed medico-legal institute, his Committee would 'resign in a body'.[61] The Home Office and the Treasury were unmoved, having long since decided that 'the resignation of the Committee would not be a very serious matter'.[62] By 1938, Trenchard saw that he was getting nowhere, and although he

> had hoped that the time had come when this country might cease to deserve the reproach of lagging behind the greater part of the civilised world in organising research and instruction in a subject of such great national importance,

he offered to adjourn his Committee indefinitely.[63] In July 1938, just over two years after the interim report had first been published, Sir Samuel Hoare (who had meanwhile succeeded Simon as Home Secretary) wrote to Trenchard: 'I welcome your view that the Committee should be ... adjourned *sine die*, in order that it may be reconstituted when circumstances permit'[64] – a pious hope which, of course, remained unfulfilled. The Advisory Committee's report thus remained a dead letter, its fate 'a sad commentary on official lassitude'.[65]

In contrast, by the outbreak of the Second World War, Dixon's Detective Committee had established forensic science laboratories at Nottingham, Birmingham, Cardiff, Bristol and Preston, and plans were in hand for a similar establishment at Wakefield. Formal detective training courses which, at least in part, offered a painless introduction to scientific aids, had been instituted at Hendon, Birmingham and in the West Riding and a permanently established Special Services Committee, together with a permanent and growing Special Services Fund, had been created within the Home Office to oversee the development of Dixon's scheme.[66]

Several reasons can be given for the contrasting fates of Dixon and Trenchard's committees. First, the Advisory Committee seemed unable to steer itself in any definite direction. Trenchard himself was incapable of distinguishing between forensic science and forensic medicine and unable as chairman to give the Committee's discussions any proper lead. The Committee members with the greatest interest in the scientific investigation of crime, notably Lord Atkin and Sir Bernard Spilsbury, in fact made few effective contributions to the discussions, while the civil servants Dixon, Sir Russell Scott and S. J. Baker contrived subtly to undermine the whole idea of a medico-legal institute.[67] Second, Trenchard's proposals were very expensive. They were costed at nearly £300,000 – more than the entire cost of the recently-established Royal Post-Graduate Medical School at Hammersmith.[68] In 1937, against a background of rapidly growing expenditure on rearmament, Scott minuted that 'It may well be doubted whether there has ever been a less auspicious moment for seeking Treasury sanction',[69] and in May 1938 Hoare believed that 'there was not the least chance of a Treasury grant in present circumstances'.[70] These expectations were indeed well-founded, for the Treasury was anxious to avoid giving any encouragement to Trenchard's proposals, and on hearing of the Advisory Committee's adjournment merely commented that 'We should ... have preferred the demise of [the] Committee to its continuance even in suspended animation.'[71]

Third, Dixon and Scott, wishing to concentrate governmental attention and funds on the developing forensic science service, undermined Trenchard's proposals for a medico-legal institute by arguing that it would concentrate on obscure or sensational cases of sudden death while neglecting more common but, for the police, more troublesome crimes against property and non-fatal assaults. Moreover, Dixon's own plans for a central forensic-scientific laboratory were in direct competition with Trenchard's proposals for a central medico-legal institute. Dixon maintained that:

> Scientific police work ... covers a very much wider field than ... medicine; in fact ... the pathological side of the work is not so important as that of the pure sciences. Whether, therefore, a Central Medico-Legal Institute, organised and developed on the lines recommended by Lord Trenchard's Committee, would be able to discharge the functions of the central organisation which this work requires, and indeed whether it is desirable that it should do so, are questions which can finally be decided only in the light of experience. On the whole, however, we incline to the view that ... the central organisation should be more intimately connected with the ordinary day-to-day work [of the police] than the contemplated Medico-Legal Institute would be.[72]

Last but not least, it no doubt suited the Baldwin and Chamberlain governments for Trenchard to remain absorbed in the work of the Advisory Committee for as long as possible at a crucial stage of their rearmament programme. As early as 1934, only three years after taking up his appointment, Trenchard had apparently decided that his work as Commissioner of the Metropolitan Police had already been accomplished and that henceforth his main interests lay elsewhere, notably in defence.[73] The Cabinet, however, wanted him to remain in post, partly, it appears, because they did not want the 'father of the Royal Air Force' sniping at them for their perceived neglect of the fighting services.[74] Towards the end of 1935, Trenchard was again determined to go, but although the Cabinet were eventually forced to accept his resignation, they were still anxious to prevent him from meddling in military affairs, especially those of the RAF.[75] Trenchard was a strong advocate of strategic bombing, while the government wanted to build up fighter defences instead. For the government, the Advisory Committee may therefore simply have been a convenient way of keeping Trenchard harmlessly occupied until it was too late for him to interfere with the overall direction of the rearmament programme. If so, it seems to have served its purpose well.

In contrast, Dixon's plans for a national forensic science service had Home Office and Treasury approval from the start. The introduction of scientific aids was seen as a direct attack on the problems of rising crime and dwindling detection rates. Nor did the scheme cost much, at least not at first; the Special Services Fund began life in 1935 with a mere £2,000, and by the outbreak of war still stood at only £40,000.[76] As a professional administrator, unlike the non-official members of the Advisory Committee, Dixon devoted his whole time to the problems of the Police Department and had very definite plans for the development of the forensic science service. Finally, whereas Trenchard was a political embarrassment, Dixon's influence was growing, and promotion to Principal Assistant Under-Secretary of State and a knighthood were only just around the corner.[77] Not surprisingly, then, by 1939 the forensic science service had firmly taken root and was rapidly developing, while Atkin and Trenchard's plans for the long-awaited medico-legal institute remained unfulfilled.

Aftermath and conclusion

The dream of establishing a medico-legal institute and chair of forensic medicine in the University of London did not entirely fade away after 1938. In February 1951, Professor Sir Sydney Smith of Edinburgh gave a paper to the Medico-Legal Society in which he called for the establishment of a broadly-based 'Institute of Forensic Medicine and Criminology' which would concern itself not only with medico-legal education and investigations but with the 'cause and prophylaxis' of the 'social disease of crime'.[78] More conventionally, in 1952 the editors of the *Medico-Legal Journal* called for the establishment of an 'Academy or Institute of Medical Jurisprudence' to help improve standards of medical evidence in the civil and criminal courts,[79] while in a symposium on 'The teaching of forensic medicine' held at Guy's Hospital in November 1954, Professor John Glaister, Jr of Glasgow once again called for the creation of a medico-legal institute to serve the needs of postgraduate training in forensic medicine.[80] An editorial of December 1960 in the *Medico-Legal Journal* still referred to an institute as 'the ultimate goal' of current attempts to improve standards of teaching and practice,[81] and as recently as 1973 Professor Keith Mant of Guy's declared that the creation of both a central medico-legal institute and a national, full-time forensic pathology service were essential for the survival of English forensic medicine.[82] However, none of these appeals has found favour either with the Home Office or the University of London. The postwar institutional development of English forensic medicine has instead focused largely on the 'mini-' medico-legal institutes created in the metropolitan and provincial teaching hospital departments of forensic medicine, while the Forensic Science Service has continued to develop under the quite separate auspices of the Home Office.[83]

For many of its leading advocates, the medico-legal institute scheme meant much more than just a reform of medico-legal education. For Trenchard, it was part and parcel of his plans for the wholesale modernization and reform of the Metropolitan Police Force, along with the Police College, the short-service commissions and the new Metropolitan Police Laboratory. The institute was to be the culmination of his plans for the organization of 'scientific jurisprudence' in the Metropolitan Police district, something which would help restore the Force's lost prestige and regain its leading position among Britain's police forces.[84] Atkin, Willcox and Spilsbury were much more concerned with the institute's potential contributions to medico-legal education and practice. But the institute also symbolized their aspirations towards a 'New Deal' for English forensic medicine which would rectify its traditional institutional weaknesses, enhance its status within general medicine and place it at the forefront of developments not only in 'police science' but in modern medicine as a whole. Viewed in this light, the failure to create a 'National Institute of Forensic Medicine' in London in the 1930s appears to mark a major turning-point in the history of modern English forensic medicine. Thereafter, 'classical' forensic medicine became, if not wholly irrelevant, at any rate increasingly marginal to the Home Office's plans for the development of the forensic science services, and of less and less importance to general medicine and surgery. While (at least, until very recently) the Forensic Science Service has enjoyed a steady growth in resources and personnel, since the 1950s English forensic medicine (or, more precisely, forensic pathology) has suffered the contraction or closure of more than half of its university and teaching hospital departments, lost all but one (Leeds) of its established chairs, and seen a steady decline in both the numbers of its accredited full-time practitioners and of new recruits to the specialty.[85] Many factors other than the lack of a strong central institution have contributed to this decline, which has itself not been uniform in its incidence, while the rapid growth of technical and professional specialization in every aspect of forensic science since 1945 makes it highly unlikely that any such institution could have succeeded in maintaining overall medical control of the development of scientific crime investigation. Nevertheless, the failure to establish a national centre of medico-legal expertise has undoubtedly been an important factor in the apparently inexorable decline of English forensic medicine. Lacking any strong institutional focus for its identity, excluded from the National Health Service at its formation and remaining isolated from the mainstreams of postwar medical research and practice, forensic medicine has languished on the fringes of general medicine and pathology and enjoyed few, if any, of the benefits which the coming of the NHS, postwar economic growth and the expansion of higher education have conferred on almost every other medical specialty.[86]

NOTES

1 For the development of medico-legal institutes worldwide during this period, see Rockefeller Foundation, Division of Medical Education, *Methods and Problems of Medical Education*, 9th Series: *Institutes of Legal Medicine* (New York, 1928).

2 Probably the best introductory surveys of the growth of 'police science' and police science laboratories are still Jürgen Thorwald, *The Marks of Cain* and *Dead Men Tell Tales (The Century of the Detective)*, trans. Richard and Clara Winston (London, 1965 and 1966).

3 Thorwald, *Dead Men Tell Tales*, p. 196.

4 For Egypt, see Sydney Smith, 'Medicolegal Institute, Ministry of Justice of the Egyptian Government, Cairo', in Rockefeller Foundation, *Institutes of Legal Medicine*, pp. 49–54, and PRO HO45/17568, sub-file 694370/10, 'Egyptian Medico-Legal Institute'. For Symons's work in Ceylon, see the account given in PRO HO45/17085, Sir Herbert Dowbiggin, Inspector-General of Police (Ceylon) to A. L. Dixon, 6 June 1934, and enclosures.

5 For Glasgow, see John Glaister, Senior, 'Forensic Medicine Department, University of Glasgow', in Rockefeller Foundation, *Institutes of Legal Medicine*, pp. 201–11, and M. Anne Crowther and Brenda M. White, *On Soul and Conscience: The Medical Expert and Crime. One Hundred and Fifty Years of Forensic Medicine in Glasgow* (Aberdeen, 1988), ch. 4. For Edinburgh, see Harvey Littlejohn, 'Department of Forensic Medicine, University of Edinburgh', in Rockefeller Foundation, *Institutes of Legal Medicine*, pp. 187–99.

6 On the state of medico-legal education in England around the turn of the century, see especially Sir William Job Collins, 'Inaugural address', *Transactions of the Medico-Legal Society* (hereafter *TMLS*), 1 (1902–4), 14–29, at pp. 20–1; Harvey Littlejohn, 'The teaching of forensic medicine', *TMLS*, 12 (1914–15), 1–12, at pp. 6–7; George Pernet, 'Remarks on the teaching of medical jurisprudence in Paris and London', *TMLS*, 4 (1906–7), 113–21, at pp. 118–21, and the comments of Drs Willcox and Cowburn in the subsequent discussion, on pp. 123–4.

7 Collins, 'Inaugural address', p. 6. For Collins, see *Who Was Who 1941–1950*, pp. 238–9.

8 Sir William Job Collins, in 'Death certification and coroners' law amendment. Deputation to the Lord Chancellor (Lord Loreburn)', *TMLS*, 4 (1906–7), 69–82, at p. 75.

9 Pernet, 'Teaching of medical jurisprudence', discussion, p. 122.

10 Littlejohn, 'Teaching of forensic medicine', p. 11.

11 Atkin became President of the Council of Legal Education in 1919 and of the Medico-Legal Society in 1923. For further details of Atkin's life and work, see *Dictionary of National Biography* (hereafter *DNB*) *1942–1950*, pp. 27–8, and Robert A. Wright, *Lord Atkin of Aberdovey 1867–1944* (London, 1951).

12 'Proposed central medico-legal institute', *British Medical Journal* (hereafter *BMJ*), 1 (1925), 1039.

13 'The proposed formation of a medico-legal institute', *TMLS*, 18/19 (1923–5), 128–62, at pp. 129–33 (Atkin's speech), pp. 133–9 (Spilsbury's) and pp. 139–42 (Willcox's).

14 Ibid., pp. 161–2.

15 Ibid., pp. 158–9. For criticisms of the committee's proposals, see pp. 148–9 (Dr Halliday Sutherland) and pp. 149–50 (Dr Morgan Finnucane).

16 'Proposed medico-legal institute', *BMJ*, 1 (1925), 1184–5, at p. 1184; 'A medico-legal institute', *Lancet*, 1 (1925), 1307.

17 *TMLS*, 18/19 (1923–5), 148.

18 'Medico-legal society', *Lancet*, 2 (1925), 1310.

19 See Willcox's and Spilsbury's contributions to the discussion of F. Temple Grey, 'The medico-legal expert in France', *TMLS*, 23 (1928–9), 172–5 (paper), 176–83 (discussion), on pp. 179–81 (Spilsbury) and pp. 181–2 (Willcox). See also Spilsbury's much later comments in his contribution to the discussion of W. G. Barnard, 'The medico-legal institute', *Medico-Legal and Criminological Review* (hereafter *ML & CR*), 5 (1937), 28–39 (paper), 39–53 (discussion), on p. 40.

20 See Temple Grey, 'The medico-legal expert in France', discussion, 176–83; T. H. Blench, 'Crime investigation in Paris', *TMLS*, 25 (1930–1), 167–83 (paper), 183–91 (discussion); and report of Lord Atkin's speech to the annual dinner of the Medico-Legal Society, 8 December 1933, in *ML & CR*, 2 (1934), 143, with the replies of Lord Dawson of Penn, President of the Royal College of Physicians, and Sir Hubert Waring, President of the Royal College of Surgeons, on pp. 145 and 151 respectively.

21 For the history of the police during this period, see T. A. Critchley, *A History of Police in England and Wales*, revd edn (London, 1978) pp. 182–201, 203–14; D. Ascoli, *The Queen's Peace: The Origins and Development of the Metropolitan Police 1829–1979* (London, 1979) pp. 192–205, 225–41; Clive Emsley, *The English Police: A Political and Social History* (Hemel Hempstead and New York, 1991), pp. 123–8, 151–6; and Norman Ambage, 'The origins and development of the Home Office Forensic Science Service, 1931–1967', unpublished Ph.D thesis, University of Lancaster, 1987, chs. 1–3. For the problem of increasing reported crime and declining detection rates in the immediate postwar period, see especially Ambage, 'Origins and development of the Forensic Science Service', pp. 33–5.

22 *Report of the Committee on the Police Service of England, Wales and Scotland* (the Desborough Committee), in *Parliamentary Papers 1919*, xxvii, 709 (Cmd. 253, Pt. 1) and *1920*, xxii, 539 (Cmd. 574, Pt. 2). See also Critchley, *History of Police*, pp. 188–94 and Ascoli, *The Queen's Peace*, pp. 151–3.

23 *Report of the Departmental Committee on Detective Work and Procedure*, 5 vols. (London: HMSO, 1939, reprinted 1947), vol. I, p. 11.

24 For Dixon's amateur scientific interests, see *DNB 1961–1970*, pp. 296–7, and Ambage, 'Origins and development of the Forensic Science Service', ch. 2.

25 Two useful surveys of scientific aids to the detection of crime available in the late 1920s are John Glaister, Sr, 'The evolution, development and application of modern medico-legal methods', *Glasgow Medical Journal*, 109 (1928), 417–37, and Sir William Willcox, 'Recent advances in toxicology and forensic medicine', *TMLS*, 22 (1927–8), 1–13.

26 On the development of toxicology in England, see especially Jürgen Thorwald, *Proof of Poison (The Century of the Detective)*, trans. Richard and Clara Winston (London, 1966) pp. 75–84, 100–101, 106–21; R. Smith, 'Forensic medicine and chemical expertise', paper to Historical Symposium of the Royal Society of Chemistry Annual Chemical Congress, Lancaster University, April 1983; Noel G. Coley, 'Alfred Swaine Taylor, MD, FRS (1806–1880): forensic toxicologist', *Medical History*, 35 (1991), 409–27.

27 See especially Glaister, 'Modern medico-legal methods', pp. 426–33; F. C. Martley, 'The importance of bloodgrouping tests in paternity cases', *TMLS*, 25 (1930–1), 25–33 (paper), 33–8 (discussion); S. C. Dyke, 'The human blood groups', *ML & CR*, 1 (1933), 99–111 (paper), 111–17 (discussion); David Harley and G. Roche Lynch, 'Blood group tests in disputed paternity', *ML & CR*, 5 (1937), 182–90; G. Roche Lynch, D. Harley and D. Harcourt Kitchin, 'The medico-legal importance of the blood groups, with special reference to non-paternity', ibid., 269–84 (paper), 284–96 (discussion). On the history of blood-grouping during the first decades of the twentieth century, see Thorwald, *Dead Men Tell Tales*, pp. 50–9; Jan Hirschfeld, 'The birth of serology and the discovery of the human ABO system', *Nordisk Medicinhistorisk Arsbok 1976* (Stockholm, 1977), pp. 163–80; A. D. Farr, 'Blood group serology – the first four decades', *Medical History*, 23 (1979), 215–26.

28 See, for example, Willcox, 'Recent advances', p. 13; C. Ainsworth Mitchell, 'The use of invisible rays in criminology', *ML & CR*, 3 (1935), 3–14, at pp. 6–10, 11–14.

29 Ibid., pp. 10–11.

30 C. Ainsworth Mitchell, 'Forgeries and their detection', *TMLS*, 24 (1929–30), 139–50; Lieut.-Col. W. W. Mansfield, 'Invisible light [*sc.*; ultra-violet radiation] and forgery detection', *ML & CR*, 7 (1939), 29–36.

31 R. Churchill, 'The examination of fire-arms and ammunition', *TMLS*, 25 (1930–1), 82–90; G. Burrard, 'The identification of firearms by microscopic examination of fired cartridge cases and fired bullets', *ML & CR*, 3 (1935), 96–8.

32 PRO HO45/20546/674932/4, memorandum by Dixon, undated [1931].

33 For the position in the provinces generally in the early and mid-1930s, see especially Symons's reports to Dixon in PRO HO45/17110; H. J. Walls, 'The Forensic Science Service in Great Britain; a short history', *Journal of the Forensic Science Society*, 16 (1976), 273–8, at pp. 274–7, and Ambage, 'Origins and development of the Forensic Science Service', chs. 2 and 3. For Roberts's police work, see HO45/16215, Chief Constable C. C. Moriarty of Birmingham to Dixon, 22 July 1935. Tryhorn later became Director of the Forensic Science Laboratory at Wakefield and Home Office Forensic Science Advisor.

34 On the use of the Home Office Analysts, the Government Chemist's Laboratory and the National Physical Laboratory, see PRO HO45/14646.

35 PRO HO45/20546/674932/4, memorandum by Dixon on 'Scientific Aids', 1931.

36 Ibid.

37 For developments at Nottingham, see PRO HO45/18103, C. T. Symons to Dixon, 16 August 1935; PRO HO45/18104, undated memorandum by Dixon, October 1936, and A. Popkess, 'Pursuit by science', *Police Journal*, 8 (1935), 199–214, especially p. 200.

38 For Trenchard and his work as Metropolitan Police Commissioner, see *DNB 1951–60*, pp. 985–9; Andrew Boyle, *Trenchard* (London, 1962), chs. 19 and 20; Ascoli, *The Queen's Peace*, pp. 225–41.

39 PRO HO45/20546/674932/1, Trenchard to Sir Russell Scott, 24 February 1934. On Trenchard's preoccupation with restoring the Metropolitan Police's leading role, see Boyle, *Trenchard*, pp. 660–1.

40 PRO HO45/20546/674932/2, Report by Colonel Drummond (Trenchard's deputy) to Trenchard, March 1934.

41 On the establishment and early days of the Metropolitan Police Laboratory, see PRO HO45/20546; HO 45/16215/488975/8; MEPOL.2/2770; Ambage, 'Origins and development of the Forensic Science Service', ch. 4.

42 'Medico-legal science', *BMJ*, 1 (1935), 833–4.

43 The fifth medical man was Mr Hugh Lett (Royal College of Surgeons). The other members of the Committee were Atkin, Sir Edwin Deller (Principal of the University of London), Sir Robert Robertson (Government Chemist), Sir Frank Smith (Secretary, Department of Scientific and Industrial Research), Sir Russell Scott and S. J. Baker (Home Office) and Trenchard himself. See 'A national medico-legal institute', *BMJ*, 2 (1936), 229–30, at p. 229; 'Medicine and crime', *Lancet*, 2 (1936), 265–6, at p. 265, note 2.

44 PRO MH 79/388, Advisory Committee on the Scientific Investigation of Crime, Minutes of the first meeting of the Advisory Committee, 3 July 1935, p. 6, para. 12 (Sir Russell Scott); ibid., Paper No. 1. Scientific Aids in Police Work. Memorandum by Mr A. L. Dixon. Many of the relevant Home Office papers are, in fact, to be found in the Ministry of Health MH 79 series rather than in the Home Office HO 45 series.

45 For the growing tension and hostility between Dixon and Trenchard, see especially PRO HO45/20546, sub-file 674932/4, and Boyle, *Trenchard*, pp. 626–7. For Symons's criticism of the approach of forensic pathologists to cases of sexual assault and drunken driving, see especially C. T. Symons, 'Development of forensic science work in England', paper dated 9 June 1936, in PRO HO45/17110, sub-file 688708/64, pp. 4–5.

46 Douglas G. Browne and E. V. Tullett, *Bernard Spilsbury: His Life and Cases* (London, 1951), especially parts 2 and 3; Thorwald, *Dead Men Tell Tales*, p. 92.

47 For Finnucane's hostile attitude to medico-legal 'experts', see note 15, above, and *TMLS*, 25 (1930–1), 187. For Ainsworth Mitchell's attitude, see C. Ainsworth Mitchell, 'Forensic chemistry in relation to medicine', *ML & CR*, 4 (1936), 1–14, especially pp. 1–5, and *ML & CR*, 5 (1937), 39.

48 *Report of the Advisory Committee on the Scientific Investigation of Crime* (London; HMSO, 1936), p. 5, para. 2.

49 See Francis H. Cowper, 'Report of the Advisory Committee on the Scientific Investigation of Crime', *ML & CR*, 4 (1936), 308–11, at p. 308, and Walls, 'The Forensic Science Service in Great Britain', p. 276.

50 *Report of the Advisory Committee*, p. 6, para. 3.

51 Ibid., p. 7, para. 5.

52 Ibid., p. 6, para. 5.
53 Ibid., p. 7, para. 6.
54 Ibid., p. 9, para. 12.
55 'A national medico-legal institute', *BMJ*, 2 (1936), 229–30; 'Medicine and crime', *Lancet*, 2 (1936), 265–6.
56 For Trenchard's approaches to these potential benefactors, see PRO MH 79/387, memorandum to MacNalty, 29 February 1936 (Rockefeller Foundation); MH 79/389, MacNalty's Minute of 21 July 1937 (Lord Nuffield); ibid., Trenchard's briefing note to members of the Advisory Committee, 23 November 1936 (Sir Henry Wellcome, Lord Nuffield, Lord Austin). Both Herbert Eason, Vice-Chancellor, and Sir Edwin Deller, Principal of the University of London and a member of the Advisory Committee up to the time of his death in December 1936, were strongly in favour of the medico-legal institute scheme, and had persuaded the University Senate conditionally to approve it shortly before the publication of the interim report. See PRO MH 79/389, Eason to Trenchard, 21 May 1936.
57 See PRO MH 79/387, memorandum by 'S.T.W.' to MacNalty, 29 February 1936; MH 79/388, comments by Scott in the minutes of the 1st, 3rd and 4th meetings of the Advisory Committee; MH 79/389, minute by E. S. Hill, 16 March 1937.
58 PRO HO45/17568, Sir Russell Scott, memorandum to Hoare, 5 July 1937, p. 2. Scott had, however, expressed very similar views more than a year earlier; ibid., minutes of 7 March and 24 July 1936. For Scott, see *Who Was Who, 1951–1960*, pp. 976–7.
59 For the debates within the Ministry of Health, see PRO MH 79/389.
60 PRO HO45/17568, Sir John Simon to Trenchard, 8 April 1937.
61 PRO HO45/17568, Trenchard to Scott, 15 June 1938.
62 PRO HO45/17568, unsigned memorandum by Scott, 13 December 1937.
63 PRO HO45/17568, Trenchard to Sir Samuel Hoare, early July 1938.
64 PRO HO45/17568, Hoare to Trenchard, 5 July 1938.
65 Boyle, *Trenchard*, p. 661.
66 *Report of the Departmental Committee on Detective Work and Procedure*, vol. V, p. 3. For the content of detective training courses at Wakefield and Hendon in the mid- and late 1930s, see PRO HO45/17491/591901/37.
67 See especially PRO MH 79/388, minutes of the first four meetings of the Advisory Committee, and related papers.
68 PRO HO45/17568, Trenchard, draft notes for Home Secretary, 6 April 1935. See also Sir Frederick Menzies's similar estimate, ibid., minutes of meeting between Trenchard, Atkin, Menzies and Kingsley Wood (then Minister of Health), 18 March 1937, pp. 4–5.
69 PRO HO45/17568, briefing note by Scott for a meeting between Hoare and Trenchard, 5 June 1937.
70 PRO HO45/17568, memorandum by Hoare, 30 May 1938.
71 PRO HO45/17568, J. A. Barlow (Treasury) to A. S. Hutchinson (Home Office), 30 June 1938.
72 *Report of the Detective Committee*, vol. V, p. 19, para. 446. See also PRO MH/79 388 and 399.
73 Boyle, *Trenchard*, p. 683.

74 Ibid., p. 650.
75 Ibid., especially ch. 21, 'The oracle'.
76 A. L. Dixon, 'The Home Office and the police between the two World Wars' (1966), unpublished manuscript, Home Office, p. 180.
77 Dixon became Principal Assistant Under-Secretary of State and was awarded a knighthood in 1941. See *DNB 1961–1970*, p. 296.
78 Sir Sydney Smith, 'The medico-legal institute and the problem of crime', *Medico-Legal Journal* (hereafter *MLJ*), 19 (1951), 57–64, at p. 64.
79 (Letitia Fairfield or Donald Norris), 'Editorial', *MLJ*, 20 (1952), 141.
80 John Glaister, Jr, 'Post-graduate teaching of forensic medicine', in 'The teaching of forensic medicine: a symposium [held at the 9th meeting of the British Association of Forensic Pathologists]', *Journal of Forensic Medicine*, 2 (1955), 135–6, at p. 135.
81 [Gavin Thurston], 'The present state of forensic medicine', *MLJ*, 28 (1960), 167–8, at p. 167.
82 A. Keith Mant, 'A survey of forensic pathology in England since 1945', *Journal of the Forensic Science Society*, 13 (1973), 17–24, at pp. 23–4. See also Gilbert Forbes, 'The organisation, staffing and equipment of an institute of forensic medicine', in C. Keith Simpson, ed., *Modern Trends in Forensic Medicine 2* (London, 1967), pp.1–27.
83 For the postwar institutional and professional development of English forensic medicine, see especially Bernard Knight, 'Legal medicine in England and Wales', *Forensic Science*, 10: 1 (July–August 1977), 13–18. For the post-1945 development of the Forensic Science Service, see Walls, 'The Forensic Science Service in Great Britain', pp. 276–8, and Ambage, 'Origins and development of the Forensic Science Service', chs. 5–7.
84 Boyle, *Trenchard*, pp. 660–1.
85 Many articles have appeared since the early 1950s bemoaning the apparent 'decline and fall' of English forensic medicine. Among the most notable have been John Glaister, Jr, 'Whither forensic medicine?', *BMJ*, 2 (1952), 473–5; Bernard Knight, 'Decline and fall', *Journal of the Forensic Science Society*, 7 (1967), 121–2; and J. Malcolm Cameron, 'The medico-legal expert and the law – past, present and future', *Medicine, Science and the Law*, 20 (1980), 3–13.
86 For an unusually prescient view of the probable consequences of English forensic medicine's exclusion from the National Health Service, see Glaister, 'Whither forensic medicine?'. See also G. Stewart Smith, 'Clinical pathology and forensic medicine', *Medicine, Science and the Law*, 2 (1961–2), 244–57, and Cameron, 'The medico-legal expert', pp. 6–8.

13

Rex v. *Bourne* and the medicalization of abortion

BARBARA BROOKES and PAUL ROTH

On 27 April 1938 a fourteen-year-old girl, Miss H, was assaulted and brutally raped by a number of guardsmen in a barracks on Horse Guards Parade, Whitehall. Popularly known as 'the case of the horse with the green tail' after the enticement which lured the young victim into the barrack's stables,[1] the assault was widely reported and sensationalized by the press. Miss H was subsequently admitted to St Thomas's Hospital for a pregnancy test, which proved to be positive. Her doctor at St Thomas's was not sympathetic to her predicament. He reportedly took the position that 'he would not interfere with life because the child may be the future Prime Minister of England' and that in any case, 'girls always lead men on'.[2] The police surgeon, the doctor at her work, and her school doctor, however, were all of the opinion that Miss H ought not to be left to carry the pregnancy to term. Miss H's parents were desperate to have the pregnancy terminated, but were said to be 'so respectable that they did not know the address of any abortionist'.[3]

Abortion was a disreputable practice in part because it was illegal. The offence of unlawfully procuring an abortion was laid down in Section 58 of the Offences Against the Person Act 1861, the relevant terms of which provided that:

> whosoever, with intent to procure the miscarriage of any woman ... shall unlawfully use any instrument or other means whatsoever ... shall be guilty of felony, and being convicted thereof shall be liable ... to be kept in penal servitude for life.

That section, while implying that there were circumstances in which abortion could be procured lawfully, contained no specific provision for abortion on humanitarian or therapeutic grounds. Although by 1920 a leading medical text declared that 'medical science' had rendered the abortion operation 'almost free from risk',[4] it was not clear whether or not doctors risked criminal prosecution for terminating pregnancy. Textbooks set out somatic indications such as heart disease, nephritis and tuberculosis, for which abortion might be performed, but uncertainty remained. Between the enactment of the 1861 Act and 1938, the issue of whether there were circumstances that would render the operation lawful was never tested in a court of law because the defence was never raised. Doctors accused of procuring abortion invariably denied that their intention was to terminate pregnancy. A typical defence to this charge was that the doctor was dealing with the results of a miscarriage induced by someone else.[5] And, since the General Medical Council only took action after criminal proceedings, the question was never raised before the Council. Throughout this period most judges and commentators on the law were agreed that abortion was justified when necessary to save the life of the mother, but even this fundamental proposition lacked the support of any judicially decided case directly on the issue.[6]

All this was to change when Aleck Bourne, a leading obstetric surgeon at St Mary's Hospital, London, was informed of the case of Miss H and decided to perform an abortion in order to invite prosecution. Bourne's confidence in his reputation, in the justice of the case, and in public support, was such that he was willing openly to test the law; an action which, if resulting in conviction, would have meant the automatic removal of his right to practise and the end to an illustrious career. The events leading up to this singular challenge to the law by a medical man, the trial itself, and its impact deserve analysis, for the outcome of the case structured medical and legal views of abortion until the 1967 reform of the law.

In particular, the Bourne trial was significant because it extended the scope of indications for abortion to include considerations of mental health. This decisively furthered the medicalization of abortion at a time when the physical indications for the operation (which made it an obviously medical matter) were actually decreasing in importance. The acceptance of an unfavourable psychiatric prognosis as an indication for therapeutic abortion established a precedent which allowed doctors thereafter to respond to the social circumstances of their patients, and to respond to women's demands for fertility control without necessarily compromising medical ethics. Provided only that they acted 'reasonably' and 'in good faith', members of the medical profession would be immune from criminal prosecution. In this way, the ethical decision as to when abortion was justified was effectively delegated to doctors. By suggesting that doctors alone were the appropriate people to decide whether to perform abortions, and that they might take mental, as well as physical, health into account, the ruling in the Bourne case effectively referred the decision about society's interest in protecting the foetus to the medical profession.

Prior to *Bourne*, those who performed abortions for purely humanitarian reasons were usually women without medical qualifications motivated by a desire 'to avoid a child being born into a state of misery'.[7] Doctors were cautioned that such considerations did 'not constitute an indication for the operation'.[8] The leaders of the profession wanted to dissociate medical practice completely from the 'methods of the illegal abortion-monger and professional abortionist'.[9] Nevertheless, since the physician's concern was with the alleviation of suffering, abortion might be performed if it could be justified on clear medical grounds. Doctors who terminated pregnancy without somatic indications were warned that they acted at their peril. Such warnings were reinforced by the occasional conviction of doctors, such as Laura Sanders-Bliss in 1936, who were thought to have terminated pregnancies without good medical reasons.[10] It was in order to clarify the circumstances in which therapeutic abortion could properly be undertaken and thus to free practitioners from the threat of criminal prosecution and ensuing professional censure, that Aleck Bourne was eager to take up a test case.

Bourne believed a test case to be necessary both from his personal experience and because of the reluctance of the medical profession to make any concrete proposals for abortion law reform. Medical-led debate over the abortion issue had been stimulated by a judge's outspoken criticism of the abortion law in 1931. McCardie J. had declined to inflict severe sentences either on amateur abortionists or on women who had procured their own miscarriages. He could not see why amateur abortionists should be accused of murder when the very last thing they intended was the death of the woman they had 'helped'. The law, he believed, should reflect changing social attitudes and since the public was now in favour of fertility control, reform of the 1861 law was necessary.[11] Following his statements, medical practitioners urged the British Medical Association to consider the abortion law at its annual meetings in 1931 and 1933. In 1934 Sir Ewen Maclean suggested that the law should make explicit provision to exempt medical men from liability to prosecution for performing abortion 'solely for the preservation of the life or health of the patient'. This would obviate the necessity for a medical man, acting according 'to the highest standards of practice', having 'to justify himself before a coroner's jury'.[12]

Nervousness about coroners' inquests may well have increased as the reputation of the Home Office forensic pathologist, Sir Bernard Spilsbury, grew in the interwar years. Spilsbury abhorred abortion and 'was merciless towards culprits of his own profession'.[13] His pursuit of abortionists was something of a crusade and he advised the police about practitioners whom he suspected of infringing the law.[14] While working as a pathologist at St Mary's Hospital, Spilsbury had taught Aleck Bourne who recalled his 'amazing attention to detail and careful recording of his observations'.[15] In

1933 Bourne challenged his old teacher's evidence in the trial of a Dr Avarne from Jersey, charged with procuring abortion. Bourne and Sydney Smith, Regius Professor of Forensic Medicine at Edinburgh, successfully refuted the prosecution's claim, based on Spilsbury's examination, that there was no evidence of foetal death preceding the operation. In the course of the trial Bourne made clear his contempt for the pathologist's understanding of clinical work. Smith later recalled that 'Bourne was a magnificent witness and the star turn of the trial'.[16] The case, which resulted in Dr Avarne's acquittal, highlighted the antipathy between the Home Office pathologist and Bourne.

Bourne and Smith, both advocates of abortion law reform, were members of the BMA Committee on the Medical Aspects of Abortion, appointed in 1934. This committee was finally set up after much discussion as to whether the BMA should attempt to lead public opinion on such a sensitive issue. The committee's report, buried in the 'Report of Council' in the *British Medical Journal* for 1936, stated that 'in its present uncompromising form, the law must be regarded as containing elements which in certain circumstances may leave the position of the doctor exposed to risks of suspicion and professional damage'.[17] It went on to discuss various indications for therapeutic abortion including mental conditions such as psychoses and psychoneuroses. Abortion was rarely indicated for the latter, the report suggested, but it made special mention of the prophylactic role abortion might play in the case of mental stress caused by pregnancy in a girl raped under the age of consent. However, since the law provided 'no specific authority for terminating pregnancy' the committee recommended clarification of the law to allow therapeutic abortion, monitored by a system of authorization.[18] Such clarification would allow doctors to respond to their patients' needs for therapeutic abortion.

'[T]he rigidity of the views of the medical profession', claimed an obstetrician in 1926, 'drove people to the abortion-mongers.'[19] Doctors were aware that medical abortions could prevent morbidity and death resulting from 'back street' abortions but they had no wish to be dictated to by their patients. This was clear in many of the objections made against publishing the BMA committee's report in 1936. Dame Louise McIlroy, a consultant and former Professor of Obstetrics and Gynaecology at London University, stated firmly that 'The medical profession were not there as servants of the public, but as advisors; they were not going to induce abortion by demand, nor for the same reasons as those of the criminal abortionist.'[20] Others, however, commended the report's call for legal clarification of the grounds for therapeutic abortion. Sir Ewen Maclean, President of the College of Obstetrics and Gynaecology, argued that publication of the report was important because whatever safeguards were in place, doctors still had 'a large measure of anxiety' about when they might legitimately perform a therapeutic abortion.[21] By this reform doctors could prevent ill-health and uphold morality by determining in what circumstances, and for whom, abortion was an acceptable therapeutic procedure. In addition, by specifying that the procedure should be done by a doctor, such a reform would expedite the conviction of unqualified abortionists. In this way the practice of abortion could be moved out of the sphere of self-medication and popular birth control and into the surgery.

Aleck Bourne was a member of the medico-legal council of the Abortion Law Reform Association, which was founded in 1936 to press for medically performed abortions to be freed from all legal restrictions.[22] It was the approach of a fellow member of the Association's medico-legal council, Dr Joan Malleson, about the situation of Miss H that led to Bourne's involvement in the case. Malleson and Bourne agreed that Miss H's predicament presented an ideal opportunity for a test case because of the public sympathy it was likely to elicit. Miss H, a healthy young woman, was clearly not at any immediate risk of dying as a result of her pregnancy, but the tragedy of her situation convinced many that abortion would be morally justified in the circumstances of her case. In a letter to Bourne later produced in the trial, Dr Malleson proposed action in the following terms:

> I understand that Dr.—, and possibly some other psychiatrists of good standing, would be prepared to sponsor 'therapeutic abortion'. I presume they must mean on grounds of prophylaxis, because there does not appear to be any nervous disorder present. All this, of course, gets us nowhere unless someone of your standing were prepared to risk a *cause célèbre* and undertake the operation in hospital.
>
> Many people hold the view that the best way of correcting the present abortion laws is to let the medical profession gradually extend the grounds for therapeutic abortion in suitable cases, until the laws become obsolete, so far as practice goes. I should imagine that public opinion would be immensely in favour of termination of pregnancy in a case of this sort.[23]

On 27 May Bourne replied:

> I am interested in the case of rape which you describe in your letter. I shall be delighted to admit her to St. Mary's and curette her. I have done this before and have not the slightest hesitation in doing it again . . . I have said that the next time I have such an opportunity I would write to the Attorney-General and invite him to take action.[24]

Four days later Miss H was taken by her mother to see Bourne, and Miss H's father wrote to him giving his consent for 'the correction to be done' on the condition that no publicity whatsoever be given to the operation.

Bourne informed Dr Malleson of this request and stated that he would have to abide by the father's wish for secrecy if he could not be persuaded to change his mind.

On 6 June Miss H was admitted to St Mary's where a second test for pregnancy proved positive. Although later in court Bourne was to admit that he had a bias in favour of performing the operation, he testified that he had never intended to operate before observing Miss H and carefully considering whether she was a 'suitable' case. To determine this, Bourne explained, at least three possibilities had to be excluded. First, he had to reassure himself that Miss H was not a 'mental defective', for if she were, he stated with a certain relentless logic, she would not suffer mental distress in the pregnancy. Second, for similar reasons he had to exclude the possibility that she belonged to the 'prostitute type' or had a 'prostitute mind';[25] in short, he had to determine whether she deserved the therapy abortion offered. Third, he had to make certain that Miss H was not infected with venereal disease, since an operation might spread the infection up the birth canal and cause serious illness.[26]

On 14 June Bourne took the swab for the infection test. He later testified that Miss H's behaviour during the carrying out of this test was decisive in confirming his decision to operate:

> He had watched her demeanour when it had been first brought home to her by this procedure that she was really pregnant and the memory of the assault had come back to her. Instead of her bearing the trifling discomfort with fortitude, she had broken down and cried.[27]

Miss H had proven herself to be deserving by having none 'of the cold indifference of the prostitute'.[28] The infection test proved negative and later that morning Bourne performed the operation.

In light of the fact that the operation was performed openly in a public hospital, and that eight days elapsed between Miss H's admission to St Mary's and the operation, Bourne's undertaking to the girl's father to spare no effort to keep the matter secret seems disingenuous. But any overt attempt by Bourne to cloak the operation in secrecy would have been tantamount to admitting that he was doing something improper. It is therefore not surprising that the matter came to the attention of the police. The different accounts of how the authorities came to be apprised of the matter suggest that the police obtained their information from more than one source.[29] According to Sir Edward Tindal Atkinson, the Director of Public Prosecutions, New Scotland Yard was informed on 12 June that a woman had been admitted to hospital for the performance of an abortion on 'humanitarian' grounds. This information was brought to the attention of the Director of Public Prosecutions, who, suspecting a possible breach of the abortion laws, advised the Commissioner of the Metropolitan Police to launch an immediate inquiry into the matter.[30]

Chief Inspector Bridger and Inspector Robinson of the Metropolitan Police did not arrive at St Mary's until the evening of 14 June, by which time the operation had already been performed. They had gone to the hospital to warn Bourne that the operation could not be performed for 'humanitarian' reasons. In his autobiography, Bourne recalled how he 'made it plain to the Inspector that I could not recognize his right to dictate to me what I, as a surgeon, should or should not decide to do in the best interests of my patient' and that it was difficult to understand what was meant by 'humanitarian grounds' since 'most of medicine is humanitarian'.[31] Bourne stated that he had already emptied the uterus and that he wanted to be arrested. He also remarked that in his professional opinion, 'it may be dangerous for a girl of her age to bear a full-term child',[32] and that in performing the operation he had only discharged his duty as an obstetric surgeon. The inspectors did not arrest Bourne, but said that they would report the matter to the proper authorities.

The Commissioner of the Metropolitan Police thereupon submitted a preliminary report to the Director of Public Prosecutions indicating that the operation had not been performed for the purpose of preserving Miss H's life, but for purely 'humanitarian' reasons. The Director of Public Prosecutions consulted with the Attorney-General as to whether to proceed against Bourne or not, and the Attorney-General agreed that it would be necessary to do so lest inaction be regarded as a tacit change in the law of abortion.[33] Accordingly, Bourne was summoned to appear before the Marylebone police court on 1 July on a charge of breaching Section 58 of the Offences Against the Person Act 1861. The object of these proceedings was to determine whether there was sufficient evidence to indict Bourne and send the case for trial before a jury. The onus resting on the Crown was to establish a *prima facie* case against Bourne.

The case for the Crown changed little between these proceedings and the eventual trial in the Central Criminal Court. Appearing for the Director of Public Prosecutions, H. A. K. Morgan contended that on such authorities as he was able to find, the premature induction of birth was lawful only where it was necessary to save the life of either the mother or the child. He maintained that Bourne was among those who believed that the law on abortion ought to be changed or relaxed, and that he had openly defied the law in order to publicize his opinion. Morgan noted that the only defence Bourne had put forward up until then was the danger to Miss H in bearing a full-term child. This, however, could not be taken seriously as a real defence, for '[i]f it were a good defence, anyone who wished to procure abortion for reasons of gain or sympathy could say that in his opinion it might be dangerous for the woman to bear a child, for childbirth was dangerous for any woman. The law of abortion would then be a dead letter.'[34] Five witnesses were called to give evidence for the Crown, the same five who were to testify in the trial proper. Miss H gave evidence of the facts. Miss H's father testified that he had given his consent to the operation subject to the condition that it be kept secret. Dr Malleson gave evidence in connection with her correspondence with Bourne. Dr P. C. F. Wingate, the resident obstetric officer at St Mary's, testified that he was present when the operation was performed and that Bourne had told him that the pregnancy was being terminated because Miss H was under age and pregnant as the result of rape. Finally, Chief Inspector Bridger testified to his conversation with Bourne and to the fact that the defendant had wanted and expected to be arrested.

The Crown clearly failed to take Bourne's therapeutic justification seriously, for neither in these proceedings nor in the trial proper did they call any expert witnesses on this point which in the end was to be vital to their case. The Crown's apparent complacency was probably reinforced by certain remarks made by the defence in the preliminary hearing which may have misled them as to the terms on which the defence would be conducted at the trial proper. Defence counsel Gerald Thesiger stated that he would advise Bourne to plead 'not guilty' and that he would reserve his defence until the trial. He did, however, make certain submissions on the law for the guidance of the presiding magistrate. He contended that on a proper view of the law the evidence presented by the Crown disclosed no felony. He pointed out that the use of the word 'unlawful' in the 1861 Act necessarily raised the implication that in certain circumstances abortion could be lawfully procured, and that Parliament with great foresight 'had left to the generations that came after 1861 to define from time to time what should be lawful'.[35] In the present case, he submitted, the fact that Miss H was both under the age of sixteen and pregnant as the result of a rape rendered the operation lawful. Up until 1929, sexual intercourse with a girl under sixteen had been a criminal offence unless she was married, and in 1929 the age for marriage had been raised to sixteen. This indicated that Parliament intended that no girl under the age of sixteen should have sexual intercourse, and that pregnancy in a girl under sixteen must perforce always be the result of a criminal act. Moreover, in the present case the girl had become pregnant as the result of a rape. Defence counsel therefore concluded that '[i]t could not be said to be unlawful to avert the consequences of a felonious trespass on a child below the age of consent and below the age at which she could be married'.[36]

Had this innovative line of defence been used at the trial proper,[37] a number of problems would have arisen. First, it would have raised the issue of whether or not it would be unlawful to perform an abortion on a woman over the age of sixteen whose pregnancy was the result of rape, for her condition was no less the product of a felonious assault. Second, the court could not have avoided dealing with a contentious moral issue, for at least on one view, the unborn child could be regarded as the entirely innocent result of an admittedly criminal act and should not be made to pay with its life for the sins of its father. Finally, the court would have had to grapple with the difficulty of defining precisely when abortion on such grounds would be lawful. Two possibilities would have been that abortion was lawful upon proof of a criminal assault, or upon the conviction of the victim's assailant. However, if the court had ruled that abortion in such circumstances was only lawful if the latter condition were fulfilled, Bourne's actions would have been unlawful, since Miss H's assailants had not yet been convicted at the time of the operation.[38] Viewed with the benefit of hindsight, such a defence was unlikely to have succeeded, and even if it had, it would in the end necessarily have restricted the applicability of the Bourne case to those instances where girls under sixteen had been raped. It would, therefore, have had little impact, as most abortions involved older, married women. The grounds eventually relied upon at the trial were potentially much wider and dealt directly with the issue of therapeutic abortion.

The magistrate overruled defence counsel's submissions on the law and held that the case was one which should properly go before a judge and jury of the high court. He remarked that this was probably also the wish of Bourne and his advisers. The trial before Macnaghten J. and a jury of ten men and two women took place on 18 and 19 July. The Attorney-General himself, Sir Donald Somervell KC, led for the prosecution. The evidence called by the Crown was identical to that presented at the police court, and in particular, the Attorney-General reiterated the Crown's position that the operation would have been lawful had it been necessary to save the life of the mother.

Before opening the case for the defence, Roland Oliver KC invited the judge to direct the jury on the law at that stage of the proceedings, stating that he did not wish to present the jury with a different view of the law from that held by the judge. Acknowledging that the case was not covered by any judicial authority whatsoever, counsel observed that the case would turn on the meaning of the word 'unlawfully' in the 1861 Act. Counsel thereupon took the opportunity to refute the Attorney-General's narrow view of when abortion would be permissible and submitted that 'anything was sufficient justification for an abortion which, in the view of a responsible and skilled surgeon, was for the benefit of the mother's health in the sense that her health would probably be seriously impaired if it was not done'.[39] The authority he cited in support of this submission – and the only authority to be referred to in the course of the trial – was the then current edition of the leading textbook *Russell on Crime*. That work stated that the word 'unlawfully' excluded from s.58 'acts done in the course of proper treatment in the interest of the life or health of the mother'.[40] Oliver further submitted that abortion should be treated no differently from any other medical operation. For example, acts of mayhem or maim were also proscribed by the 1861 Act, yet surgeons who amputated limbs or removed an eye acted lawfully if the procedure was in the interests of the patient's health; there was no requirement in either logic or law that such operations had to be limited only to the saving of life. Therefore, the same legal standard should apply to all medical procedures. Accordingly, the proper test in the present case was 'When Dr Bourne used the instrument on June 14, was he acting in the honest and reasonable belief, based on adequate knowledge and experience, that it was in the best interests of the girl's health that her pregnancy should be terminated?'[41]

Macnaghten J. thereupon directed the jury on the law. First, he concurred with both prosecution and defence counsel that 'the word "unlawfully" is not a meaningless word in this section, and it necessarily follows that there may be a procurement of abortion which is lawful'.[42] Although it had long been thought that this was the proper significance of the word in the context of s.58,[43] it was still open to the judge to hold otherwise by treating the word as pleonastic. In that case 'unlawfully' could be regarded as having been employed by the draftsman merely to indicate 'contrary to the terms of the section following that word',[44] and that the procurement of abortion was always unlawful. This step in the judge's reasoning, therefore, was significant, even if it only confirmed what many had previously believed. It would be all the more difficult for another judge to hold thereafter that s.58 imposed a blanket prohibition on all abortions without exception.

Second, once the judge had decided that s.58 did allow the possibility that in certain circumstances abortion could be lawfully procured, it fell to him to specify what those circumstances were. This task was rendered difficult by the absence of any aid to interpretation in s.58 itself and by the lack of any relevant case law on this provision. It was at this point that the judge chose to accept the Crown's submission on the law and directed that in cases where 'it is reasonably impossible for a woman to be delivered of her child and survive', the procuring of an abortion 'by a skilled person, without any risk to the patient' was plainly lawful. The judge stated that he had no doubt that 'that has always been the view of the judges of this country'.[45] In support of this view, however, the judge referred only to the Infant Life (Preservation) Act 1929, which had hitherto been cited by neither the Crown nor the defence. The judge regarded this statute as rendering the position 'greatly simplified' and 'of tremendous value in throwing light on the law of this subject'.[46]

The 1929 Act had been enacted to plug a loophole in the law of infanticide, not for the purpose of clarifying the law on abortion. While it was murder to kill an unwanted child once it had been delivered and had an existence independent of its mother, and while it was an offence against s.58 of the 1861 Act unlawfully to procure a miscarriage, it was theoretically possible to escape criminal liability by killing a child while it was being delivered and before it had an existence independent of its mother. Accordingly, s.1(1) of the 1929 Act provided that

> any person who with intent to destroy the life of a child capable of being born alive, by any wilful act causes a child to die before it has an existence independent of its mother, shall be guilty of felony, to wit, of child destruction, and shall be liable on conviction thereof on indictment to penal servitude for life.

Although the judge did not explicitly say upon what basis he felt it proper to invoke the aid of the 1929 Act in interpreting the 1861 Act, it is clear that the later statute was relevant to the issue either by way of providing an analogy to or in being *in pari materia* (on the same subject)[47] as s.58 of the earlier statute. The intention behind the 1929 Act could reasonably be regarded as similar to that of the 1861 Act, its function being to complete the protection of the unborn child during the period before it had an existence independent of its mother. Furthermore, s.1(2) of the 1929 Act provided that

> [f]or the purposes of this act, evidence that a woman had at any material time been pregnant for a period of twenty-eight weeks or more shall be prima facie proof that she was at that time pregnant of a child capable of being born alive.

Therefore, the procuring of an abortion after the twenty-eighth week of a pregnancy could fall under either s.58 of the 1861 Act or s.1(1) of the 1929 Act, or both if the intentionality required by the later statute was proved, and if the presumption set out in s.1(2) was not rebutted. To the extent that the two statutes overlapped, at least, they were certainly *in pari materia*, which would have required the judge to consider the 1929 Act.

For Macnaghten J., the particular relevance of the 1929 Act to the point at issue lay in the proviso to s.1(1), which specified in what circumstances a person would avoid criminal liability for destroying a child:

> no person shall be found guilty of an offence under this section unless it is proved that the act which caused the death of the child was not done in good faith for the purpose only of preserving the life of the mother.

The judge thought it reasonable to construe s.58 of the 1861 Act as if it contained precisely the same proviso, and he accordingly directed the jury:

> If you are satisfied by the evidence, when we have heard it all, that Mr Bourne did not terminate the pregnancy of this girl in good faith for the purpose of preserving the life of the girl; if you are satisfied that the Crown have proved that negative, you should find him Guilty. If you think that the Crown have not proved the negative that the law requires them to prove, then you should find him Not Guilty.[48]

The legal effect of this direction was to place squarely on the Crown the burden of proving beyond reasonable doubt that Bourne had not performed the operation in good faith for the purpose of preserving the girl's life, instead of requiring Bourne to raise a specific defence.[49] This direction, therefore, required the Crown to prove a negative proposition, one that would inevitably be more difficult to prove in relation to physicians than it would be in the case of 'back street' abortionists. In practical terms, however, the defence would have to adduce sufficient evidence to raise a reasonable doubt in the Crown's case.

The judge's basic exposition of the law has been labelled 'orthodox'[50] and 'conservative',[51] but it is difficult to see how he could reasonably have gone any further than he did when the case was the first of its kind and raised controversial issues. The submissions on the law offered by the defence were not particularly persuasive. Abortion differed from other medical procedures in that society had an interest in the unborn child, whereas the same could not be said of a diseased limb or eye.[52] While the law might well require the same standard of reasonable care and skill in all medical procedures, including abortion, this begged the legal and ethical question of how this standard should apply when the interest in preserving a woman's health, as opposed to her life, conflicted with the interest in preserving unborn life. Moreover, the textbook cited by the defence in support of the contention that therapeutic abortion was permissible in the interests of the mother's health merely reflected what could be found in a number of medical textbooks as a matter of professional understanding rather than as an indubitable proposition supported by the weight of legal authority.[53]

The judge, then, could not fairly be criticized for taking a cautious approach at this stage of the proceedings. He was having to deal with a highly controversial subject upon which there was a great diversity of opinion, and which was therefore best left for Parliament to reconsider. In these circumstances, with a dearth of legal authority from which to proceed and a lack of detailed argument in court to consider, it was reasonable that he should provide an exposition of the law based on the albeit minimal common ground shared between the prosecution and the defence. On the one hand, he might have thought that if he took a wider view he would be accused of playing fast and loose with the law and opening a floodgate, with the Crown having no right of appeal if Bourne were acquitted.[54] On the other, it is clear that he took into consideration the fact that if Bourne were convicted upon this strict view of the law, an appellate court would be able to rectify the matter if his view was mistaken.[55] Moreover, the judge would have known that Bourne was financially able to lodge a possible appeal against conviction, since his defence was supported by the London and Counties Medical Protection Society.

At this point in the proceedings the legal issue had thus been narrowed down to the meaning of 'preserving the life of the mother'. This the judge left as a question of fact depending upon the particular circumstances of each case. He did leave open the possibility, however, that the operation might lawfully be performed in cases where the threat of death was not imminent, but where 'the sooner it is done the better', observing that '[t]here are many considerations which influence the decision of the doctor on what should be done in the particular case'.[56]

Immediately after Macnaghten J.'s direction to the jury, defence counsel seized the opportunity it presented to submit that he could not 'altogether separate the questions of what is necessary to preserve life and what is necessary to preserve health'. The judge agreed, and he reiterated that it was for the jury to decide on the basis of the facts whether the Crown had discharged its burden of proof. 'Nobody', he said, 'can say without knowing the facts of the case whether the abortion was lawful or unlawful.'[57] By allowing that the preservation of life and the preservation of health were not always separable issues, the judge enabled the defence to adduce evidence that serious danger to the girl's health would have resulted had the operation not been performed, and to have that evidence considered by the jury in deciding whether or not the operation was lawfully performed. In effect the judge was leaving the interpretation of 'preserving the life of the mother' to the jury, which would no doubt be predisposed to acquit a doctor who operated for good medical reasons, especially a doctor of Bourne's eminence.

Opening the case for the defence, Bourne's counsel accordingly set out to emphasize the *bona fides* of the defendant in performing the operation. Stating twice that Bourne had acted out of the 'purest charity', he explained that the defendant had operated in the belief that he was only 'carrying out his duty under the law, which was to look after his patient to the best of his ability'.[58] In particular, he had wished to save Miss H from mental or nervous breakdown. Bourne, counsel observed, belonged to that great body of medical men and women who believed that the operation ought to be performed by persons with skill, knowledge and experience in order to minimize the danger to the patient, whereas s.58 was directed against professional abortionists who operated for other reasons. Indeed, counsel declared, Bourne was to be praised for his gallantry and courage in risking martyrdom in order to have the law on this matter clarified.

Bourne himself was the first witness for the defence. Three main points were emphasized in his evidence. First, although he admitted that he had been biased in favour of performing the operation on Miss H after hearing the circumstances of her case, he explained that he had never intended to terminate her pregnancy before verifying that she was a suitable subject for the operation. Second, he drove home the vital point that had been raised shortly before in counsel's submission to the judge, stating that he could not draw a clear distinction between danger to life and danger to health. 'If we waited for danger to life', Bourne asserted, 'the woman is past assistance.'[59] Cross-examined by the Attorney-General on this point, Bourne denied that a clear distinction could be made and explained that

> there is a large group whose health may be damaged, but whose life almost certainly will not be sacrificed. There is another group at the other end whose life will be definitely in very great danger . . . There is a large body of material between those two extremes in which it is not really possible to say how far life will be in danger, but we find, of course, that the health is depressed to such an extent that life is shortened, such as in cardiac cases, so that you may say that their life is in danger, because death might occur within measurable distance of the time of their labour.[60]

Bourne suggested that Miss H's case fell into this middle group of cases; although the operation had not been necessary to save Miss H from imminent death, her health would have been so seriously affected by bringing the pregnancy to term that the possibility existed that her life would have been shortened. Had the Crown called any expert medical witnesses this argument might have been weakened substantially, in particular the seemingly arbitrary way Miss H's case was ranked alongside cardiac cases rather than among cases belonging to the first group described by Bourne.

Third, Bourne maintained that the operation in this particular case was indicated by the likely harm to Miss H's nervous system and mental health if the termination were not carried out. This accorded with Bourne's understanding of the law. He viewed the law as being based on the everyday practice of reputable members of the profession, which, he affirmed, held that it was justifiable to terminate a pregnancy '[i]f there were adequate medical reasons in the widest sense'.[61] While conceding that any physical harm received by Miss H in the course of the assault or likely to be caused by giving birth at her tender age did not in themselves constitute sufficient indications for an abortion, Bourne asserted that '[t]he circumstances of her conception were ... such as to implant in her mind seeds of terror'. In his experience the mental and nervous injury in such cases was the more difficult to cure: '[i]t would have been a source of nervous, psychoneurotic, and other troubles, and there would perhaps have been secondary physical illnesses all her life'.[62]

Bourne had a deep interest in psychological factors in relation to gynaecology, and he may well have wanted the case to stand on his evidence as to the nervous trauma facing Miss H if her pregnancy was allowed to continue. His counsel, however, believed he would be convicted 'unless further evidence of physical risks as well as mental were forthcoming'.[63] This proved to be sound advice, as Bourne's testimony on this point was somewhat weakened by the Crown in cross-examination. Questioned by the Attorney-General, Bourne 'could not recall personally any instances of nervous or mental damage, but he had had many brought to his knowledge by reading and by conversation in the general way of collecting experience by contact with medical men'.[64] When asked by the Attorney-General why he did not therefore obtain a second opinion, Bourne stated that as he was usually appealed to himself as an expert on such matters, he considered his own opinion sufficient.

In fact, there was little English data on the psychological consequences of rape that could be used to support Bourne's case. The BMA Committee on the Medical Aspects of Abortion had recommended in 1936 that therapeutic abortion should be available in cases of pregnancy resulting from rape under the age of consent because of the physical difficulties and 'severe *mental* injury' attendant on labour in young girls.[65] The leading psychiatric textbook of the day, however, contained no discussion of either rape or abortion until after the Bourne judgement.[66] A 1933 survey of ninety-five British alienists on the effects of pregnancy on insanity had revealed that most regarded the induction of abortion for the treatment of mental disease 'with little favour' or 'unqualified disapproval'.[67] Because the mother's life was rarely at stake, the author of the survey concluded that mental disease would 'rarely form an indication for termination of pregnancy' unless it could be demonstrated that there were cases where conception led to permanent insanity. Even though the 'calamity' of pregnancy following rape claimed 'universal sympathy', the need for therapeutic abortion was only considered, and rejected, on eugenic grounds.[68]

Dr John Rawlings Rees, the first expert witness for the defence, provided justification for Bourne's action in striking new terms. Rees was Medical Director of the Tavistock Clinic where research focused on the link between psychological and somatic aspects of illness.[69] He likened the impact of rape to shell-shock, stating that the 'girl had been in fact wounded, one might say she had been blown up' and that she would 'be buried by having to continue pregnancy'.[70] Although it is not clear that Rees had actually examined Miss H, his knowledge of similar cases convinced him that she would suffer a mental breakdown. He suggested that such cases resulted in a syndrome 'which was in some sense unique', thus foreshadowing the 'Rape Trauma Syndrome' described by Burgess and Holmstrom in 1974.[71] Rees cited cases and research on child assault to support his contention that 'the danger of mental disturbance was reduced if pregnancy was terminated'. He advocated a broad view of the words 'to preserve life', arguing that '[p]reserving life ... meant preserving health; it was not possible to let a person drift into a mental breakdown in the future and say one was preserving life'.[72]

If Rees's association with the Tavistock Clinic made him slightly unorthodox, the two other expert witnesses for the defence were solidly mainstream. Mr William Gilliat, a leading obstetric and gynaecological surgeon and a member of the medical staff of the Royal household,[73] detailed the higher risks of death in childbirth facing young girls. The maternal mortality rate in the fifteen to twenty age group was, he suggested, one per thousand higher than the average. Furthermore, in a study he had made of thirty-five young women giving birth between the ages of fifteen and sixteen, 45 to 50 per cent of the women showed some abnormality in labour, a figure consistent with the findings of another study. The principal difficulty that arose in such cases was 'ineffective action of the uterus and delay', making surgical interference necessary and thus increasing the likelihood of sepsis. Such infection, he asserted, would not eventually disappear if it occurred in childbirth, but remained permanently.[74] Finally, Lord Horder, doctor to Royalty and a popular figure with wide interests, testified on the psychiatric aspect of the case. He considered abortion justifiable in cases where 'severe mental or nervous breakdown seemed likely to occur if pregnancy were not terminated'.[75] Although he had not personally seen the patient, he considered the operation justifiable in view of Miss H's age and the fact that she had been raped.

After the closing arguments by counsel, Macnaghten J. summed up the case for the jury.[76] Consistent with his direction of the previous day, his exposition of the law rested on the proviso to s.1(1) of the Infant Life (Preservation) Act 1929. In order to secure a conviction, the Crown would have to prove beyond reasonable doubt that the operation 'was not done in good faith for the purpose only of preserving the life of the mother'. Despite this restrictive legal basis for the direction, emphasizing the threat to life, the tenor of the judge's speech was clearly favourable to Bourne and in fact adopted much of what had been submitted for the defence. In particular, the significance of the judge's summing-up lay first in its emphasis on the requirement of *bona fides* on the part of the person performing the abortion. In practical terms this amounted to the decisive legal test of the lawfulness of the operation. Second, Macnaghten's broad interpretation of the words 'for the purpose only of preserving the life of the mother' allowed a large subjective component to enter into a complex clinical matter. This meant that the principal basis upon which juries might infer good faith could be generously interpreted. Cumulatively, these two aspects of the judge's direction served to uphold the absolute medicalization of the operation, placing those without medical qualifications automatically beyond the pale of the law. If it was a licensed doctor who performed the operation, and if that doctor appeared to be acting honestly, the operation would be legal. *Bona fides* in this context meant that the doctor's practice raised no suspicions and that there were no unexplained deviations from acceptable practice.

Early in his direction, Macnaghten J. compared Bourne's case with one he had presided over only six days before:

> I mention that case only to show you how different the case now before you is from the type of case which usually comes before a criminal court. In that case, a woman without any medical skill or any medical qualifications did what is alleged against Mr Bourne here: she unlawfully used an instrument for the purpose of procuring the miscarriage of a pregnant girl. She did it for money. £2 5s was her fee, and she came from a distance to a place in London to do it. £1 had to be paid to make the appointment. She came, she used her instrument, and, within an interval of time measured not by minutes but by seconds, the victim of her malpractice was dead on the floor.[77]

This was the case of Mary Gray who was sentenced to three years penal servitude for performing an unlawful abortion by means of 'a syringe or some other unknown means'.[78] Macnaghten J. remarked that unlike Gray, Bourne was a 'man of the highest skill' who had performed the operation 'openly in one of our great hospitals'. The judge accepted defence counsel's submissions on Bourne's *bona fides* without question, observing that Bourne had performed the operation 'as an act of charity ... believing that he was doing the right thing, and that he ought, in the performance of his duty as a member of a profession devoted to the alleviation of human suffering, to do it'.[79]

Similarly, at the close of his direction to the jury, the judge emphasized that doctors 'alone could properly perform such an operation', and expressed the hope that no doctors 'would ever lend themselves to the malpractices of professional abortionists'. One sure indication of a doctor's *bona fides*, Macnaghten J. added, was seeking a second opinion from a colleague 'of high standing'.[80] The fact that Bourne himself had not done this went unremarked by the judge.

As to the crucial question of a doctor acting *in good faith* 'for the purpose only of preserving the life of the mother', the judge directed the jury to take a 'reasonable' view of those words.[81] He remarked that

> There has been much discussion in this case as to the difference between danger to life and danger to health. It may be that you are more fortunate than I am, but I confess that I have found it difficult to understand what the discussion really meant, since life depends upon health, and it may be that health is so gravely impaired that death results.[82]

Macnaghten J. then went on to cite Bourne's testimony, casting doubt on the Attorney-General's suggestion that a clear distinction existed between danger to health and danger to life. Bourne had observed that a great number of intermediate cases, including the one at issue, fell in between the group whose 'health may be damaged, but whose life almost certainly will not be sacrificed', and the group 'whose life will be definitely in very great danger'. The judge left it to the jury whether or not to accept this contention and stated that 'If that view commends itself to you, you will not accept the suggestion that there is a clear line of distinction between danger to health and danger to life.'[83] This part of the judge's summing-up, therefore, indicated that while the operation should be restricted to those cases where the mother's longevity might otherwise be affected,[84] in view of the difficulty of distinguishing danger to life from danger to health, doctors should normally be allowed the benefit of the doubt.

Later in his summing-up, however, Macnaghten J. took a more expansive view of what a 'reasonable' interpretation entailed:

> As I have said, I think those words ought to be construed in a reasonable sense, and, if the doctor is of opinion, on reasonable grounds and with adequate knowledge, that the probable consequence of the continuance of the pregnancy will be to make the woman a physical or mental wreck, the jury are quite entitled to take the view that the doctor who, under those circumstances and in that honest belief, operates, is operating for the purpose of preserving the life of the mother.[85]

Here the judge clearly drew upon the defence counsel's submission on the proper legal test to be applied, that is, whether the doctor was 'acting in the honest and reasonable belief, based on adequate knowledge and experience, that it was in the best interests of the girl's health that her pregnancy should be terminated'.[86] Moreover, he accepted that a doctor could be acting lawfully if he operated to prevent the patient from becoming a 'mental wreck', a condition which Dr Rees had testified would have been the likely result had Bourne not performed the operation. In short, this part of the judge's direction was tantamount to inviting the jury to acquit Bourne, which they duly did after forty minutes' deliberation.

If this part of the judge's summing-up was unrecognizable as a gloss on the proviso to s.1(1) of the Infant Life (Preservation) Act 1929,[87] it was nevertheless welcome in many quarters for placing a very liberal interpretation upon that proviso.[88] One commentator, attempting to reconcile the internal contradictions in the direction, confidently remarked that

> The decision ... should bring comfort to the mind of the practitioner who is confronted with a problem of terminating pregnancy to preserve the life of his patient. To preserve surely means to keep intact, to maintain in its proper state and to guard from such dangers as may beset it. What is the life of an individual either to herself or to the community if she is a permanent physical or mental wreck?[89]

Such interpretations of the summing-up did not marry well with the actual wording of the proviso to s.1(1) of the 1929 Act. However, even the Director of Public Prosecutions recognized that the Bourne case 'extended the possible circumstances in which the operation may be regarded as lawful', in that 'sufficiently grave danger to health mental or physical would render the operation lawful'.[90]

Despite its logical weaknesses, the summing-up as a whole was approved by many for clarifying the law, even though it was sufficiently ambiguous to allow subsequent judges to adopt either a restrictive or permissive view of the legal requirements for a therapeutic abortion. One newspaper stated that the case was 'one of the most important in medico-legal history' because of the issues involved. To the *Yorkshire Observer* the judgement, by placing the burden on the Crown to prove that the operation was not done in good faith, 'appeared to establish a revolution in medical practice'.[91] And, in some quarters, Bourne himself was regarded as a hero.[92]

Not all were as sanguine about the possible consequences of the greater freedom in medical practice that Macnaghten J.'s direction seemed to indicate. The Attorney-General voiced his anxiety 'that medical practitioners generally might be encouraged by it to extend the operation to all cases where the health of the woman was concerned, and that the defence that the operation was necessary on grounds of health might be open to professional abortionists.'[93] In fact, uncertainty persisted within the medical profession, despite the *BMJ*'s confident assertion that 'the law, hitherto vague, has now been clarified'.[94] Doctors continued to seek the advice of their local and central Ethical Committees about the propriety of 'non-medical' abortions.[95] The British Medical Association's 1949 publication *Ethics and Members of the Medical Profession* made special reference to 'Termination of pregnancy', stating that 'This should only be done on purely medical grounds and it is essential to obtain a confirmatory second opinion before recommending or undertaking such action.'[96] 'Purely medical grounds' was not glossed, but psychiatric indications were coming to play an increasingly important role and were under scrutiny in two subsequent and important trials involving doctors.

The interwar years saw a 'profound transformation' which extended psychiatry's role in society and helped secure the discipline's position as an integral part of medicine.[97] That the law was taking increased cognizance of psychiatric factors is evident in the 1922 Infanticide Act which reduced the offence from murder to manslaughter if a woman killed her newly born child when 'she had not fully recovered from the effect of giving birth to such child, but by reason thereof the balance of her mind was then disturbed'.[98] A further Act in 1938 added a consideration of 'the effect of lactation' which, it has been argued, 'made explicit the medicalisation of the crime' of infanticide.[99] The use of psychiatric evidence in the Bourne trial testified to the growing importance attached to psychological matters in medicine. After the Bourne ruling practitioners were much more likely to consider psychiatric reasons as a possible indication for abortion. No doubt as a direct outcome of Macnaghten J.'s summing-up, the 1940 edition of Henderson and Gillespie's standard *Textbook of Psychiatry* included a section on abortion for the first time. It stated:

> Abortion, especially in cases of rape and incest, meets with a large measure of public approval. It is also entirely justifiable in those cases where the mother becomes seriously ill mentally during her pregnancy. In Britain it is customary for the family doctor to call for a psychiatrist's opinion before finally allowing the operation. He thereby secures both the patient's welfare and his own reputation.[100]

This interpretation went beyond the law which, according to the 1939 Inter-Departmental Committee on Abortion, remained ill-defined and required legislation to put the matter beyond doubt.[101] The Home Office, however, saw no need to amend the law,[102] and such legislation was not forthcoming until the Abortion Act was enacted in 1967.

Any uncertainties that the medical profession had about the law were reinforced after the Bourne case by increased policing of abortion. Fourteen doctors were convicted of procuring abortion between 1939 and 1944, more than a quarter of the fifty-three doctors struck off the medical register for the offence during the period from 1900 to 1958.[103] Conviction invariably resulted in erasure from the medical register by the General Medical Council.[104] Many doctors were reluctant to act in this atmosphere although the advocates of abortion law reform sought to reassure them. In 1950 Dr Eustace Chesser called on his colleagues to fight backstreet abortion by taking pleas for termination seriously. Doctors, he argued, had 'not only a right, but a duty' to advise termination when it was indicated, and fulfilment of that duty was 'an honourable, not a shady thing'.[105] The Bourne case remained the leading legal authority on abortion, a status it enjoyed largely because it was the only relevant case to have been officially reported in the *Law Reports*.[106] Two subsequent important but unreported[107] cases followed the trend set by *Bourne* in placing emphasis on the doctor's *bona fides* and the need to follow regular medical practice. Both these cases also involved psychiatric indications.

In the first one, the 1948 case of *R.* v. *Bergmann and Ferguson*, Morris J. confirmed that 'different considerations apply' when determining the lawfulness of an abortion performed by a doctor rather than by an unqualified person and he directed the jury to apply Macnaghten J.'s test from *Bourne*.[108] Dr Eleonore Bergmann was charged with four counts of unlawfully procuring a miscarriage, and Mary Bell Ferguson, a psychiatrist on the medical staff of the Tavistock Clinic, was charged with two counts as an accessory before the fact for having given second opinions supporting the decision to perform two of those abortions.

The Crown contended that the justifications given for the operations performed by Bergmann went beyond the limits set out in the Bourne case.[109] Indeed, the prosecution was able to present some evidence suggesting that the operations were not performed in good faith, but for 'sympathetic' reasons. The first count involved a married maternity nurse known personally to Bergmann. Her husband did not want the child, and the couple had difficulties in finding accommodation. Bergmann had initially refused to perform the operation, but eventually relented. Counts two and three involved women who had first consulted their own family doctors to ascertain pregnancy before going to Bergmann, who then referred them to Ferguson for a second opinion. One of these women was a student who was separated from her husband and feared for her career. The other woman was unmarried, and the father was a married man. The fourth count concerned a married woman who had borne an earlier child just six months before. In each of the latter three cases, Bergmann had asked for large payments in cash: £75, £55 and 50 guineas, respectively. The Crown was also able to point to certain other matters which put the operations in a dubious light, such as the number of inaccuracies in Bergmann's accounts and appointment book, and the fact that all of the procedures had been undertaken privately in Bergmann's surgery.

The defence was able to raise a reasonable doubt in the Crown's case against the two doctors. Regarding the first case, Bergmann testified that she had believed the foetus was already dead from the woman's own attempts to produce a miscarriage. The second woman was characterized by Ferguson as being mentally too unstable to be a mother and sure to have become 'mentally crippled'. There was also haemophilia in her family and she was possibly epileptic. The third woman, according to Bergmann, was 'very distraught and very unbalanced', and she also suffered from jaundice and chronic exhaustion.[110] She had in fact been invalided out of the WRNS. Ferguson regarded her as a neurotic and a suicide risk. As for the fourth woman, there was some doubt whether she had been pregnant at all, and it came down to being an issue of her word against that of Bergmann, who testified that she had merely cleared up a uterine condition and fitted a birth control device. As for the other matters which appeared to undermine the doctors' *bona fides*, it was contended that Bergmann's fees were not excessive, while Ferguson had charged the 'modest fee' of three guineas for her services. Moreover, Ferguson had in fact declined to recommend abortion in six cases referred to her by Bergmann, and the two had never actually met, thus effectively dispelling the suspicion of collusion between them.

The jury took just seven minutes to find both doctors not guilty,[111] despite the fact that none of the patients whom the Crown produced as witnesses against them had been in any apparent danger of dying. This trial clearly revealed the difficulties facing the prosecution in obtaining convictions against doctors. And it indicated that, for most jurors, an earnest concern to avert serious harm to a woman's mental or physical health would suffice to render the operation lawful.[112] Throughout his summing-up, Morris J. emphasized that the vital issue to be determined by the jury was the doctor's honesty in performing or advising the operations.

Between the Bergmann–Ferguson trial and the 1958 case of Newton and Stungo, medical uncertainty about psychiatric indications for abortion continued. The author of a 1948 text, *Modern Psychiatry in Practice*, cited *Bourne* but warned that it was difficult to separate 'social and economic factors from purely psychological ones'.[113] The difficulties surrounding the law led the BMA to issue a press release in 1953 stating that 'if, as is sometimes believed, therapeutic abortion is in fact permissible under the existing law, it is highly desirable that the legal position should be made clear'.[114] The Psychiatry Section of the Royal Society of Medicine organized a meeting to discuss the psychiatric indications for the termination of pregnancy in February 1957. The meeting resulted in 'complete lack of agreement on what constituted grounds for advising termination in women suffering from mental illness'.[115] The lack of agreement over psychiatric indications meant that practice varied widely, such indications comprising 40 per cent of the reasons for therapeutic abortion in one hospital in the late 1950s and not featuring at all in others.[116]

In the 1958 case of *R.* v. *Newton and Stungo*,[117] the Crown succeeded in obtaining a conviction against Dr Newton for unlawfully procuring a miscarriage and, because his patient died two weeks after the operation, for constructive manslaughter. The patient, an unmarried Australian nurse, had been seen by two psychiatrists, the second of whom, Dr Stungo,[118] referred her to Newton in the belief that she was suicidal. The judge directed the jury to find Dr Stungo not guilty since there was no evidence of bad faith on his part and, indeed, one of the prosecution's expert witnesses had corroborated the difficulty of assessing suicidal symptoms. More questionable was the good faith of Dr Newton. If Newton had operated 'merely in order to oblige the woman, or to relieve her of embarrassment, or for a substantial reward' then, the judge stated, 'he is just as guilty of the criminal offence of abortion as would be the woman in a back street'.[119]

Newton's good faith was undermined by a number of suspicious departures from the standards of good medical practice. He had the misfortune of being the fourth and last in a line of medical men to whom the patient was successively referred, which the Crown suggested 'was a convenient set-up under the cloak of medical attention whereby the law is dodged. You send the woman from one doctor to another, who eventually does it for £75.'[120] Newton was in fact not a specialist in either obstetrics or gynaecology, but described himself as an endocrinologist. As a nurse, the patient would ordinarily have been charged less than £75.[121] Newton's somewhat lame explanation for this high fee was that he had wished to dissuade the woman from going through with the abortion. Once the woman had decided to undergo the operation, Newton performed it privately and without assistance in his own surgery. This was contrary to the professional etiquette expected of a male doctor when examining or treating a woman in this manner. More damaging to Newton's defence was the testimony of an expert witness for the Crown, who said that the particular procedure performed by Newton on the woman, who was already three months pregnant, would normally be done in a hospital operating theatre with the patient kept in hospital for five to seven days. Despite the woman having been very ill and thought to be suicidal, Newton sent her back to her hotel. When her condition deteriorated, Newton did not put her in hospital or get a second opinion at once, but waited for five days. Particularly prejudicial to Newton's case was the fact that he lied when eventually he had to send her to hospital. He did not tell the hospital registrar what he had done, and when contacted by the registrar, initially denied that he had performed the abortion, telling him that the woman had seen him about her flu and menstrual irregularity, and that he had merely given her some tablets and sent her away.

Newton was convicted because he appeared to have been too ready to perform the operation, overly reliant on the referring doctors' opinions, greedy, and secretive to a degree that went beyond mere discretion. The jury found these factors convincing evidence that Newton lacked the good faith that might have rendered the operation lawful. The verdict, therefore, was more a judgement on the doctor's honesty than anything else. Neither in this case, nor that of Bergmann, was the judgement of the psychiatrists involved seriously questioned.

The test of *bona fides*, successfully defended in the Bergmann trial and found wanting in Newton's case, reinforced the elements of the Bourne case which emphasized that consultation with a medical colleague, reasonable fees, and openness in procedure were evidence of good faith in performing the abortion operation. But the crux of the abortion issue remained the definition of 'purely medical grounds', and on this *Bourne* remained the authoritative case until the 1967 reform of the law. In its light, medical grounds were seen to cover danger to health as well as to life. Moreover, the use of psychiatric grounds, recognized by the Bourne trial to include the need to protect *future* mental health, enabled doctors to respond to patients' demands for abortion while remaining within the law. This was evident in the *BMJ*'s advice that terminations for pregnant women who had rubella were legally sanctioned when it could 'be shown that worry over potential foetal abnormality [was] adversely affecting the mother's health'.[122]

Bourne's 'courageous episode'[123] made a clear legal distinction between abortions performed by doctors and those performed by people without medical qualifications. The effect of these legal developments was to prevent the ethical question abortion raised from being answered by women themselves; it was placed firmly in doctors' hands. Prior to *Bourne*, doctors had been advised that the 'essential difference' between therapeutic and criminal abortion was that 'medical abortion was open, clean, and in the interests of the mother's health' while 'criminal abortion was secret, dirty, and for the convenience of the mother'.[124] The Bourne trial reinforced the priority of medical opinion over the judgement of the mother. Bourne himself was 'strongly opposed to abortion for purely social and trivial indications'.[125] In 1943 he resigned from the Abortion Law Reform Association, arguing that the problem of abortion could be treated more constructively by measures such as an increase in family allowances and removal of the stigma of illegitimacy.[126]

The Bourne case remained authoritative and, in 1967 when the abortion law was reformed, it confirmed the medicalization of abortion which *Bourne* had established. The 1967 Abortion Act enabled a registered medical practitioner, acting in good faith, and with consultation, to terminate pregnancy in an approved hospital. The grounds for termination included the protection of the physical or mental health of the pregnant woman or her family. Parliament thereby sanctioned the accepted practice of responsible medical practitioners, reflecting the approval of the wider community for the practical *modus vivendi* hammered out by judges, juries and doctors between 1938 and 1967. With the passage of the 1967 Act, the role of doctors as society's arbiters on a contentious moral issue, signalled by *Bourne*, received statutory confirmation.

NOTES

1 Lilian Wyles, *A Woman at Scotland Yard* (London, 1952), p. 221.
2 'Charge of procuring abortion: Rex v. Bourne', *British Medical Journal* [hereafter *BMJ*], 2 (1938), 199–205, at p. 199.
3 Ibid. Miss H had apparently recently started work and was seen by both a school doctor and the chief medical officer of the firm where she worked: Wyles, *A Woman at Scotland Yard*, p. 224.
4 F. J. Smith, ed., *Taylor's Principles and Practice of Medical Jurisprudence*, 7th edn (London, 1920), vol. II, p. 143.
5 For example, 'Rex v. H. Windsor Bell', *BMJ*, 1 (1929), 1061–2; *R.* v. *Sanders–Bliss* reported in 'Woman doctor convicted of procuring abortion', *BMJ*, 2 (1936), 102.
6 For example, Grantham J. in 'Regina v. Collins', *BMJ*, 2 (1898), 59–65, 122–30, at p. 129, and McCardie J. in 'Rex v. H. Windsor Bell', p. 1061, suggested that doctors might act lawfully when saving the mother's life, but these observations were not directly relevant to the decisions of the cases at hand and so were *obiter dicta*.
7 'Two views of criminal abortion', *Medico-Legal and Criminological Review*, 4:4 (1936), 317.
8 J. Ellison, A. Goodwin, C. Read and L. C. Rivett, *Sex Ethics: The Principles and Practice of Contraception, Abortion and Sterilization* (London, 1934), p. 161.
9 Beckwith Whitehouse, 'A paper on the indications for the induction of abortion', *BMJ*, 2 (1932), 337–41, at p. 340.
10 'Illegal operations: woman doctor sent to penal servitude', *The Times*, 1 July 1936, p. 18; 'When is abortion lawful?', *BMJ*, 1 (1937), 393–4, at p. 393.
11 *The Times*, 12 December 1931, p. 12.
12 'Proposed special committee on the law relating to abortion', *BMJ*, 1, Supplement (1934), 150–1, at p. 151.
13 D. G. Browne and E. V. Tullett, *Bernard Spilsbury: His Life and Cases* (London, 1951), p. 33.
14 Ibid., and p. 120.
15 A. Bourne, *A Doctor's Creed* (London, 1962), p. 21.
16 S. Smith, *Mostly Murder* (London, 1961), p. 253.
17 'Report of the Committee on Medical Aspects of Abortion', *BMJ*, 1, Supplement (1936), 230–8, p. 232.
18 Ibid., p. 237. The Committee drew attention to inconsistency between the terms of the Infant Life (Preservation) Act 1929 and the law relating to abortion, commenting that the latter was 'uncompromising' in its language: Ibid., para. 18, at p. 232.
19 'Discussion on indications and methods for termination of pregnancy before the viability of the child', *BMJ*, 2 (1926), 237–48, at p. 248.
20 'Medical aspects of abortion', *BMJ*, 2, Supplement (1936), 51–5, at p. 51.
21 Ibid., p. 52.
22 B. Brookes, *Abortion in England, 1900–1967* (London, 1988), ch. 4.

23 'Charge of procuring abortion', p. 199.
24 Ibid.
25 Ibid.; *R.* v. *Bourne* [1939], 1 *King's Bench Reports* [hereafter *KB*], 687–96, at 688. Throughout this essay, we use legal conventions when citing law reports.
26 'Charge of procuring abortion', p. 202.
27 Ibid.
28 Bourne, *A Doctor's Creed*, p. 99.
29 The Attorney-General, Sir Donald Somervell, who led the prosecution for the Crown, stated at the trial that the authorities had learned of the matter not through any act by Bourne, and that the defendant did nothing inconsistent with his undertaking to Miss H's father: 'Charge of procuring abortion', p. 199. However, an anonymous colleague of Bourne interviewed by John Keown stated that Bourne told him that he had informed the police: *Abortion, Doctors, and the Law. Some Aspects of the Legal Regulation of Abortion in England from 1803 to 1982* (Cambridge, 1988), pp. 188, 189n. According to Lilian Wyles, the police received an anonymous letter on 14 June stating that the operation would be performed that day and asking whether the authorities proposed to take any action to stop it: Wyles, *A Woman at Scotland Yard*, p. 230. In his case note, R. W. Durand states that the police learned of the matter through Miss H being required for evidence in connection with the proceedings against her assailants: 'Abortion: medical aspects of *Rex* v. *Bourne*', *Modern Law Review*, 2:3 (1938), 236–9, at p. 237.
30 'Further memorandum of the Director of Public Prosecutions', approved by the Attorney-General and submitted to the Inter-Departmental Committee on Abortion on 3 October 1938, Public Record Office [hereafter PRO], MH71/27/161/2.
31 Bourne, *A Doctor's Creed*, p. 99.
32 'Further memorandum', PRO MH71/27/161/2; cf. 'Charge of procuring abortion', p. 200.
33 'Further memorandum', pp. 2–3.
34 'Artificial abortion following rape', *Lancet*, 2 (1938), 99–100, at p. 99; cf. 'Charge of procuring abortion. Mr. Aleck Bourne at Marylebone Police Court', *BMJ*, 2 (1938), 97–8, at p. 97.
35 'Artificial abortion following rape', *Lancet*, 2 (1938), 99.
36 Ibid., p. 100.
37 For brief discussions of such a defence, see 'The Bourne case: a legal viewpoint', *BMJ*, 2 (1938), 262–3, and 'Abortion "to preserve life"', *Justice of the Peace and Local Government Review*, 102:31 (1938), 492–3. Indeed, in his opening address to the jury, defence counsel acknowledged that it would not be lawful to perform an abortion 'merely because an unfortunate child had been raped': 'Charge of procuring abortion', p. 201.
38 During cross-examination by defence counsel at the trial proper, Dr Joan Malleson remarked that she thought it right that doctors should take pity on a woman who was raped. The judge thereupon asked her whether she meant pity for a woman where the rape had been established in a court of law, or where the woman concerned merely alleged that a rape had taken place: 'Charge of procuring abortion', p. 200. One of Miss H's assailants, found guilty of rape, received a sentence of four years' penal servitude. A second, found guilty of

aiding and abetting, received the same sentence while the third, found guilty of attempted rape, was sentenced to hard labour for twenty-two months. 'Penal servitude for two troopers', *The Times*, 30 June 1938, p. 11.

39 'Charge of procuring abortion', p. 200.

40 9th edn, ed. R. E. Ross (London, 1936), vol. I, p. 517.

41 'Charge of procuring abortion', p. 200.

42 Ibid.

43 See above, note 6; F. J. Smith, ed., *Taylor's Principles and Practice of Medical Jurisprudence*, 5th edn (London, 1905), vol. II, p. 154, citing the opinion given by Sir Edward Clarke QC and Mr Horace Avory to the Royal College of Physicians in 1895; 'The ethical, legal, and medical aspects of abortion', *Lancet*, 1 (1927), 230–3, at p. 231; and 'The law relating to abortion', *BMJ*, 1 (1938), 408–10, at p. 410.

44 'Further memorandum'; cf. *Report of the Inter-Departmental Committee on Abortion* (Chairman, Norman Birkett KC) (London, 1939), p. 29, para. 72; and Glanville Williams, 'Legal and illegal abortion', *British Journal of Criminology*, 4:4 (1964), 557–69, at p. 559.

45 'Charge of procuring abortion', pp. 200–1.

46 Ibid.

47 This principle of statutory interpretation enables different statutes upon the same subject 'to be taken together as forming one system, and as interpreting and enforcing each other': *R.* v. *Palmer* [1785], 1 *Leach* 352–6, 168 *English Reports* 279–81; cf. *R.* v. *Loxdale* [1758], 1 *Burrows* 445–52, 97 *English Reports* 394–8. While as a general rule it is not proper to refer to a later statute in determining the meaning of an earlier one, it is permissible to do so when the terms of the earlier statute are 'obscure or ambiguous' and 'fairly and equally open to divers meanings': *Ormond Investment Co Ltd* v. *Betts* [1928], *Appeal Cases*, 143–73, per Lord Atkinson at 164 and Lord Buckmaster at 156 respectively; cf. *Kirkness* v. *John Hudson & Co Ltd* [1955], *Appeal Cases*, 696–739.

48 'Charge of procuring abortion', p. 201.

49 Cf. the proviso to the law of abortion suggested in 1846, but not adopted in the 1861 Act, by the Commissioners for Revising and Consolidating the Criminal Law: 'Provided that no act specified in the last preceding Article shall be punishable where such act is done in good faith with the intention of saving the life of the woman whose miscarriage is intended to be procured': *Parliamentary Papers* (1846), vol. XXIV, p. 148, art. 16. Such a provision would have placed the obligation of raising the defence on the defendant.

50 'Abortion. *R.* v. *Bourne*', *Journal of Criminal Law*, 2 (1938), 536–40, at p. 537.

51 Keown, *Abortion, Doctors and the Law*, p. 57.

52 In a comment written after the trial, Lord Horder, one of the expert medical witnesses for the defence, distanced himself from this analogy: 'Abortion: a question of diagnosis', *The Spectator*, 22 July 1938, p. 135.

53 Cf. D. Seaborne Davies, 'The law of abortion and necessity', *Modern Law Review*, 2:2 (1938), 126–38, at p. 136.

54 Section 36 of the Criminal Justice Act 1972 now gives the Attorney-General the right to refer a point of law to the Court of Appeal, but such a reference does not affect a previous acquittal.

55 See *R.* v. *Bourne* [1938], 3 *All England Reports* [hereafter *All ER*], 615–21, at 616E: 'If I err in stating to you what the law is, and if you find the accused guilty, there is a Court of Criminal Appeal which will put the matter right.' This passage was omitted (and there were a number of other changes to the text) in the edited version of the judge's direction to the jury reported in the official *Law Reports*.
56 'Charge of procuring abortion', p. 201.
57 Ibid.
58 Ibid.
59 'Charge against surgeon: Judge on "lawful" operations', *The Times*, 19 July 1938, p. 4.
60 *R.* v. *Bourne* [1939], 1 *KB* 692; *R.* v. *Bourne* [1938], 3 *All ER* 617H–618A.
61 'Charge of procuring abortion', p. 202.
62 Ibid.
63 Obituary of Aleck William Bourne, *BMJ*, 1 (1975), 99.
64 'Charge of procuring abortion', p. 202.
65 'Report of the Committee on Medical Aspects of Abortion', *BMJ*, 2, Supplement (1936), 235.
66 D. K. Henderson and R. D. Gillespie, *A Textbook of Psychiatry*, 4th edn (London, 1936).
67 A. Leyland Robinson, 'The effect of reproduction upon insanity', *Journal of Obstetrics and Gynaecology of the British Empire*, 40:1 (1933), 39–66, at p. 54.
68 Ibid., p. 58.
69 H. V. Dicks, *Fifty Years of the Tavistock Clinic* (London, 1970), p. 4.
70 'Charge of procuring abortion', p. 202.
71 Ibid., p. 203; A. Wolbert Burgess and L. Lytle Holmstrom, 'Rape trauma syndrome', *American Journal of Psychiatry*, 131 (1974), 981–6.
72 'Charge of procuring abortion', p. 203.
73 Obituary, *The Times*, 28 September 1956.
74 'Charge of procuring abortion', p. 203.
75 Ibid.
76 This was the direction to the jury reported at *R.* v. *Bourne* [1939], 1 *KB* 687–96 and *R.* v. *Bourne* [1938], 3 *All ER* 615–21. The version reported in the official *Law Reports* was an edited version of the summing-up actually given, for which see the version reported in the *All England Reports*; cf. 'Charge of procuring abortion', p. 203.
77 *R.* v. *Bourne* [1938], 3 *All ER* 616A–B; cf. *R.* v. *Bourne* [1939], 1 *KB* 689–90.
78 PRO/CRIM 4/1641/16. Gray had also been charged with manslaughter, but that count was not proceeded with, the penalties for breaches against s.58 and manslaughter being the same. Sir Bernard Spilsbury appeared as an expert witness for the Crown.
79 *R.* v. *Bourne* [1939], 1 *KB* 690; *R.* v. *Bourne* [1938], 3 *All ER* 616C.
80 *R.* v. *Bourne* [1939], 1 *KB* 695; *R.* v. *Bourne* [1938], 3 *All ER* 621D.
81 *R.* v. *Bourne* [1939], 1 *KB* 692; *R.* v. *Bourne* [1938], 3 *All ER* 618B, 619A. Although Macnaghten J. was purporting to interpret the words of the proviso to s.1(1) of the Infant Life (Preservation) Act 1929, he did not consider the word 'only'.
82 *R.* v. *Bourne* [1939], 1 *KB* 692; cf. *R.* v. *Bourne* [1938], 3 *All ER* 617E.

83 *R.* v. *Bourne* [1939], 1 *KB* 692; cf. *R.* v. *Bourne* [1938], 3 *All ER* 618A–B.
84 Glanville Williams limited his interpretation of the significance of the Bourne case to what the judge directed in this part of his summing-up: see 'The law of abortion', *Current Legal Problems*, 5 (1952), 128–47, at p. 132 and his book *The Sanctity of Life and the Criminal Law* (London, 1958), p. 153.
85 *R.* v. *Bourne* [1939], 1 *KB* 693–4; cf. *R.* v. *Bourne* [1938], 3 *All ER* 619B–C.
86 'Charge of procuring abortion', p. 200.
87 Cf. Lord Diplock's comment on Macnaghten J. in connection with the Bourne case in *Royal College of Nursing of the United Kingdom* v. *Department of Health and Social Security* [1981], 1 *All ER* 545–78 at 567: 'No disrespect is intended to that eminent judge and former head of my old chambers if I say that his reputation is founded more on his sturdy common sense than on his lucidity of legal exposition.'
88 For the continuing relevance of the Bourne case to the offence of child destruction, see P. D. G. Skegg, *Law, Ethics, and Medicine* (Oxford, 1984), pp. 12–19.
89 Durand, 'Abortion', *Modern Law Review*, 2:3 (1938), 238.
90 PRO MH 71/27/161/2 8.
91 Unattributed press clipping, Abortion Law Reform Association Collection, SA/ALR, Contemporary Medical Archives Centre [hereafter CMAC], Wellcome Institute for the History of Medicine, London.
92 'Aleck Bourne's contribution to history', *Time and Tide*, 28 July 1938, p. 1046.
93 PRO MH 71/27/157.
94 'Charge of procuring abortion', p. 227.
95 CMAC SA/BMA/D 153, Wellcome Institute, London.
96 British Medical Association, *Ethics and Members of the Medical Profession* (London, 1949), p. 16.
97 M. Stone, 'Shell-shock and the psychologists', in W. F. Bynum, R. Porter and M. Shepherd, eds., *The Anatomy of Madness: Essays in the History of Psychiatry* (London, 1985), vol. II, p. 247. See also J. Busfield, *Managing Madness: Changing Ideas and Practice* (London, 1986), p. 330.
98 Infanticide Act 1922, s.1(1).
99 K. O'Donovan, 'The medicalisation of infanticide', *Criminal Law Review* (1984), 259–64 at p. 262.
100 5th edn (London, 1940), p. 43.
101 *Report of the Inter-Departmental Committee on Abortion* (London, 1939), pp. 70–2.
102 CMAC SA/ALR/3/4/59, Wellcome Institute, London.
103 CMAC SA/ALR/A3/8, Wellcome Institute, London.
104 Russell Smith, written communication 20 April 1990. See Russell G. Smith, *Medical Discipline: The Professional Conduct Jurisdiction of the General Medical Council 1858–1990* (Oxford: Clarendon, 1994).
105 *Medical World*, 16 June 1950.
106 It was also highly influential elsewhere in the Commonwealth: cf. Rebecca J. Cook and Bernard M. Dickens, 'Development of Commonwealth abortion laws', *International and Comparative Law Quarterly*, 28 (1979), 424–57, at p. 425.
107 For criticism in this regard, see 'The law relating to therapeutic abortion: an instance of the inadequacy of law reporting', *Law Society's Gazette*, 58 (1961),

539; cf. J. D. J. Havard, 'Therapeutic abortion. *R.* v. *Newton and Stungo*', *Criminal Law Review* (1958), 600–13.

108 Rex v. Eleonore Bergmann and Mary Bell Ferguson, Central Criminal Court, 13 May 1948, Morris J. Transcript of summing-up, CMAC SA/ALR/A2/3,6,4–5, Wellcome Institute, London; cf. 'Alleged conspiracy to procure miscarriages: two doctors acquitted', *BMJ*, 1 (1948), 1008–9.

109 'Alleged conspiracy to procure miscarriages', *BMJ*, 1 (1948), 762–3, at p. 762.

110 Transcript, *R.* v. *Bergmann and Ferguson*, pp. 16, 19.

111 Bergmann, however, pleaded guilty to attempted suicide and was sentenced to eleven days' imprisonment.

112 Cf. Denning L. J. in *Bravery* v. *Bravery* [1954], 1 *Weekly Law Reports* 1169–81 at 1180, who stated by way of *obiter dictum* that abortion is unlawful 'unless it is necessary to prevent serious injury to health'.

113 W. L. Neustatter, *Modern Psychiatry in Practice*, 2nd edn (London, 1948), pp. 242–3.

114 CMAC SA/ALR/A3/2, Wellcome Institute, London.

115 'Psychiatric indications for terminating pregnancy', *BMJ*, 1 (1957), 457.

116 T. N. A. Jeffcoate, 'Indications for therapeutic abortion', *BMJ*, 1 (1960), 581–8, at p. 585.

117 'Criminal abortion and manslaughter: five-year sentence on doctor', *BMJ*, 1 (1958), 1242–8; cf. 'Abortion', *Criminal Law Review* (1958), 469–70; and Havard, 'Therapeutic abortion', *Criminal Law Review* (1958), 600–13.

118 Dr Stungo was discharged during the trial on the basis of insufficient evidence. He had kept careful notes of his consultation with the woman and charged a reasonable fee.

119 'Criminal abortion and manslaughter: five-year sentence on doctor', *BMJ*, 1 (1958), 1247.

120 Ibid., 1243.

121 For example, Dr Bergmann had not asked for a fee at all from the nurse who had been treated by her, but suggested that she could donate £10 to the staff Christmas Fund. Transcript, *R.* v. *Bergmann and Ferguson*, p. 9.

122 T. N. A. Jeffcoate, 'Indications for therapeutic abortion', *BMJ*, 1 (1960), 588.

123 Obituary of Aleck William Bourne, *Lancet*, 1 (1975), 116.

124 'Worcester and Herefordshire branch: Worcester and Bromsgrove division, branch report', *BMJ*, 1, Supplement (1934), 247.

125 Obituary of Aleck W. Bourne, *BMJ*, 1 (1975), 99.

126 Aleck Bourne to the secretary, ALRA, 4 December 1943, CMAC SA/ALR/17/3/3, Wellcome Institute, London.

Index

Cambridge History of Medicine

Health, medicine and morality in the sixteenth century EDITED BY CHARLES WEBSTER

The Renaissance notion of woman: A study in the fortunes of scholasticism and medical science in European intellectual life IAN MACLEAN

Mystical Bedlam: madness, anxiety and healing in sixteenth century England MICHAEL MACDONALD

From medical chemistry to biochemistry: The making of a biomedical discipline ROBERT E. KOHLER

Joan Baptista Van Helmont: Reformer of science and medicine WALTER PAGEL

A generous confidence: Thomas Story Kirkbride and the art of asylum-keeping, 1840–1883 NANCY TOMES

The cultural meaning of popular science: Phrenology and the organization of consent in nineteenth-century Britain ROGER COOTER

Madness, morality and medicine: A study of the York Retreat, 1796–1914 ANNE DIGBY

Patients and practitioners: Lay perceptions of medicine in pre-industrial society EDITED BY ROY PORTER

Hospital life in enlightenment Scotland: Care and teaching at the Royal Infirmary of Edinburgh GUENTER B. RISSE

Plague and the poor in Renaissance Florence ANNE G. CARMICHAEL

Victorian lunacy: Richard M. Bucke and the practice of late-nineteenth-century psychiatry S. E. D. SHORTT

Medicine and society in Wakefield and Huddersfield 1780–1870 HILARY MARLAND

Ordered to care: The dilemma of American nursing, 1850–1945 SUSAN M. REVERBY

Morbid appearances: The anatomy of pathology in the early nineteenth century RUSSELL C. MAULITZ

Professional and popular medicine in France, 1770–1830: The social world of medical practice MATTHEW RAMSEY

Abortion, doctors and the law: Some aspects of the legal regulation of abortion in England 1803–1982 JOHN KEOWN

Public health in Papua New Guinea: Medical possibility and social constraints, 1884–1984 DONALD DENOON

Health, race and German politics between national unification and Nazism, 1870–1945 PAUL WEINDLING

The physician-legislators of France: Medicine and politics in the early Third Republic, 1870–1914 JACK D. ELLIS

The science of woman: Gynaecology and gender in England, 1800–1929 ORNELLA MOSCUCCI

Science and empire: East Coast fever in Rhodesia and the Transvaal PAUL F. CRANEFIELD

The colonial disease: A social history of sleeping sickness in northern Zaire, 1900–1940 MARYINEZ LYONS

Quality and quantity: The quest for biological regeneration in twentieth-century France WILLIAM H. SCHNEIDER

Bilharzia: A history of imperial tropical medicine JOHN FARLEY

Preserve your love for science: Life of William A. Hammond, American neurologist BONNIE E. BLUSTEIN

Patients, power, and the poor in eighteenth-century Bristol MARY E. FISSELL

AIDS and contemporary history EDITED BY VIRGINIA BERRIDGE AND PHILIP STRONG

Mission and method: The early nineteenth-century French public health movement ANN F. LA BERGE

The meanings of sex difference in the middle ages: Medicine, natural philosophy and culture JOAN CADDEN

Medicine before the plague: Practitioners and their patients in the Crown of Aragon, 1285–1345 MICHAEL R. MCVAUGH

Public health and preventive medicine in British India, 1859–1914 MARK HARRISON

Legal history in medicine EDITED BY MICHAEL CLARK AND CATHERINE CRAWFORD

Printed in the United States
By Bookmasters